Study Guide for

Fundamentals of Nursing
The Art and Science of Nursing Care

Seventh Edition

CAROL R. TAYLOR, PhD, MSN, RN
Center for Clinical Bioethics
Professor of Nursing
Georgetown University
Washington, DC

CAROL LILLIS, MSN, RN
Faculty Emerita, Assistant to the Provost
Delaware County Community College
Media, Pennsylvania

PRISCILLA LeMONE, DSN, RN, FAAN
Associate Professor Emerita, Sinclair School of Nursing
University of Missouri
Columbia, Missouri
Adjunct Associate Professor, College of Nursing
Ohio State University
Columbus, Ohio

PAMELA LYNN, MSN, RN
Instructor
School of Nursing
Gwynedd-Mercy College
Gwynedd Valley, Pennsylvania

MARILEE LeBON, BA
Editor/Writer
Brigantine, New Jersey

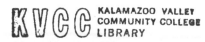
Wolters Kluwer | Lippincott Williams & Wilkins
Health
Philadelphia • Baltimore • New York • London
Buenos Aires • Hong Kong • Sydney • Tokyo

Executive Acquisitions Editor: Carrie Brandon
Senior Product Manager: Betsy Gentzler
Editorial Assistants: Shawn Loht, Amanda Jordan
Design Coordinator: Holly McLaughlin
Illustration Coordinator: Brett MacNaughton
Manufacturing Coordinator: Karin Duffield
Prepress Vendor: Aptara, Inc.

7th Edition

9 8 7 6 5 4 3 2 1

Printed in the United States of America.

ISBN: 978-0-7817-9386-5

LWW.com

Preface

Marilee LeBon, in close consultation with the authors of the seventh edition of *Fundamentals of Nursing: The Art and Science of Nursing Care*, has carefully developed this Study Guide. We recognize that beginning students in nursing must learn an enormous amount of information and skills in a short period of time. The Study Guide is structured to help you integrate the knowledge you have gained and begin to apply it to the practice of nursing. To help you accomplish this goal, the following types of exercises are provided in each chapter of the Study Guide.

PRACTICING FOR NCLEX

Multiple Choice Questions: Each chapter contains a section of multiple choice questions presented in the NCLEX-RN exam format.

Alternate-Format Questions: The alternate-format-style questions for the NCLEX-RN exam include the types of questions described below. Several of these types are provided in each chapter to help you become familiar with this NCLEX format. They are:

- Multiple Response Questions: questions with a detailed stem that require you to select more than 1 correct answer
- Prioritization Questions: questions with a detailed stem that require you to place the options provided in the correct order
- Hot Spot Questions: questions that require you to identify a specific area on an illustration or a graph
- Fill-in-the-Blank Questions: questions that require you to perform a calculation that results in a very specific number answer
- Chart/Exhibit Questions: multiple choice questions with a detailed stem that require you to review information in a chart or an exhibit in order to select the correct answer

DEVELOPING YOUR KNOWLEDGE BASE

These exercises group similar types of questions together to help you learn the information in a variety of formats. The types of questions included follow the same format in each Study Guide chapter, but not every type of question is used in each chapter. The format includes:

- Fill-in-the-Blanks
- Identification Questions
- Matching Exercises
- Correct the False Statements
- Short Answer

APPLYING YOUR KNOWLEDGE

These questions challenge you to reflect on the critical thinking and blended skills developed in the classroom and apply them to your own practice of the *art and science of nursing care*.

- Critical Thinking Questions: these questions offer an exciting and practical means to challenge the assumptions you bring to nursing and to "stretch" your application of new theoretical concepts.
- Reflective Practice Using Critical Thinking Skills: these exercises offer opportunities to use your critical thinking ability and knowledge of blended skills to respond to real-life scenarios, similar to those that may occur in your practice.
- Patient Care Studies: These studies in the clinical nursing care chapters provide a unique opportunity for you to "encounter" an actual patient, and to use the nursing process to assess and diagnose the patient's nursing needs and brainstorm ways to best meet these needs.

The answers to the Practicing for NCLEX, Developing Your Knowledge Base, and Patient Care Study questions are included in the Answer Key at the back of the book so that you can immediately assess your own learning as you complete each chapter.

We hope you find this Study Guide to be helpful and enjoyable, and we wish you every success as you begin the exciting journey toward becoming a nurse.

Carol R. Taylor
Carol Lillis
Priscilla LeMone
Pamela Lynn
Marilee LeBon

Contents

CHAPTER 1

Introduction to Nursing

PRACTICING FOR NCLEX

MULTIPLE CHOICE QUESTIONS

Circle the letter that corresponds to the best answer for each question.

1. Which of the following statements most clearly defines the role of the nurse in the early Christian period?

   a. The nurse was viewed as a slave, carrying out menial tasks based on the orders of the priest-physician.

   b. Women called deaconesses made the first organized visits to the sick, and members of male religious groups gave nursing care and buried the dead.

   c. The nurse was usually the mother who cared for her family during sickness by providing physical care and herbal remedies.

   d. Women who had committed crimes were recruited into nursing in lieu of serving jail sentences.

2. Which of the following nursing advocates elevated the status of nursing to a respected occupation, improved the quality of nursing care, and founded modern nursing education?

   a. Jane Addams

   b. Clara Barton

   c. Dorothea Dix

   d. Florence Nightingale

3. Which of the following statements is an accurate description of nursing's role, according to the American Nurses Association (ANA)?

   a. Nursing is a profession dependent upon the medical community as a whole.

   b. It is the role of the physician, not the nurse, to assist patients in understanding their health problems.

   c. It is the role of nursing to provide a caring relationship that facilitates health and healing.

   d. The essential components of professional nursing care are strength, endurance, and cure.

4. The various definitions of nursing provided in this chapter conclude that the central focus of nursing is based on which of the following?

   a. The care provided by the nurse

   b. The patient receiving care

   c. The nurse as the caregiver

   d. Nursing as a profession

5. Who established the Red Cross in the United States in 1882?

   a. Clara Barton

   b. Dorothea Dix

   c. Jane Addams

   d. Florence Nightingale

6. When a nurse helps a patient make an informed decision about his/her own health and life, which of the following nurse's roles has been performed?

   a. Advocate

   b. Counselor

   c. Caregiver

   d. Communicator

1

7. Which of the following developments had the greatest influence on the development of nursing as a profession since the 1950s?

   a. Large numbers of women began to work outside the home, asserting their independence.

   b. Nursing practice was broadened to include practice in a wide variety of healthcare settings.

   c. Male dominance in the healthcare profession slowed the progress of professionalism in the nursing practice.

   d. Hospital schools were established to provide more easily controlled and less expensive staff for the hospital.

8. Learning how to use a new piece of hospital equipment would most likely occur in which type of educational setting?

   a. Continuing education

   b. Graduate education

   c. In-service education

   d. Undergraduate studies

9. Which of the following nursing education programs attracts more men, minorities, and nontraditional students and prepares nurses to give care to patients in various structured settings?

   a. Diploma in nursing

   b. Associate degree in nursing

   c. Baccalaureate degree in nursing

   d. Graduate education in nursing

10. Which of the following is used by the nurse to identify the patient's healthcare needs and strengths and to establish and carry out a plan of care to meet those needs?

    a. Nursing standards

    b. Nursing orders

    c. Nurse practice acts

    d. Nursing process

ALTERNATE-FORMAT QUESTIONS

Multiple Response Questions

Circle the letters that correspond to the best answers for each question.

1. Which of the following nursing actions demonstrate the aim of nursing to promote health? *(Select all that apply.)*

   a. Increasing student awareness of sexually transmitted diseases by distributing informational pamphlets at a college health center

   b. Performing diagnostic measurements and examinations in an outpatient setting

   c. Serving as a role model of health for patients by maintaining a healthy weight

   d. Helping a person with paraplegia learn how to use a wheelchair

   e. Facilitating decisions about lifestyles that would enhance the well-being of a teenager

   f. Administering an insulin shot to a diabetic patient

2. Which of the following nursing actions demonstrate the aim of nursing to facilitate coping? *(Select all that apply.)*

   a. Teaching a class on the nutritional needs of pregnant women

   b. Changing the bandages of a patient who has undergone heart surgery

   c. Teaching a patient and his/her family how to live with diabetes

   d. Assisting a patient and his/her family to prepare for death

   e. Starting an intravenous line for a malnourished elderly person

   f. Providing counseling for the family of a teenager with an eating disorder

3. Which of the following criteria define nursing as a profession? *(Select all that apply.)*

   a. A well-defined body of specific and unique knowledge

   b. Standards of performance determined by the medical community

   c. An established code of ethics

   d. Commitment to ongoing research

   e. Selective membership

   f. Recognized authority by a professional group

4. Which of the following are professional nursing organizations that are operating in the United States? *(Select all that apply.)*

   a. ANA

   b. NNO

   c. ICN

   d. AACN

   e. NASN

   f. ANO

5. Which of the following statements accurately describe a nurse practice act? *(Select all that apply.)*

   a. A nurse practice act regulates the practice of nursing.

   b. Nurse practice acts are regulated by the federal government.

   c. Nurse practice acts exclude untrained and unlicensed people from practicing nursing.

   d. The enforcement of rules and regulations does not fall within the scope of nurse practice acts.

   e. Nurse practice acts establish the criteria for the education and licensure of nurses.

   f. Legal requirements and titles for RNs and LPNs are not specifically defined by the nurse practice acts.

6. Which of the following statements regarding nursing licenses are accurate? *(Select all that apply.)*

   a. The board of nursing for each state or province has the legal authority to allow graduates of approved schools of nursing to take the licensing examination.

   b. The licensed nurse is approved to practice nursing in any state.

   c. The nursing license is valid during the life of the holder.

   d. The nursing license can be denied due to criminal actions.

   e. The nursing license cannot be revoked or suspended for professional misconduct.

   f. A license is not necessary to practice nursing in nursing homes.

Prioritization Questions

1. The role of medicine developed from the pre-civilization era, through the eras signifying the beginning of civilization, the beginning of the 16th century, the 18th and 19th centuries, and the World War II era to the present. Place the events that defined these eras listed below in the correct chronologic order to follow this timeline.

   a. An explosion of knowledge in medicine and technology occurred.

   b. Focus on religion was replaced by a focus on warfare, exploration, and expansion of knowledge.

   c. Belief in good and evil spirits bringing health or illness existed; medicine men were physicians.

   d. Hospital schools were organized; female nurses were under control of male hospital administrators and physicians; males dominated the healthcare setting.

   e. Varied healthcare settings developed.

   f. Temples were the centers of medical care; belief that illness is caused by sin and gods' displeasure existed; priests were physicians.

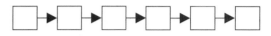

2. The role of the nurse developed from the pre-civilization era, through the eras signifying the beginning of civilization, the beginning of the 16th century, the 18th and 19th centuries, and the World War II era to the present. Place the following roles of the nurse listed below in the correct chronologic order to follow this timeline.

   a. There was a shortage of nurses; criminals were recruited as nurses; nursing was viewed as disreputable.

   b. Nursing was broadened in all areas and was practiced in a wide variety of settings; nursing was viewed as a profession.

   c. Nurses were portrayed as a mother, caring for family and delivering physical care and health remedies.

   d. Nurses were viewed as slaves, carrying out menial tasks based on the orders of the priest.

   e. Florence Nightingale elevated nursing to a respected occupation and founded modern methods in nursing education.

   f. Efforts were made to upgrade nursing education, and women were more assertive and independent.

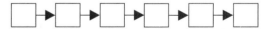

DEVELOPING YOUR KNOWLEDGE BASE

FILL-IN-THE-BLANKS

1. The _____, founded in 1899, was the first international organization of professional women.

2. Founded in the late 1800s, the _____ is a professional organization for registered nurses in the United States.

3. The _____, developed by the ANA, define the activities of nurses that are specific and unique to nursing.

4. _____ are laws established in each state in the United States to regulate the practice of nursing.

5. One of the major guidelines for nursing practice, the _____, integrates both the art and science of nursing.

CORRECT THE FALSE STATEMENTS

Circle the word "true" or "false" that follows the statement. If you circled "false," change the underlined word or words to make the statement true. Place your answer in the space provided.

1. A <u>nurse practice</u> act is a law that regulates the practice of nursing.

   True   False _____

2. The ANA defines <u>continuing education</u> as those professional development experiences designed to enrich the nurse's contribution to health.

   True   False _____

3. The legal right to practice nursing is termed <u>professional standards</u>.

   True   False _____

4. When a nurse completes a diploma, associate degree, or baccalaureate program, he or she becomes licensed as a <u>licensed practical nurse</u>.

   True   False _____

5. In early civilizations influenced by the theory of animism, the roles of physician and nurse were <u>interchangeable</u>.

   True   False _____

6. The <u>ANA</u>, founded in 1899, was the first international organization of professional women, with nurses from both the United States and Canada as charter members.

   True   False _____

7. All nursing actions focus on the <u>orders of the physician</u>.

   True   False _____

8. <u>Practical nursing</u> was developed to prepare nurses to give bedside nursing care to patients.

   True   False _____

9. When the major goals of healthcare—promoting, maintaining, or restoring health—can no longer be met, <u>the nurse's duties are terminated</u>.

   True   False _____

10. Nursing has evolved through history from a technical service to a <u>knowledge-centered process</u> that allows maximizing of human potential.

    True   False _____

SHORT ANSWER

Nursing has been defined in many ways, but there are essential elements present in most thoughtful perspectives. Use your own words to expand the following short definitions of nursing.

1. Nursing is caring. _____

2. Nursing is sharing. _____

3. Nursing is touching. _____

4. Nursing is feeling. _____

5. Nursing is listening. _____

6. Nursing is accepting. _____

7. Nursing is respecting. _____

_____

_____

8. Give an example in which a nurse may incorporate the following broad aims of nursing into a nursing care plan for a patient who is undergoing diagnostic tests for lung cancer and who smokes two packs of cigarettes a day.

   a. Promoting health: _____

   _____

   _____

   b. Preventing illness: _____

   _____

   c. Restoring health: _____

   _____

   _____

   d. Facilitating coping: _____

   _____

   _____

9. List the criteria that define the following concepts:

   a. A profession: _____

   _____

   _____

   b. A discipline: _____

   _____

   _____

10. Describe how the following issues are affecting nursing in transition:

   a. Technologic advances: _____

   _____

   b. Nursing actions: _____

   _____

   _____

11. Give an example of a nursing action that might be performed by a nurse relying on the following four competencies:

   a. Cognitive skills: _____

   b. Technical skills: _____

   c. Interpersonal skills: _____

   d. Ethical/legal skills: _____

12. Complete the following table with the correct word or phrase to differentiate among the nursing roles that are listed.

Title	Education/Preparation	Role Description
Example: Nurse researcher	Advanced degree	Conducts research relevant to practice and education
Nurse midwife		
Nurse practitioner		
Nurse anesthetist		
Nurse administrator		
Nurse entrepreneur		

APPLYING YOUR KNOWLEDGE

CRITICAL THINKING QUESTIONS

1. Think of nursing situations in which the nurse involved promoted each of nursing's aims.

   a. Describe an instance of each.

      Promoting health:

      Preventing illness:

      Restoring health:

      Facilitating coping:

   b. Describe the factors that might warrant a particular nursing aim in each case.

   c. How would you evaluate whether your nursing aims were successful?

2. Research a historical figure in nursing whom you respect and admire. Write a nursing philosophy that best expresses his/her nursing goals. Then interview a modern-day nurse about his/her nursing philosophy. Note how the two philosophies are similar or different. Form your own nursing philosophy based on your results.

REFLECTIVE PRACTICE USING CRITICAL THINKING SKILLS

Use the following expanded scenario from Chapter 1 in your textbook to answer the questions below.

Scenario: Albert Rowlings, a 62-year-old man, presents to the ER with chest pain and shortness of breath. On assessment, the nurse notes blood pressure of 139/90. Mr. Rowlings is 45 pounds overweight and says he smokes a pack of cigarettes a day and drinks a six-pack of beer each evening while watching TV. After Mr. Rowlings is admitted and treated for hypertension, the nurse attempts to teach him lifestyle modifications such as diet, exercise, and stress reduction. He says, "Just save your breath. Why should I bother about all that? I'd be better off dead than living like I am now, anyway!" Mr. Rowlings then turns his back to the nurse and clicks on the TV.

1. What might be causing Mr. Rowlings to respond negatively to patient teaching related to lifestyle modification and stress reduction?

   _____

   _____

   _____

2. What would be a successful outcome for this patient?

   _____

   _____

   _____

3. What intellectual, technical, interpersonal, and/or ethical/legal competencies are most likely to bring about the desired outcome?

   _____

   _____

   _____

4. What resources might be helpful for Mr. Rowlings?

   _____

   _____

   _____

Cultural Diversity

PRACTICING FOR NCLEX

MULTIPLE CHOICE QUESTIONS

Circle the letter that corresponds to the best answer for each question.

1. The use of eye contact varies from culture to culture. Which of the following assumptions may be accurate when eye contact is used as nonverbal communication by different cultural groups in the following situations?

   a. A Native American stares at the floor while talking with the nurse. Assumption: He is embarrassed by the conversation.

   b. A Hasidic Jewish man listens intently to a male physician, making direct eye contact with him, but refuses to make eye contact with a female nursing student. Assumption: Jewish men consider women inferior to men.

   c. A Muslim-Arab woman refuses to make eye contact with her male nurse. Assumption: She is being modest.

   d. An African American man rolls his eyes when asked how he copes with stress in the workplace. Assumption: He may feel he has already answered this question and has become impatient.

2. Which one of the following statements about food accurately reflects foods that are edible for various cultural groups?

   a. For some Asians, Hispanics, and Seventh-Day Adventists, religious beliefs prohibit the consumption of pork.

   b. Patients following a vegetarian diet generally eat chicken.

   c. Vietnamese patients will not eat beans.

   d. French patients consider corn to be animal feed.

3. Nursing is a subculture of which of the following larger cultures in our society?

   a. Healthcare providers

   b. Organizations of nurses

   c. Institutions

   d. Healthcare systems

4. An African American patient complains of gas after eating a bedtime snack of cheese and crackers. This may be a symptom of which of the following conditions?

   a. Lactose intolerance

   b. Keloid formation

   c. Thalassemia

   d. G6PD deficiency

5. Which of the following best describes the type of health promotion practiced by Hawaiians?

   a. One should eat a diet balanced with yin and yang foods and maintain harmony with friends and family.

   b. Past illness is viewed as part of the whole and there is an emphasis on preventive medicine with treatment using medicinal plants and minerals.

   c. Proper diet, proper behavior, and exercise in fresh air are prescriptions for maintaining health.

   d. Illness is seen as preventable; nutrition is important, but not physical activity.

6. If a patient refuses to allow the nurse to draw blood for a test because he believes blood is the body's life force and cannot be regenerated, it is likely that he belongs to which of the following ethnic groups?

   a. Hispanic–Puerto Rican

   b. Asian

   c. Hispanic–Mexican

   d. African American

7. Which of the following statements would best apply to Native American cultures?

   a. The family is not expected to be part of nursing care.

   b. Direct eye contact is preferred when speaking to healthcare professionals.

   c. A low tone of voice is considered respectful.

   d. Careful notes are kept regarding home care and medications.

8. In which of the following ethnic groups would folk-healing practices and home remedies be used by some families for particular illnesses?

   a. African American

   b. White middle class

   c. Asian

   d. Jewish descent

9. A 79-year-old Native American woman is placed in a nursing home by her son, who is no longer able to care for her. She appears disoriented and complains of the "bright lights and constant activity." Her feelings are likely to be a result of which of the following conditions?

   a. Culture assimilation

   b. Culture disorientation

   c. Culture blindness

   d. Culture shock

ALTERNATE-FORMAT QUESTIONS

Multiple Response Questions

Circle the letters that correspond to the best answers for each question.

1. Which of the following disorders might you screen for in an African American man? *(Select all that apply.)*

   a. Keloid formations

   b. Tay-Sachs disease

   c. Gout

   d. Lactase deficiency

   e. Sickle cell anemia

   f. Cystic fibrosis

2. Which of the following statements accurately describe the characteristics of culture? *(Select all that apply.)*

   a. Culture guides behavior into acceptable ways for people in a specific group.

   b. Culture is not affected by a group's social and physical environment.

   c. Cultural practices and beliefs are constantly evolving and changing over time to satisfy a group's needs.

   d. Culture influences the way people of a group view themselves.

   e. There are differences both within cultures and among cultures.

   f. Subcultures exist within most cultures.

3. Which of the following statements concerning dominant and minority groups are true? *(Select all that apply.)*

   a. The dominant group is always the largest group in a society.

   b. The dominant group in the United States is currently composed of white middle-class people of European ancestry.

   c. The values of a dominant group have little influence on the value system of society as a whole.

   d. A minority group usually has some physical or cultural characteristic that identifies the people within it as different.

   e. When minority groups live within a dominant group, many of their members lose the cultural characteristics that once made them different.

   f. When a minority group and a dominant group trade some characteristics, the process is known as cultural imposition.

4. Which of the following is a value or belief commonly shared by members of the African American culture? *(Select all that apply.)*

   a. Oriented to the present

   b. Frequently highly religious

   c. Youth valued over age

   d. Praise of self or others considered poor manners

   e. Respect given according to sex (male)

   f. Clergy members highly respected

5. Which of the following cultural characteristics are consistent with the Appalachian culture? *(Select all that apply.)*

    a. Belief is in a divine existence rather than attending a particular church.

    b. Illness is considered a punishment from God.

    c. Isolation is an accepted way of life.

    d. Feelings about losses or death may be fatalistic.

    e. Independence and self-determination are valued.

    f. Youth is valued over age.

DEVELOPING YOUR KNOWLEDGE BASE

FILL-IN-THE-BLANKS

1. An overgrowth of connective tissue occurring during the healing process is known as

    _____.

2. A _____ is a large group of people who are members of a larger cultural group but have certain characteristics not common to the larger culture.

3. The sense of identification that a cultural group has collectively, based on the group's common heritage, is known as its

    _____.

4. The idea that one's own ideas, practices, and beliefs are superior to, or are preferred to, those of others is termed _____.

5. _____ is a disorder that occurs when the shape of the red blood cells causes them to break down more rapidly than normal-shaped red blood cells.

6. _____ occurs when one ignores differences in cultures and proceeds as though they do not exist.

7. The feelings a person experiences when placed in a different culture that the person perceives as strange are known as _____ and may result in psychological discomfort or disturbances.

8. _____ exists when a person assumes that all members of a culture or ethnic group act alike.

MATCHING EXERCISES

Match the cultural group listed in Part A with a major concept of their healthcare practice listed in Part B. Answers may be used more than once.

PART A

a. White middle class

b. African American

c. Asian

d. Hispanic

e. Native American

f. Hawaiian

g. Appalachian

PART B

1. ___ Healthcare may include spiritualists, herb doctors, root doctors, conjurers, skilled elder family members, voodoo, and faith healing.

2. ___ Good health is achieved by the proper balance of yin and yang.

3. ___ "Granny" woman or folk healer provides care and may be consulted even if the patient is also receiving traditional care.

4. ___ Self-diagnosis and use of over-the-counter medications often occurs.

5. ___ Dieting and extensive use of exercise and exercise facilities are common practices.

6. ___ The secret of good health is to balance cold and hot within the body.

7. ___ Medicine men are frequently used.

8. ___ Use of acumassage, acupressure, and acupuncture is common.

9. ___ The patient's illness is viewed as part of the whole. Emphasis is placed on preventive medicine.

10. ___ Folk healers frequently base treatments on humoral pathology (curanderas).

SHORT ANSWER

1. Describe how you would advise impoverished patients who are not meeting their healthcare needs due to the following conditions:

    a. Lack of transportation to clinic, hospital, or doctor's office:

    _____

    _____

b. Living in overcrowded conditions; absence of running water and adequate sanitation:

_____

_____

c. Use of drugs or alcohol to escape reality of situation:

_____

_____

2. Explain how the following cultural factors may affect the interaction of a nurse with a patient in this situation: A nurse attempts to perform a nursing history on an Appalachian woman admitted to the hospital with chest pain.

a. Patient refuses to answer questions and refers to her "granny" woman as a source of information.

_____

_____

b. Patient's extended family is present during the interview and answers each question before the patient has a chance to speak.

_____

_____

c. Patient states that she has always taken a special herb prepared by her folk healer to alleviate her chest pains. She tells you she does not trust modern medications.

_____

_____

3. Using the *Transcultural Assessment: Health-Related Beliefs and Practices* located in your textbook, assess the health-related beliefs of a patient of a different culture. How do this patient's beliefs differ from yours? What nursing actions could you take to help this patient express and practice his or her beliefs?

Patient, culture, and medical condition: _____

_____

_____

Health-related beliefs: _____

_____

_____

How my beliefs differ: _____

_____

_____

Nursing actions for patient: _____

_____

_____

4. Explain why the following groups of people are at high risk for living in poverty.

a. Families headed by single women: _____

_____

_____

b. Older adults: _____

_____

_____

c. Future generations of those now in poverty:

_____

_____

APPLYING YOUR KNOWLEDGE

CRITICAL THINKING QUESTIONS

1. How would you respond to the individual nursing needs of the following patients?

a. A Jewish man refuses to let a female nurse perform a nursing history and asks for a male doctor to examine him instead.

b. An African American girl, age 13, delivers her first baby. She tells you she had an abortion earlier but is ready for this new baby.

c. An Asian American who speaks halting English brings his grandfather (who speaks no English) to the emergency room. The grandfather presents with the warning signs of a myocardial infarction.

2. Interview fellow classmates and friends representing different cultures to determine how they respond to an illness in the family. Ask them what type of home remedies they use for the common cold. Identify any risk factors they may have for serious illness, including culturally related diseases.

REFLECTIVE PRACTICE USING CRITICAL THINKING SKILLS

Use the following expanded scenario from Chapter 2 in your textbook to answer the questions below.

Scenario: Danielle Dorvall, a 45-year-old Haitian woman, has been in the United States for approximately 8 months. She recently had a surgical repair of a fractured femur and is now confined to bed in skeletal traction. When the nurse appears to change Ms. Dorvall's dressings, she asks that a Haitian folk healer from her neighborhood be allowed to come to the hospital to help heal her broken leg.

1. How might the nurse respond to Ms. Dorvall's request for a Haitian folk healer?

_____

_____

_____

2. What would be a successful outcome for this patient?

_____

_____

_____

3. What intellectual, technical, interpersonal, and/or ethical/legal competencies are most likely to bring about the desired outcome?

_____

_____

_____

4. What resources might be helpful for Ms. Dorvall?

_____

_____

_____

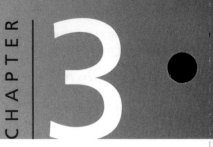

CHAPTER 3

Health and Illness

PRACTICING FOR NCLEX

MULTIPLE CHOICE QUESTIONS

Circle the letter that corresponds to the best answer for each question.

1. Immunizing children against measles is an example of which of the following levels of preventive care?
   a. Primary
   b. Secondary
   c. Tertiary

2. Referring an HIV-positive patient to a local support group is an example of which of the following levels of preventive care?
   a. Primary
   b. Secondary
   c. Tertiary

3. In which of the following stages of acute illness does the patient decide to accept the diagnosis and follow the prescribed treatment plan?
   a. Stage 1
   b. Stage 2
   c. Stage 3
   d. Stage 4

4. Which of the following best describes a period of remission in a patient with a chronic illness?
   a. The symptoms of the illness reappear.
   b. The disease is no longer present.
   c. New symptoms occur at this time.
   d. Symptoms are not experienced.

5. During the recovery and rehabilitation stage of illness, the person who is ill is expected to do which of the following?
   a. Give up the dependent role.
   b. Assume a dependent role.
   c. Seek medical attention.
   d. Recognize symptoms of illness.

6. Needs are an integral part of each person's human dimension. Which needs are met when a person feels a sense of belonging to a group or community and being loved by others?
   a. Spiritual needs
   b. Sociocultural needs
   c. Intellectual needs
   d. Emotional needs

ALTERNATE-FORMAT QUESTIONS

Multiple Response Questions

Circle the letters that correspond to the best answers for each question.

1. Which of the following are stages of illness behaviors according to Suchman (1965)? *(Select all that apply.)*
   a. Experiencing symptoms
   b. Assuming the sick role
   c. Determining the degree of illness
   d. Assuming a dependent role
   e. Preparing for recovery or death
   f. Achieving recovery and rehabilitation

2. Which of the following statements accurately describe Suchman's stages of illness? *(Select all that apply.)*

   a. In stage 1, the person defines himself or herself as being sick, seeks validation of this experience from others, and gives up normal activities.

   b. In stage 2, most people focus on their symptoms and bodily functions.

   c. When help from a healthcare provider is sought, the person becomes a patient and enters stage 3, assuming a dependent role.

   d. When a patient decides to accept a diagnosis and follow a prescribed treatment plan, he or she is in stage 4, achieving recovery and rehabilitation.

   e. In stage 1, pain is the most significant symptom indicating illness, although other symptoms, such as a rash, fever, bleeding, or cough, may be present.

   f. Most patients complete the final stage of illness behavior in the hospital or a long-term care setting.

3. Which of the following examples of basic human needs would be considered within the sociocultural dimension? *(Select all that apply.)*

   a. Fear

   b. Thinking

   c. Support systems

   d. Circulation

   e. Housing

   f. Feeling loved by others

4. Which of the following are characteristics of a chronic illness? *(Select all that apply.)*

   a. It is a permanent change.

   b. It causes, or is caused by, irreversible alterations in normal anatomy and physiology.

   c. It is characterized by stages of illness behaviors, which may occur rapidly or slowly.

   d. It generally has a rapid onset of symptoms and lasts only a relatively short time.

   e. It requires special patient education for rehabilitation.

   f. It requires a short period of care or support.

5. Which of the following statements accurately describe existing models of health and illness? *(Select all that apply.)*

   a. In the agent–host–environment model of health and illness developed by Leavell and Clark (1965) for community health, the agent, host, and environment react separately to create risk factors.

   b. The health–illness continuum model views health as a constantly changing state, with high-level wellness and death being on opposite ends of a graduated scale.

   c. In his high-level wellness model, Halbert Dunn (1980) described wellness as "good health."

   d. The processes of being, belonging, becoming, and befitting are defined in Halbert Dunn's high-level wellness model.

   e. The health belief model (Rosenstock, 1974) is concerned with what people perceive or believe to be true about themselves in relation to their health.

   f. The health promotion model developed by Pender (2006) incorporates the characteristics, experiences, and beliefs of generalized populations to motivate health-promoting behaviors and establish behavioral norms.

6. Which of the following actions exemplify the focus of secondary preventive care? *(Select all that apply.)*

   a. Scheduling immunizations for a child

   b. Teaching parents about child safety in the home

   c. Performing range-of-motion exercises on a patient

   d. Assessing a child for normal growth and development

   e. Dispensing medications on a pediatric ward

   f. Referring a patient with a new colostomy to a support group

Chart/Exhibit Questions

Refer to the chart below to determine the type of human dimension that is represented by the examples listed.

Human Dimensions	Basic Human Needs	Examples
Physical Dimension	Physiologic needs	Circulation
Environmental Dimension	Safety and Security needs	Climate
Sociocultural Dimension	Love and Belonging needs	Support systems
Emotional Dimension	Self-esteem needs	Loneliness
Intellectual and Spiritual Dimension	Self-actualization needs	Values

1. An older adult must live with and control his diabetes. _____

2. Worried about losing his job, a 35-year-old executive exacerbates his ulcer. _____

3. The mother of a toddler must learn how to childproof her house. _____

4. An older woman has a raised toilet seat installed in her bathroom. _____

5. A homeless man does not seek treatment for pneumonia. _____

6. A Catholic woman refuses treatment for cancer and arranges a pilgrimage to a holy site where miraculous cures have been recorded by her religious leaders. _____

7. A 15-year-old pregnant woman must learn how to care for her baby when it is born. _____

8. A woman with rheumatoid arthritis improves her mobility with the use of pain medications. _____

DEVELOPING YOUR KNOWLEDGE BASE

FILL-IN-THE-BLANKS

1. _____ is a medical term meaning that there is a pathologic change in the structure or function of the body or mind.

2. Arthritis is an example of a(n) _____ illness.

3. A(n) _____ illness generally has a rapid onset of symptoms and lasts only a relatively short time.

4. The reappearance of symptoms of a chronic disease in a patient who has been in remission is known as a period of _____.

5. A landscaper's increased risk for developing skin cancer because of excessive exposure to the sun is considered a(n) _____ risk factor.

MATCHING EXERCISES

Match the risk factors listed in Part A with their appropriate examples listed in Part B. Answers may be used more than once.

PART A

a. Age

b. Genetic composition

c. Physiologic factors

d. Health habits

e. Lifestyle

f. Environment

PART B

1. ____ A mother and her school-aged child are concerned about increasing gang-related violence in their neighborhood.

2. ____ A teenager who is a new driver is admitted to the emergency room with multiple fractures after wrecking his car.

3. ____ A woman with multiple sex partners tests positive for HIV.

4. ____ A woman is worried about breast cancer because it "runs in the family."

5. ____ An overweight executive presents with high blood pressure.

6. ____ An alcoholic man develops a liver abscess.

7. ____ A patient tells you his father died of colon cancer.

8. ____ A smoker develops a chronic cough.

9. ____ A toddler presents with a mild concussion following a fall.

10. ____ A pregnant woman has toxemia in her fifth month.

11. ___ A 40-year-old man has a father and brother who died of heart attacks at an early age.

12. ___ An elderly man fractures a hip and ankle bone when falling down a flight of stairs in his home.

Match the model of health and illness listed in Part A with the correct definition in Part B.

PART A

a. Agent–host–environment model
b. Health belief model
c. Health–illness continuum
d. High-level wellness model
e. Health promotion model

PART B

13. ___ This model views health as a constantly changing state, with high-level wellness and death being on opposite ends of a graduated scale.

14. ___ Halbert Dunn's model of health is based on a person functioning to maximum potential while maintaining balance and a purposeful direction in the environment.

15. ___ This model, developed by Leavell and Clark for use in community health, is helpful for examining the causes of disease in an individual by looking at and understanding risk factors.

16. ___ Rosenstock's model of health is based on three components of disease perception: (1) perceived susceptibility to a disease, (2) perceived seriousness of a disease, and (3) perceived benefits of action.

17. ___ This model, developed by Pender, illustrates the multidimensional nature of persons interacting with their environment as they pursue health.

SHORT ANSWER

1. Describe how your own self-concept has been influenced by the following factors:

a. Interpersonal interactions: _____

_____

_____

b. Physical and cultural influences: _____

_____

_____

c. Education: _____

_____

_____

d. Illness: _____

_____

_____

2. Compare and contrast the two types of illnesses listed below:

a. Acute illness: _____

_____

_____

b. Chronic illness: _____

_____

_____

3. Describe where you personally fit on the health–illness continuum, and why:

_____

_____

_____

_____

4. List two examples of nursing actions that would be performed at each of the following levels of preventive care.

a. Primary preventive care: _____

_____

_____

b. Secondary preventive care: _____

_____

_____

c. Tertiary preventive care: _____

_____

_____

5. Describe Dunn's processes (high-level wellness health model) that are a part of each individual's perception of his/her own wellness state and help that person know who and what he/she is.

a. Being: _____

_____

_____

b. Belonging: _____

_____

_____

c. Becoming: _____

_____

_____

d. Befitting: _____

_____

_____

APPLYING YOUR KNOWLEDGE

CRITICAL THINKING QUESTIONS

1. Identify and compare the factors affecting the health and illness of the following patients:

a. A 39-year-old pregnant woman who has been in good health throughout her pregnancy is admitted to the obstetrics unit for vaginal bleeding in her 16th week of pregnancy. Her husband is at her bedside.

b. A 20-year-old woman in her 23rd week of pregnancy, who is addicted to crack cocaine, is brought to the emergency room by her boyfriend. She is having contractions.

Determine the nurse's role in assisting these patients and their families.

2. Interview two patients: one who has recently experienced an acute illness and one who is chronically ill. Identify the individual health risk factors, basic human needs, and self-concepts of each patient. Explore and compare the different ways acute and chronic illnesses affect patients and their families.

REFLECTIVE PRACTICE USING CRITICAL THINKING SKILLS

Use the following expanded scenario from Chapter 3 in your textbook to answer the questions below.

Scenario: Ruth Jacobi is a 62-year-old woman who was hospitalized after a "mini-stroke." While hospitalized, she was prescribed medication for high blood pressure and was referred to a smoking cessation support group. She has now returned to her pre-event level of functioning and is being prepared for discharge. She says, "I know I have an increased risk for a major stroke, so I want to do everything possible to stay as active and healthy as I can."

1. How might the nurse respond to Ms. Jacobi's stated desire for a higher level of wellness?

_____

_____

_____

2. What would be a successful outcome for this patient?

_____

_____

3. What intellectual, technical, interpersonal, and/or ethical/legal competencies are most likely to bring about the desired outcome?

_____

_____

_____

4. What resources might be helpful for Ms. Jacobi?

_____

_____

_____

Health of the Individual, Family, and Community

PRACTICING FOR NCLEX

MULTIPLE CHOICE QUESTIONS

Circle the letter that corresponds to the best answer for each question.

1. Which of the following needs has the highest priority?
   a. The need to be loved by someone
   b. The need to be the best nurse you possibly can
   c. The need to live in a safe environment
   d. The need for a balanced intake and output of fluids

2. Which of the following theorists identified stages of the family cycle and critical family developmental tasks?
   a. Duvall
   b. Erickson
   c. Maslow
   d. Johnson

3. A change in body image, such as the loss of a body part, may affect which of the following type of human needs?
   a. Love and belonging needs
   b. Safety and security needs
   c. Self-actualization needs
   d. Self-esteem needs

4. Which of the following would be considered a community risk factor?

   a. A woman finds out that she is genetically inclined to develop crippling arthritis.
   b. An 80-year-old man is at risk for falls in his home due to clutter in his hallways and stairways.
   c. Children of a low-income family are kept inside the home on a sunny summer day because of lack of recreational opportunities in their neighborhood.
   d. A child is born with severe mental retardation.

ALTERNATE-FORMAT QUESTIONS

Multiple Response Questions

Circle the letters that correspond to the best answers for each question.

1. Which of the following are examples of physiologic needs according to Maslow's hierarchy of needs? *(Select all that apply.)*
   a. A nurse washes her hands and puts on gloves before inserting a catheter in a patient.
   b. A nurse invites a patient's estranged son to visit him.
   c. A nurse counsels an overweight teenager about proper nutrition.
   d. A nurse administers pain medication to a postoperative patient.
   e. A nurse attains a master's degree in nursing by going to school in the evening.
   f. A home care practitioner requests a quiet environment so her elderly patient can get some rest.

2. Which of the following are examples of self-actualization needs according to Maslow's hierarchy of needs? *(Select all that apply.)*

   a. A nurse attains a master's degree in nursing by going to school in the evening.

   b. A nurse refers a patient's spouse to an Al-Anon group meeting.

   c. A student nurse takes a course in communication to improve her ability to relate to patients.

   d. A nurse raises the side rails on the bed of a patient at risk for falls.

   e. A nurse administers insulin to a diabetic patient.

   f. A nurse subscribes to several nursing journals to stay abreast of developments in the profession.

3. Which of the following statements about the family unit are accurate? *(Select all that apply.)*

   a. According to Friedman (2003), the members of a group home would not be considered a family.

   b. The family is a buffer between the needs of individual members and society.

   c. The family should not be concerned with meeting the needs of society.

   d. Duvall (1977) identified critical family developmental tasks and stages in the family life cycle.

   e. The nuclear family is composed of two parents and their children.

   f. A blended family exists when parents adopt a child from another culture.

4. Which of the following is a developmental task of the family with middle-aged adults? *(Select all that apply.)*

   a. Adjust to the cost of family life

   b. Maintain ties with younger and older generations

   c. Prepare for retirement

   d. Adjust to loss of spouse

   e. Support moral and ethical family values

   f. Cope with loss of energy and privacy

Prioritization Question

1. Place the following list of human needs in order from highest-level needs to lower-level needs according to Maslow's hierarchy of basic human needs:

a. A nurse includes family members in the care of a patient.

b. A nurse places a no smoking sign on the door of a patient who is receiving oxygen.

c. A nurse provides nutrition for a patient through a feeding tube.

d. A nurse prepares a room for a clerical visit requested by a patient.

e. A nurse helps a patient focus on her strengths following a diagnosis of breast cancer.

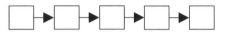

DEVELOPING YOUR KNOWLEDGE BASE

FILL-IN-THE-BLANKS

1. The most important of all basic human needs is _____.

2. According to Maslow's hierarchy of basic human needs, physical activity and rest are considered to be _____ needs.

3. Relatives such as aunts, uncles, and grandparents are part of what is known as the _____ family.

4. The function of the family that helps a family member meet his or her basic needs by providing emotional comfort and helping to establish and maintain an identity in times of stress is _____.

5. The number and availability of healthcare institutions and services would be considered a(n) _____ risk factor.

MATCHING EXERCISES

Match the correct risk factor category listed in Part A with the appropriate example of family risks listed in Part B. (Some answers will be used more than once.)

PART A

a. Lifestyle

b. Psychosocial

c. Developmental

d. Environmental

e. Biologic

PART B

1. ____ A child with severe birth defects is born into a family.

2. ____ A teacher reports to a teenage boy's parents that drugs have been found in his locker.

3. ____ A recently divorced single parent of a 2-year-old must return to work but cannot afford adequate childcare.

4. ____ Two families are forced to live together in cramped conditions to make ends meet.

5. ____ Families in a city ghetto area fear walking to school/work because of gang activity on their street.

6. ____ An older adult living with her son's family cannot tolerate what she feels is inadequate discipline of her grandchildren.

7. ____ A mother returns home from the hospital with a premature baby for whom she must provide care.

8. ____ A 13-year-old in her first trimester of pregnancy tells you she didn't think she could become pregnant the first time she had sexual relations.

9. ____ A family vacationing in Mexico becomes ill after drinking the local water.

10. ____ An elderly man who lives alone cannot afford his prescriptions.

11. ____ A couple learns that their infant has sickle cell anemia.

12. ____ A 5-year-old girl accuses her uncle of touching her inappropriately.

13. ____ A 3-month-old infant fails to thrive because of malnutrition.

14. ____ A woman whose mother died of breast cancer finds a lump in her breast during her monthly breast examination.

SHORT ANSWER

1. Give an example of the following family functions and explain how each meets the needs of individual family members and society as a whole.

   a. Physical: _____

   _____

   _____

   b. Economic: _____

   _____

   _____

   c. Reproductive: _____

   _____

   _____

   d. Affective and coping: _____

   _____

   _____

   e. Socialization: _____

   _____

   _____

2. A first-time mother-to-be is taken to the surgical unit for an emergency cesarean birth. Her husband is standing nearby, with a look of confusion and apprehension on his face. Give an example of how each of the following basic needs can be met by the nurse in caring for this couple.

   a. Physiologic needs: _____

   _____

   _____

   b. Safety and security needs: _____

   _____

   _____

   c. Love and belonging needs: _____

   _____

   _____

   d. Self-esteem needs: _____

   _____

   _____

   e. Self-actualization needs: _____

   _____

   _____

3. List three types of families you have dealt with in your life experience. Describe how each family differs from one another. Which families do you feel have been most effective in preparing their members to meet individual, family, and community needs? Explain your choices.

a. _____
_____
_____
_____
_____
_____

b. _____
_____
_____
_____
_____
_____

c. _____
_____
_____
_____
_____
_____

4. List typical questions that should be part of a family assessment.

a. _____
_____

b. _____
_____

c. _____
_____

APPLYING YOUR KNOWLEDGE

CRITICAL THINKING QUESTIONS

1. Volunteer some of your time at a local homeless shelter or any other service-oriented organization. Identify the individual immediate and long-term needs of the individuals served. List each of these needs in order of importance. What can be done to help promote health in these individuals? Explain how you could attempt to provide

the following basic needs for the individuals served:

a. Physiologic needs:

b. Safety and security needs:

c. Love and belonging needs:

d. Self-esteem needs:

e. Self-actualization needs:

2. Review the lifestyles of some of the characters in your favorite TV dramas. Identify their risk factors, and give an example of a character at risk for each of the following:

a. Lifestyle

b. Social/psychological

c. Environmental

d. Biologic

Describe an appropriate nursing response for each example noted above.

REFLECTIVE PRACTICE USING CRITICAL THINKING SKILLS

Use the following expanded scenario from Chapter 4 in your textbook to answer the questions below.

Scenario: Samuel Kaplan is an 80-year-old man who walks with a cane after recent knee surgery. His wife, aged 76 years, was diagnosed with Alzheimer's disease 1 year ago. The couple has no family living nearby, but a son lives with his wife and children about 200 miles away. After it is suggested that his wife be admitted to a nursing home, Mr. Kaplan breaks into tears and says, "I don't think I can continue to care for my wife at home anymore. But how can I even consider putting her in a nursing home?"

1. What basic human needs should be addressed by the nurse to provide individualized, holistic care for Mr. Kaplan?

_____
_____
_____

2. What would a successful outcome be for this patient?

_____
_____
_____

3. What intellectual, technical, interpersonal, and/or ethical/legal competencies are most likely to bring about the desired outcome?

_____

_____

_____

4. What resources might be helpful for Mr. Kaplan?

_____

_____

_____

CHAPTER 5

Theory, Research, and Evidence-Based Practice

PRACTICING FOR NCLEX

MULTIPLE CHOICE QUESTIONS

Circle the letter that corresponds to the best answer for each question.

1. Which of the following statements accurately describes a characteristic of a theory?
   a. A theory is based on facts and contains absolute or direct proof.
   b. A theory is a single statement or concept that gives meaning to a series of events.
   c. Theories cannot be tested or changed.
   d. A theory is a group of concepts that form a pattern of reality.

2. When a nursing theorist identifies a specific idea or action and then makes conclusions about general ideas, he/she is using which of the following methods?
   a. Inductive reasoning
   b. Nursing process
   c. Deductive reasoning
   d. General systems theory

3. Which of the following theories is based on the breaking down of whole things into parts and then learning how these parts work together as a whole?
   a. Adaptation theory
   b. Developmental theory
   c. General systems theory
   d. Psychosocial theory

4. Which of the following statements accurately describes a characteristic of a system?
   a. A system is an entity in itself and cannot communicate with or react to its environment.
   b. Boundaries separate systems from each other and from their environments.
   c. All systems are closed in that they do not allow energy, matter, or information to move between systems and boundaries.
   d. Each system is independent of its subsystems in that a change in one element does not affect other systems.

5. According to Eric Erikson's developmental theory, psychosocial development is accomplished through which of the following processes?
   a. Socialization
   b. Human needs
   c. Heredity
   d. Health status

6. Of the four common components in theories of nursing, which of the following should be the focus of nursing?
   a. Environment
   b. Health
   c. Nursing
   d. Person

7. Which of the following theorists believed that a person is a biopsychosocial being who is basically good?

a. Imogene M. King

b. Madeline Leininger

c. Sister Callista Roy

d. Jean Watson

8. According to Levine's theory of nursing, nursing practice should focus on which of the following?

a. The art and science of a human-to-human care process with a spiritual dimension

b. The human and the complexity of his or her relationships with the environment

c. The balance within an individual, specific to the behavioral system, when illness occurs

d. The variables affecting human response to stressors, with primary concern for the total person

9. Which of the following would best define the environment in Orem's self-care model?

a. Modern society's values and expectations

b. All the patterns that exist external to the individual

c. The culture of each individual group, or society

d. The healthcare system, including the nurse

ALTERNATE-FORMAT QUESTIONS

Multiple Response Questions

Circle the letters that correspond to the best answers for each question.

1. Which of the following statements regarding quantitative research are accurate? *(Select all that apply.)*

a. Basic research is designed to directly influence or improve clinical practice.

b. The types of quantitative research depend on the level of current knowledge about a research problem.

c. Data that researchers collect from subjects are called variables.

d. A hypothesis is based on the independent variables that the researcher finds.

e. Independent variables are the causes or conditions that are manipulated or identified to determine the effects of the dependent variable.

f. Instruments are the devices used to collect and record data.

2. Which of the following are qualitative research methods? *(Select all that apply.)*

a. Phenomenology

b. Grounded theory

c. Ideology

d. Democracy

e. Ethnography

f. Historical

3. Which of the following are accurate guidelines when using the quantitative research process? *(Select all that apply.)*

a. State the research problem as a general problem, as opposed to focusing narrowly on the problem being studied.

b. Do not define the purpose of the study until conclusions have been made.

c. Review related literature for information.

d. Formulate hypotheses and variables.

e. Select a research design that is loosely determined and can be manipulated as information is collected.

f. Collect and analyze data from various sources, including people, literature, documents, and findings.

4. Which of the following are types of quantitative research? *(Select all that apply.)*

a. Exploratory research

b. Descriptive research

c. Correlational research

d. Outcome research

e. Experimental research

f. Evidence-based research

5. Which of the following statements are accurate descriptions of nursing theorists and their central themes? *(Select all that apply.)*

a. Hildegard Peplau: Nursing is a therapeutic, interpersonal, and goal-oriented process.

b. Faye Abdullah: The patient is an individual who requires help to reach independence.

c. Ernestine Weidenbach: Emphasis is on the ill person in the healthcare setting; describes detailed nursing skills and actions.

d. Martha Rogers: A focus on rehabilitation, encompassing nursing's autonomy in the therapeutic use of cure and care.

e. Dorothea Orem: Self-care is a human need; self-care deficits require nursing actions.

f. Madeline Leininger: Caring is the central theme of nursing care, nursing knowledge, and nursing practice.

6. Which of the following are key points in the general systems theory? *(Select all that apply.)*

   a. A system is a set of separate and distinct elements.

   b. The whole system is always greater than the sum of its parts.

   c. Systems are hierarchical in nature and are composed of interrelated subsystems that work together to effect change.

   d. Systems are not separated from each other by boundaries.

   e. A system communicates with and reacts to its environment through input and output.

   f. A closed system allows input from or output to the environment.

DEVELOPING YOUR KNOWLEDGE BASE

FILL-IN-THE-BLANKS

1. _____ research involves the concepts of basic and applied research.

2. _____ are abstract impressions organized into symbols of reality.

3. The _____ theory describes the process by which living matter adjusts to other living things and to environmental conditions.

4. _____ is the patient's right to agree knowledgeably, to participate in a study without coercion, or to refuse to participate without jeopardizing the care he/she will receive.

5. _____ is nursing care provided that is supported by reliable research-based evidence.

MATCHING EXERCISES

Match the term in Part A with the correct definition listed in Part B.

PART A

a. Adaptation theory

b. General systems theory

c. Philosophy

d. Concept

e. Theory

f. Process

g. Developmental theory

h. Nursing theory

i. System

j. Knowledge system

PART B

1. ____ The action phase of a conceptual framework; a series of actions, changes, or functions that bring about a desired goal

2. ____ The study of wisdom, fundamental knowledge, and the processes used to develop and construct our perceptions of life

3. ____ A set of interacting elements, all serving the common purpose of contributing an overall goal

4. ____ Differentiates nursing from other disciplines and activities in that it serves the purposes of describing, explaining, predicting, and controlling desired outcomes of nursing care practices

5. ____ Abstract impressions from the environment organized into symbols of reality; describes objects, properties, and events and the relationships among them

6. ____ A statement that explains or characterizes an action, occurrence, or event that is based on observed facts but lacks absolute or direct proof

7. ____ Emphasizes relationships between the whole and the parts and describes how parts function and behave

8. ____ Defines a continuously occurring process that effects change and involves interaction and response

9. ____ Outlines human growth as a predictable and orderly process beginning with conception and ending with death

SHORT ANSWER

1. Nursing theories are often based on, and influenced by, other broadly applicable processes and theories. Briefly describe the ideas and principles of the following theories that are basic to many nursing concepts.

   a. General systems theory: _____

   _____

   _____

b. Adaptation theory: _____

_____

_____

c. Developmental theory: _____

_____

_____

2. List four basic characteristics of nursing theories:

a. _____

_____

b. _____

_____

c. _____

_____

d. _____

_____

3. Explain how the following factors have influenced the nursing profession.

a. Cultural influences on nursing: _____

_____

_____

_____

b. Educational influences on nursing: _____

_____

_____

_____

c. Research and publishing in nursing: _____

_____

_____

_____

d. Improved communication in nursing: _____

_____

_____

_____

e. Improved autonomy of nursing: _____

_____

_____

_____

4. Which nursing theorist(s) best defines your own personal beliefs about nursing practice, and why?

_____

_____

_____

APPLYING YOUR KNOWLEDGE

CRITICAL THINKING QUESTIONS

1. Describe how three different theories of nursing would direct the nursing care (identification and management of health/nursing needs) of the family described here: A 15-year-old girl who self-mutilates by cutting is admitted to the psychiatric ward for evaluation. Her family is anxious about her behavior and worried about her prognosis. A teacher who reported the incident is close to the girl and asks to speak to the attending physician.

2. Write the theories discussed in this chapter on a piece of paper, along with a brief description of their basic tenets (refer to Table 5-1 in the textbook). Interview your faculty, nurses you know, and classmates and have them rank the theories in order of importance based on their own system of beliefs. Ask the participants to give you an example of their personal philosophy that they would like to incorporate into their nursing practice. Note which theory was most widely respected, and determine its value to your own practice.

REFLECTIVE PRACTICE USING CRITICAL THINKING SKILLS

Use the following expanded scenario from Chapter 5 in your textbook to answer the questions below.

Scenario: Charlotte Horn, the daughter of a 57-year-old patient being discharged with an order for intermittent nasogastric tube feedings, is being taught how to perform the procedure. During one of the teaching sessions, Charlotte asks several questions: "How will I know the tube is in the right place? Will someone be available if I have a problem inserting the tube? What can I do to keep my mother comfortable with this tube in her?"

1. How might the nurse respond to Ms. Horn's concerns regarding the care of her mother?

_____

_____

_____

2. What would be a successful outcome for this patient?

_____

_____

_____

3. What intellectual, technical, interpersonal, and/or ethical/legal competencies are most likely to bring about the desired outcome?

_____

_____

_____

4. What resources might be helpful for Ms. Horn?

_____

_____

_____

Values, Ethics, and Advocacy

PRACTICING FOR NCLEX

MULTIPLE CHOICE QUESTIONS

Circle the letter that corresponds to the best answer for each question.

1. When a nurse is able to recognize that an ethical moment has occurred with a patient, he/she is experiencing which of the following ethical abilities?
   a. Ethical responsiveness
   b. Ethical reasoning
   c. Ethical sensibility
   d. Ethical valuing

2. A nurse who is caring for a new mother realizes that the woman is not prepared to go home with her newborn after a hospital stay of only 24 hours, but hospital policy dictates that the mother be discharged. This nurse may be faced with which of the following moral problems?
   a. Ethical uncertainty
   b. Ethical distress
   c. Ethical dilemma
   d. Ethical dissatisfaction

3. Which of the following principles applies to utilitarian action guiding theory?
   a. The rightness or wrongness of an action depends on the consequences the action produces.
   b. An action is right or wrong independent of the consequences it produces.

   c. An action is right or wrong depending on the process used to arrive at the action.
   d. The rightness or wrongness of an action is not dependent on the process used to arrive at the action.

4. Which of the following guidelines was developed by the American Hospital Association to enumerate the rights and responsibilities of patients while receiving hospital care?
   a. Code of Ethics
   b. Patient Bill of Rights
   c. Biomedical ethics
   d. Hospital patient advocacy

5. Which of the following elements of ethical agency could be described as the cultivated dispositions that allow one to act as one believes one ought to act?
   a. Ethical sensibility
   b. Ethical responsiveness
   c. Ethical character
   d. Ethical valuing

6. When a nurse provides the information and support that patients and their families need to make the decision that is right for them, he/she is practicing which of the following principles of bioethics?
   a. Autonomy
   b. Nonmaleficence
   c. Justice
   d. Fidelity

7. Nurses who value patient advocacy follow which of the following guidelines?

   a. They value their loyalty to an employing institution or to a colleague over their commitment to their patient.

   b. They give priority to the good of the individual patient rather than to the good of society in general.

   c. They choose the claims of the patient's well-being over the claims of the patient's autonomy.

   d. They make decisions for patients who are uninformed concerning their rights and opportunities.

ALTERNATE-FORMAT QUESTIONS

Multiple Response Questions

Circle the letters that correspond to the best answers for each question.

1. Which of the following statements reflect the mode of value transmission known as laissez-faire? *(Select all that apply.)*

   a. A boy says a prayer before meals that he learned from his parents.

   b. A boy is taken for ice cream to celebrate his good report card.

   c. A teenage boy explores the religions of his friends in hopes of developing his own faith.

   d. A boy is taught how to behave in public by his schoolteacher.

   e. A teenage girl is punished for staying out too late with her friends.

   f. A teenage girl tries alcohol at a party with her friends.

2. Which of the following actions best describe the use of the professional value of autonomy? *(Select all that apply.)*

   a. A nurse stays later than his/her shift to continue caring for a patient in critical condition.

   b. A nurse researches a new procedure that would benefit his/her patient.

   c. A nurse keeps her promise to call a patient's doctor regarding pain relief.

   d. A nurse reads the Patient Bill of Rights to a visually impaired patient.

   e. A nurse collaborates with other healthcare team members to ensure the best possible treatment for his patient.

   f. A novice nurse seeks the help of a more experienced nurse to insert a catheter in a patient.

3. Which of the following actions best describe the use of the professional value of altruism? *(Select all that apply.)*

   a. A nurse demonstrates an understanding of the culture of his/her patient.

   b. A nurse becomes a mentor to a student nurse working on her floor.

   c. A nurse is accountable for the care provided to a mentally challenged patient.

   d. A nurse lobbies for universal access to healthcare.

   e. A nurse respects the right of a Native American to call in a shaman for a consultation.

   f. A nurse protects the privacy of a patient with AIDS.

4. Which of the following actions best describes the use of the professional value of human dignity? *(Select all that apply.)*

   a. A nurse plans nursing care together with his/her patient.

   b. A nurse provides honest information to a patient about his/her illness.

   c. A nurse provides privacy for an elderly patient.

   d. A nurse reports an error made by an incompetent coworker.

   e. A nurse plans individualized nursing care for his/her patients.

   f. A nurse refuses to discuss a patient with a curious friend.

5. Which of the following statements accurately represent the basic principles of ethics? *(Select all that apply.)*

   a. The term "ethics" generally refers to personal or communal standards of right or wrong.

   b. The ability to be ethical begins in childhood and develops gradually.

   c. An action that is legal or customary is ethically right.

   d. Ethics is a systematic inquiry into the principles of right and wrong conduct, of virtue and vice, and of good and evil, as they relate to conduct.

   e. A commitment to developing one's ability to act ethically is known as one's ethical agency.

f. Most nurses are born with a natural ability to behave in an ethically professional way.

6. Which of the following are key principles of the Beauchamp/Childress principle-based approach to bioethics? *(Select all that apply.)*

　a. Autonomy

　b. Nonmaleficence

　c. Human dignity

　d. Beneficence

　e. Altruism

　f. Justice

DEVELOPING YOUR KNOWLEDGE BASE

FILL-IN-THE-BLANKS

1. When a young boy is left to explore values on his own with no guidance from his parents, the parents are using a(n) _____ approach to value transmission.

2. Parents who encourage their children to seek more than one solution to a problem and weigh the consequences of each are practicing the _____ mode of value transmission.

3. When a nurse analyzes her feelings regarding choices that need to be made when several alternatives are presented and decides whether these choices are rationally made, she is engaging in the practice of _____.

4. A nurse who is proud and happy about his decision to further his education is involved in the _____ step of the process of valuing.

5. A(n) _____ is an organization of values in which each value is ranked along a continuum of importance, often leading to a personal code of conduct.

6. _____ is the protection and support of another's rights.

MATCHING EXERCISES

Match the term in Part A with the correct definition listed in Part B.

PART A

a. Value

b. Ethical agency

c. Advocacy

d. Values clarification

e. Ethics

f. Morals

g. Ethical dilemma

h. Value system

i. Ethical distress

PART B

1. ___ Two (or more) clear moral principles apply, but they support mutually inconsistent courses of action.

2. ___ A process of discovery allowing a person to discover what choices to make when alternatives are presented and to identify whether these choices are rationally made or the result of previous conditioning

3. ___ A personal belief about worth that acts as a standard to guide one's behavior

4. ___ Personal or communal standards of right and wrong

5. ___ Ethical problem in which the person knows the right thing to do, but institutional constraints make it nearly impossible to pursue the right actions

6. ___ A commitment to developing one's ability to act ethically

7. ___ A systematic inquiry into the principles of right and wrong conduct, of virtue and vice, and of good and evil, as they relate to conduct

8. ___ The protection and support of another's rights

Match the mode of value transmission in Part A with the appropriate example listed in Part B. Answers may be used more than once.

PART A

a. Modeling

b. Moralizing

c. Laissez-faire

d. Rewarding and punishing

e. Responsible choice

PART B

9. ___ A boy receiving good grades in school is taken to a video arcade to celebrate.

10. ___ A girl is encouraged by her parents to explore all aspects of her own personal code of ethics.

11. ____ A child whose parents smoke decides to give it a try.

12. ____ A boy is left to his own devices when confronted with moral issues.

13. ____ A child is taught by teachers and parents that premarital sex is sinful.

14. ____ A child is encouraged to interact with people of various cultures to explore different values.

15. ____ A boy is sent to his room following an altercation with his sibling.

16. ____ A boy learns to eat a healthy diet by following his parents' example.

17. ____ A boy is allowed to determine his own bedtime.

SHORT ANSWER

1. Describe how you, as a nurse, would help the following patient to define her values and choose a plan of action using the steps listed in your text: A 36-year-old mother of a 10-year-old child with cystic fibrosis works during the day as a cashier and is going to school at night to study nursing. Her husband is a salesman who has constant overnight travel. The child needs more attention than the mother has time to supply, and the mother feels guilty for spending time to better herself. She cannot afford to hire a full-time caretaker for her child.

   a. Values clarification: _____
   _____

   b. Choosing: _____
   _____

   c. Prizing: _____
   _____

   d. Acting: _____
   _____

2. Identify four ethical issues confronted by nurses in their daily nursing practice. How would you deal with these issues in your own practice?

   a. _____
   _____

   b. _____
   _____

   c. _____
   _____

   d. _____
   _____

3. Briefly describe the five principles of bioethics, and give an example of each.

   a. Autonomy: _____
   _____
   _____

   b. Nonmaleficence: _____
   _____
   _____

   c. Beneficence: _____
   _____
   _____

   d. Justice: _____
   _____
   _____

   e. Fidelity: _____
   _____
   _____

4. Describe how a nurse might react in this situation according to the elements of ethical agency: You overhear a nurse on your ward discussing with her patient another patient's HIV status. This is not the first time this nurse has been indiscreet. You are afraid to confront the nurse because she is your superior and has been known to punish coworkers who displease her by assigning them the most difficult cases.

   a. Ethical sensibility: _____
   _____

   b. Ethical responsiveness: _____
   _____

   c. Ethical reasoning: _____
   _____

   d. Ethical accountability: _____
   _____

   e. Ethical character: _____
   _____

f. Ethical valuing: _____

_____

g. Transformative ethical leadership: _____

_____

5. Describe how you, as a nurse, would act as an advocate for the following patients:

a. An infant born addicted to crack cocaine whose mother wants to take him home:

_____

_____

b. A 12-year-old girl who seeks a pregnancy test at a Planned Parenthood clinic without her parents' knowledge: _____

_____

_____

c. A 15-year-old girl who is anorexic and who refuses to eat anything during her hospital stay: _____

_____

_____

d. A 28-year-old man, who contracted AIDS from an infected male partner, and who tells you that the other nurses have been avoiding him: _____

_____

_____

e. A 48-year-old mother with emphysema who refuses to quit smoking: _____

_____

_____

f. A 78-year-old woman in a nursing home who is dying of cancer and asks you to help her "end the pain" through assisted suicide:

_____

_____

_____

6. List the qualities you possess that you feel are most important in developing your own personal code of ethics: _____

_____

_____

7. Use the five-step model of ethical decision making listed in your text to resolve the following moral distress: You believe that a homeless patient, diagnosed with high blood pressure, needs a psychological work-up. She appears confused and unable to care for herself or manage her medication. She is alternately withdrawn and combative. You suspect she may have early Alzheimer's disease. Your superiors insist she be discharged without further treatment, and you are told there is no room for her on the psychiatric ward.

a. Assess the situation: _____

_____

b. Diagnose the ethical problem: _____

_____

c. Plan: _____

_____

d. Implement your decision: _____

_____

e. Evaluate your decision: _____

_____

8. Give an example of an ethical problem that may occur between the following healthcare personnel, patients, and institutions.

a. Nurse/patient: _____

_____

b. Nurse/nurse: _____

_____

c. Nurse/physician: _____

_____

d. Nurse/institution: _____

_____

APPLYING YOUR KNOWLEDGE

CRITICAL THINKING QUESTIONS

1. Describe how you would respond in an ethical manner to the requests of the following patients:

a. A patient with end-stage pancreatic cancer confesses to you that the only relief he can get from his pain is from smoking marijuana. He asks you to look the other way while he lights up a joint.

b. The anxious father of a 17-year-old gay patient asks you to perform an HIV test on his son without his son's knowledge.

c. A woman who presents with contusions and marks consistent with domestic abuse tells you that her husband pushed her down the steps. She asks you not to tell anyone. When her husband arrives, he hovers over her in an obsessive and overly protective manner.

2. Describe what you would do in the following situations:

a. A doctor asks you to falsify a report that he prescribed medicine contraindicated for a patient's condition.

b. A nurse coworker refuses to bathe an HIV-positive patient.

c. Due to administrative cutbacks, there are not enough nurses scheduled to cover the critical care unit in which you work.

Share your responses with a classmate and explore the difference in your responses. What competencies and character traits promote ethical behavior?

REFLECTIVE PRACTICE USING CRITICAL THINKING SKILLS

Use the following expanded scenario from Chapter 6 in your textbook to answer the questions below.

Scenario: William Raines, a homeless 68-year-old man diagnosed with schizophrenia, developmental delays, and uncontrolled hypertension, was admitted for control of moderately severe elevation of his blood pressure. A review of his medical record reveals that Mr. Raines, who has no medical insurance, was getting samples of medications for blood pressure treatment from the pharmaceutical representatives at the clinic. A recent policy change stopped this practice approximately 4 weeks ago. Mr. Raines is about to be discharged with several prescriptions for medications, but he refuses to take the prescriptions, saying, "Why take that useless paper? I haven't got any money to buy those pills with, anyway."

1. How might the nurse react to Mr. Raines response to filling his prescriptions?

_____

_____

_____

2. What would be a successful outcome for this patient?

_____

_____

_____

3. What intellectual, technical, interpersonal, and/or ethical/legal competencies are most likely to bring about the desired outcome?

_____

_____

_____

4. What resources might be helpful for Mr. Raines?

_____

_____

_____

CHAPTER 7

Legal Implications of Nursing

PRACTICING FOR NCLEX

MULTIPLE CHOICE QUESTIONS

Circle the letter that corresponds to the best answer for each question.

1. A body of law that has evolved from accumulated judiciary decisions is known as which of the following?
   a. Statutory law
   b. Administrative law
   c. Common law
   d. Constitutional law

2. A nurse who misrepresents the outcome of a procedure or treatment may have committed which of the following torts?
   a. Slander
   b. Fraud
   c. Libel
   d. Assault

3. Which of the following is the process in which specialty knowledge, experience, and clinical judgment are validated by many U.S. professional organizations?
   a. Certification
   b. Accreditation
   c. Licensure
   d. Litigation

4. Which of the following is the primary reason for filling out an incident report?
   a. To document everyday occurrences
   b. To document the need for disciplinary action
   c. To improve quality of care
   d. To initiate litigation

5. The Good Samaritan laws would protect which of the following actions performed by a healthcare practitioner?
   a. Any emergency care where consent is given
   b. Negligent acts performed in an emergency situation
   c. Medical advice given to a neighbor regarding her child's rash
   d. Emergency care for a choking victim in a restaurant

6. Protection of employees from discrimination based on race, color, religion, sex, and national origin is provided under which of the following government agencies?
   a. OSHA
   b. EEOC
   c. HUD
   d. NAACP

7. When a nurse has met all the criteria necessary for recognition by the ANA, he/she is said to have undergone which of the following processes?
   a. Licensure
   b. Accreditation
   c. Certification
   d. Registration

8. A nurse who comments to her coworkers at lunch that her patient with a sexually transmitted disease has been sexually active in the community may be guilty of which of the following torts?

   a. Slander

   b. Libel

   c. Fraud

   d. Assault

9. What is the process by which an educational program is evaluated and recognized as having met certain predetermined criteria?

   a. Licensure

   b. Registration

   c. Accreditation

   d. Certification

10. Which of the following actions would be recommended for a nurse who is named as a defendant?

   a. Discuss the case with the plaintiff to ensure understanding of each other's positions.

   b. If a mistake was made on a chart, change it to read appropriately.

   c. Be prepared to tell your side to the press, if necessary.

   d. Do not volunteer any information on the witness stand.

ALTERNATE-FORMAT QUESTIONS

Multiple Response Questions

Circle the letters that correspond to the best answers for each question.

1. Which of the following are sources of laws at the federal and state level? *(Select all that apply.)*

   a. Constitutions

   b. Mandates

   c. Criminal law

   d. Common law

   e. Statutes

   f. Administrative law

2. Which of the following statements accurately describe the process of litigation? *(Select all that apply.)*

   a. The person bringing suit against another is called the defendant.

   b. Litigation is the process of bringing and trying a lawsuit.

   c. The defendant is presumed guilty until proven innocent.

   d. The appellate court, the first-level court, hears all the evidence in a case and makes a decision based on facts.

   e. The opinions of appellate judges are published and become common law.

   f. Common law is based on the principle of *stare decisis*.

3. Which of the following are examples of voluntary standards in nursing? *(Select all that apply.)*

   a. State nurse practice acts

   b. Rules and regulations of nursing

   c. American Nurses Association Standards of Practice

   d. Professional standards for certification of individual nurses in general practice

   e. Process of certification

   f. Process of licensure

4. Which of the following statements accurately describe the components of the judicial system? *(Select all that apply.)*

   a. A crime is a wrong against a person or his or her property, but the act is considered to be against the public as well.

   b. People who break certain laws are not guilty of a crime if they did not intend it.

   c. In most cases, criminal law is statutory law.

   d. A misdemeanor is a more serious crime than a felony.

   e. Misdemeanors are commonly punishable with fines.

   f. A tort is punishable by the state.

5. Which of the following are considered intentional torts in nursing practice? *(Select all that apply.)*

   a. Negligence

   b. Malpractice

   c. Assault and battery

   d. Fraud

   e. False imprisonment

   f. Defamation

6. Which of the following are elements that must be established to prove that malpractice or negligence has occurred? *(Select all that apply.)*

   a. Duty

   b. Intent to harm

c. Breach of duty

d. Causation

e. Punitive damages

f. Fraud

7. Which of the following are steps that occur when a malpractice suit is being litigated? *(Select all that apply.)*

   a. The basis for the claim is appropriate and timely, and at least one element of liability is present.

   b. All parties named as defendants, as well as insurance companies and attorneys, work toward a fair settlement.

   c. If the case is presented to a malpractice arbitration panel, the decision of the panel must be accepted by both parties.

   d. The defendants contest allegations, and pretrial discovery begins.

   e. A review of medical records is not allowed in pretrial discovery.

   f. If a verdict from a trial court is not accepted by both sides, it may be appealed to an appellate court.

8. Which of the following are legal safeguards for the nurse? *(Select all that apply.)*

   a. Informed consent

   b. Incompetent practice

   c. Patient education

   d. Executing physician orders without questioning them

   e. Documentation

   f. Inadequate staffing

Prioritization Question

1. Place the following steps involved in malpractice litigation in the order in which they would normally occur:

   a. Decision or verdict is reached.

   b. The basis for the claim is appropriate and timely; all elements of liability are present.

   c. Trial takes place.

   d. Pretrial discovery activities and review of medical records and deposition of plaintiff, defendants, and witnesses are performed.

   e. All parties named as defendants, as well as insurance companies and attorneys, work toward a fair settlement.

f. If the verdict is not accepted by both sides, it may be appealed to an appellate court.

g. The case is presented to a malpractice arbitration panel. The panel's decision is either accepted or rejected, in which case a complaint is filed in trial court.

h. The defendants contest allegations.

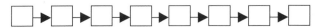

DEVELOPING YOUR KNOWLEDGE BASE

FILL-IN-THE-BLANKS

1. _____ law is law in which the government is involved directly.

2. A state's _____ protects the public by broadly defining the legal scope of nursing practice.

3. _____ is a specialized form of credentialing based on laws passed by a state legislature.

4. A nurse called by either attorney to explain to the judge and jury what happened, based on the patient's record, and to offer an opinion about whether the nursing care met acceptable standards is called a(n) _____.

5. When the nurse participates in establishing, maintaining, and improving healthcare environments and conditions of employment, he/she is participating in a practice known as _____.

6. When a nurse documents the fall of an elderly patient, he or she is filing a(n) _____ report.

7. The Joint Commission defines a(n) _____ as an unexpected occurrence involving death or serious or psychological injury, or the risk thereof.

MATCHING EXERCISES

Match the type of tort listed in Part A with an example of the tort listed in Part B.

PART A

a. Assault

b. Battery

c. Slander

d. Liability

e. Invasion of privacy

f. False imprisonment

g. Fraud

h. Negligence

i. Libel

PART B

1. ____ A nurse seeking a middle-management position in long-term care claims to be certified in gerontologic nursing, which is not the case.

2. ____ A nurse tapes an interview with a patient without his knowledge.

3. ____ A nurse threatens to slap an elderly patient who refuses to clean up after herself.

4. ____ A nurse spreads a rumor that a patient is a compulsive gambler.

5. ____ A nurse forgets to replace an IV bag that is empty.

6. ____ A nurse uses restraints on a patient unnecessarily.

7. ____ A nurse physically attacks a patient who complains that she is not being cared for properly.

8. ____ A nurse circulates a petition among her coworkers in an attempt to remove a coworker from her unit who has engaged in inappropriate behavior with a patient. This behavior is described at the top of the petition.

Match the terms listed in Part A with their definitions listed in Part B.

PART A

a. Litigation

b. Plaintiff

c. Defendant

d. Crime

e. Credentialing

f. Felony

g. Tort

h. Contract

i. Testator

j. Beneficiary

k. Misdemeanor

l. Precedent

PART B

9. ____ The person who makes a will

10. ____ The exchange of promises between two parties

11. ____ The process of a lawsuit

12. ____ The case that first sets down the rule by decision

13. ____ The one being accused in a lawsuit

14. ____ A wrong against a person or his/her property, considered to be against the public as well

15. ____ Crimes that are commonly punishable with fines or imprisonment for less than 1 year, or with both, or with parole

16. ____ The person or government bringing suit against another

17. ____ A crime punishable by imprisonment in a state or federal penitentiary for more than 1 year

18. ____ A wrong committed by a person against another person or his/her property that generally results in a civil trial

19. ____ A person who receives money or property from a will

Match the type of law listed in Part A with an example of the law listed in Part B.

PART A

a. Administrative law

b. Common law

c. Public law

d. Private law

e. Criminal law

f. Constitutional law

g. Statutory law

PART B

20. ____ Laws regulating relationships between individuals and the government

21. ____ Nurse practice acts

22. ____ Rules and regulations of boards of nursing

23. ____ Malpractice law

24. ____ Laws regulating relationships among people

25. ____ Laws involving murder, manslaughter, criminal negligence, theft, and illegal possession of drugs

SHORT ANSWER

1. Give an example of how nurses could avoid the following common allegations of malpractice.

   a. Failure to ensure patient safety: _____
   _____

   b. Improper treatment or performance of treatment: _____
   _____

   c. Failure to monitor and report: _____
   _____

   d. Medication errors and reactions: _____
   _____

   e. Failure to follow agency procedure: _____
   _____

   f. Equipment misuse: _____
   _____

   g. Adverse incidents: _____
   _____

   h. Improper use of infection control techniques: _____
   _____

2. Explain the difference between voluntary standards of nursing practice and legal standards, and give an example of each.

   a. Voluntary standards: _____
   _____

      Example: _____

   b. Legal standards: _____

      Example: _____

3. List four cases in which informed consent is needed from a patient:

   a. _____

   b. _____

   c. _____

   d. _____

4. Give three examples of invasion of privacy in a nurse–patient relationship:

   a. _____

   b. _____

   c. _____

5. List three strengths a nurse must possess to testify competently as an expert witness:

   a. _____

   b. _____

   c. _____

6. What conditions are necessary for a contract to be valid?
   _____
   _____

7. Describe what conditions you, as a nurse, would require to accept a telephone order from a physician:
   _____
   _____
   _____

8. List two cases in which it would be appropriate to question a physician's order:

   a. _____

   b. _____

9. Mrs. Toole, age 85, is recovering from a hip replacement at home. When bathing Mrs. Toole, a visiting nurse practitioner forgets to replace her bed rails, and Mrs. Toole falls out of bed. Mrs. Toole is shaken up and sore from her fall, but there appears to be no further damage to her hip.

   a. What is the nurse's liability in this situation?
   _____
   _____

   b. What information should be included in the incident report?
   _____
   _____
   _____

c. Do you feel the patient has a case for neg-ligence? Explain why or why not, using the four elements of liability that must be present to prove that negligence has occurred (duty, breach of duty, causation, damages):

_____

_____

_____

APPLYING YOUR KNOWLEDGE

CRITICAL THINKING QUESTIONS

1. Think about how you would respond in the following situation, and discuss your responsi-bilities with your classmates. Are there ever differences between the legally prudent and morally right response?

   a. Another student tells you she inadvertently gave medications to the wrong patient. She is terrified of your nurse supervisor and has decided not to inform anyone.

   b. An elderly resident in a nursing home tells you that the evening nurses are mean and sometimes push and hit her, but she begs you not to tell anyone.

   c. You observe a surgeon contaminate a sterile field; when you inform him, he tells you not to be so squeamish.

2. Watch a TV show or movie that depicts a courtroom drama. Write down all the legal jar-gon you hear and see if you can define it. Note whether the jury delivers the same verdict that you would deliver. Describe your reaction to the proceedings and verdict, and state how your conscience would dictate your resolution of the conflict.

3. Stage a mock jury with your peers. Have each person take a turn suggesting a legal issue. Let the jury deliberate and return a verdict in each case.

4. Interview someone in the legal department of the institution where you will be practicing. Ask them about the legal issues that face novice nurse practitioners and what the hospi-tal does to prevent problems from arising. Dis-cuss with this administrator what you perceive to be your legal responsibilities to patients in terms of patient safety, informed consent, equipment use, incident reports, and medica-tion errors.

REFLECTIVE PRACTICE USING CRITICAL THINKING SKILLS

Use the following expanded scenario from Chapter 7 in your textbook to answer the questions below.

Scenario: Meredith Bedford is the mother of a terminally ill young boy diagnosed with a brain tumor who is admitted to the pediatric oncology unit for a pain management program. One morning she comes out to the nurses' sta-tion and firmly says, "I'm very unhappy with the care my son is receiving. I'm going to talk with my attorney as soon as possible to press charges against the hospital." The nurse currently in charge of the boy's care is under investigation for malpractice in another case.

1. How might the nurses involved in this scenario respond to Ms. Bedford's disclosure that she will be pressing charges against the hospital?

   _____

   _____

   _____

2. What intellectual, technical, interpersonal, and/or ethical/legal competencies are most likely to be used in this situation?

   _____

   _____

   _____

3. What resources might be helpful for the nurses in this case?

   _____

   _____

   _____

CHAPTER 8

Healthcare Delivery Systems

PRACTICING FOR NCLEX

MULTIPLE CHOICE QUESTIONS

Circle the letter that corresponds to the best answer for each question.

1. In which of the following health insurance plans is the patient most limited in choice of healthcare provider?
   a. HMO
   b. PPO
   c. POS
   d. LTC

2. Which of the following types of health plans allows a third-party payer to contract with a group of healthcare providers to provide services at a lower fee in return for prompt payment and volume guarantee?
   a. HMO
   b. PPO
   c. POS
   d. LTC

3. In which of the following types of care can patients move to a living space, such as an apartment, while they are still physically able to care for themselves, and then have access to progressively more healthcare services, as needed, as long as they live?
   a. Aging in place
   b. Rest homes
   c. Nursing homes
   d. Aging gracefully

4. Diagnosis-related groups were implemented by the federal government to meet what healthcare problem?
   a. Increasing numbers of ill elderly
   b. Increasing fragmentation of care
   c. Increasing consumer complaints
   d. Increasing healthcare costs

5. Which of the following abilities would be most important for a nurse who works in a crisis intervention center?
   a. Well-developed technical skills
   b. Low tolerance for frustration
   c. Strong communication and counseling skills
   d. Ability to relate to coworkers on a professional level

6. Which of the following programs illustrates a focus on health in our society?
   a. Research on the treatment of AIDS
   b. Incarceration of drug addicts
   c. Antismoking ads on television
   d. Aggressive therapy for cancer

7. What does the term *fragmentation of care* mean?
   a. Care is provided only on certain days, such as Monday through Friday.
   b. Care is provided only to those with the resources to pay for it.

c. The healthcare provider performs total care.

d. Care is given by many different providers.

8. Which of the following nursing functions would most likely be found in an ambulatory care facility?

a. Serving as an administrator or manager

b. Providing direct patient care

c. Educating individuals or groups

d. Assessing the home environment

9. Which of the following patients would be covered by Medicare?

a. People who have kidney failure

b. Infants of low-income families needing immunizations

c. All people with disabilities

d. Dependents of people who are 65 years or older

10. Which of the following statements describes a characteristic of case management?

a. The primary objective is to identify specific protocols and timetables for care.

b. In many of these cases, the cost of services has skyrocketed.

c. Nurses who are case managers give direct care to patients.

d. Continuity of care is sacrificed under the case management system.

ALTERNATE-FORMAT QUESTIONS

Multiple Response Questions

Circle the letters that correspond to the best answers for each question.

1. Which of the following are methods used to ensure continuity of care and cost-effective care as a patient moves through the healthcare system? *(Select all that apply.)*

a. Managed care

b. Case management

c. Rural health centers

d. Parish nursing

e. Primary healthcare

f. Primary care centers

2. Which of the following would be a typical role of a nurse in a primary care center? *(Select all that apply.)*

a. Managing members of the healthcare team

b. Performing in-service education

c. Making health assessments

d. Performing technical procedures

e. Researching nursing issues

f. Providing health education

3. Which of the following statements accurately describe home healthcare in the healthcare system? *(Select all that apply.)*

a. Nurses who provide care in the home provide physical care but are unable to administer medications.

b. The importance of home healthcare is evidenced by the growing number of older people with chronic illnesses.

c. Providing for a dignified death at home is not within the realm of home healthcare.

d. Home healthcare agencies provide many different health-related services, including nursing assessment, teaching and support of patients and family, and direct care.

e. One disadvantage of home healthcare is the nurse's inability to collaborate with other healthcare providers.

f. Home healthcare is one of the most rapidly growing areas of the healthcare system, owing in part to systems of reimbursement.

4. Which of the following statements accurately describe types of payment plans for healthcare services? *(Select all that apply.)*

a. Medicare is a federally funded public assistance program for people of any age who have low incomes.

b. HMOs are prepaid managed care plans that allow subscribers to receive medical services through a group of affiliated providers.

c. Private insurance is always financed through for-profit organizations.

d. PPOs allow a third-party payer to contract with a group of healthcare providers to provide services at a lower fee in return for prompt payment and guaranteed volume of patients.

e. Most long-term insurance is paid for by Medicare.

f. The premiums of private insurance plans tend to be higher than those for managed care plans, but members can choose their own physician and services.

DEVELOPING YOUR KNOWLEDGE BASE

FILL-IN-THE-BLANKS

1. A(n) _____ is a person who enters a healthcare facility and stays there for more than 24 hours.

2. _____ centers are often located in convenient areas, such as shopping malls, often offer walk-in services without appointments, and are often open at times other than traditional office hours.

3. _____ care is a type of care provided for caregivers of homebound ill, disabled, or elderly patients.

4. _____ is a program of palliative and supportive care services providing physical, psychological, social, and spiritual care for dying persons and their families and loved ones.

5. Alcoholics Anonymous is an example of a(n) _____ agency.

6. A(n) _____ is a member of the collaborative team trained in techniques that improve pulmonary function and oxygenation.

MATCHING EXERCISES

Match the type of healthcare listed in Part A with its definition in Part B.

PART A

a. Respite care

b. Hospice services

c. Mental health centers

d. Voluntary agencies

e. Rehabilitation centers

f. Daycare centers

g. Parish nursing centers

h. Ambulatory care centers

i. Homeless shelters

j. Public health agencies

k. Long-term care facilities

l. Rural health centers

m. Hospitals

n. Schools

o. Home care

p. Industry

q. Primary care centers

PART B

1. ____ Care for infants and children whose parents work, elderly who cannot be home alone, and patients with special needs who do not need to be in a healthcare institution

2. ____ Not-for-profit community agencies financed by private donations, grants, or fundraisers

3. ____ Community health nursing practice that emphasizes holistic healthcare, health promotion, and disease prevention, with the aim of reaching people before they are sick; often volunteer and church oriented

4. ____ Special services available to terminally ill individuals and their families, providing inpatient and home care committed to maintaining quality of life and dignity in the dying person

5. ____ Provides services for patients requiring psychological or emotional rehabilitation and for treatment of chemical dependency

6. ____ Local, state, or federal agencies that provide public health services to communities of various sizes

7. ____ Urgent care center that provides walk-in emergency care services

8. ____ Often located in geographically remote areas with few healthcare providers; many of these centers are run by nurse practitioners

9. ____ Provide 24-hour services and hot lines for people who are suicidal, who are abusing drugs or alcohol, and who require psychological or psychiatric counseling

10. ____ Living units that provide housing for people who do not have regular shelter

11. ____ The traditional acute care provided for people who were too ill to care for themselves at home, who were severely injured, who required surgery or complicated treatments, or who were having babies

12. ____ Healthcare services are provided by physicians and advanced practice nurses in offices and clinics offering the diagnosis and treatment of minor illnesses, minor surgical procedures,

obstetric care, well-child care, counseling, and referrals.

13. ___ The type of care provided to homebound ill, disabled, or elderly patients to allow the primary caregiver to have some time away from the responsibilities of day-to-day care

14. ___ Nurses in this setting are often the major source of health assessment, health education, and emergency care for the nation's children.

15. ___ Occupational health nurses practicing in these settings focus on preventing work-related illnesses and injuries by conducting health assessments, teaching health promotion, and caring for minor injuries and illnesses.

Match the team member in Part A with their role in the healthcare system listed in Part B.

PART A

a. Physician

b. Physician assistant

c. Physical therapist

d. Respiratory therapist

e. Occupational therapist

f. Speech therapist

g. Dietitian

h. Pharmacist

i. Social worker

j. Unlicensed assistive personnel

k. Chaplain

PART B

16. ___ Licensed to formulate and dispense medications

17. ___ Trained to help hearing-impaired patients speak more clearly

18. ___ Responsible for the diagnosis of illness and medical or surgical treatment of that illness

19. ___ Help nurses provide direct care to patients; titles include nursing assistants, orderlies, attendants, or technicians

20. ___ Responsible for managing and planning for dietary needs of patients

21. ___ Licensed to assist physically challenged patients to adapt to limitations

22. ___ Has completed a specific course of study and a licensing examination in preparation for providing support to the physician

23. ___ Seeks to restore function or prevent further disability in a patient after an injury or illness

24. ___ Counsels patients and family members and informs them of, and refers them to, various community resources

25. ___ Has been trained in techniques that improve pulmonary function and oxygenation

SHORT ANSWER

1. List four factors that have influenced the need for increased home healthcare.

   a. _____

   b. _____

   c. _____

   d. _____

2. Describe the role of the nurse in the following healthcare centers:

   a. Primary care offices: _____

   _____

   b. Ambulatory care centers and clinics: _____

   _____

   c. Mental health centers: _____

   _____

   d. Rehabilitation centers: _____

   _____

   e. Long-term care centers: _____

   _____

3. How have recent changes in the healthcare system affected the role of the hospital as a provider of healthcare services?

   _____

   _____

4. List six services that can be performed during outpatient care.

   a. _____

   b. _____

c. _____

d. _____

e. _____

f. _____

5. Explain the term *DRG* and how it is implemented in hospitals:

_____

_____

_____

_____

6. Define the term *fragmentation of care* and its effect on the healthcare system:

_____

_____

_____

_____

APPLYING YOUR KNOWLEDGE

CRITICAL THINKING QUESTIONS

1. Think about a group of individuals in your community that is underserved and lacks access to nursing resources. How might the needs of this group be addressed?

2. Visit a healthcare clinic in your community. Find out what types of services are performed and the backgrounds of the patients seeking these services. Research how the clinic is funded and how the staff is reimbursed for its services. Would you feel comfortable being cared for in this clinic? Explain why or why not.

3. Look at the promotional materials for a local healthcare plan and interview people on the plan. Which features of the plan are most important for the insured? What does the plan lack? Is the insured party free to choose his/her own doctors or treatment plans?

4. Compare the roles and responsibilities of a physical therapist versus an occupational therapist, a physician versus a physician assistant, and a social worker versus a chaplain. Write down the responsibilities of each professional, where they overlap to provide continuity of care for the patient, and where they diverge to

meet the specific needs of each patient. How will this information help you as a nurse to coordinate the efforts of the interdisciplinary team?

REFLECTIVE PRACTICE USING CRITICAL THINKING SKILLS

Use the following expanded scenario from Chapter 8 in your textbook to answer the questions below.

Scenario: Margaret Ritchie, age 63, is caring at home for her 67-year-old husband, who is diagnosed with amyotrophic lateral sclerosis (ALS, or Lou Gehrig's disease). She says, "All the help from the home care agency has been a blessing, but I need more help and some other equipment now, and our insurance company doesn't cover these things. Plus, now the doctor says that his condition has really worsened and he probably has 6 months or less to live." On further assessment, the nurse notes that Mrs. Ritchie appears overwhelmed with her home situation and may be suffering from "caregiver burnout."

1. What nursing interventions might the nurse employ to assist Mrs. Ritchie with her caregiver duties?

_____

_____

_____

2. What would be a successful outcome for this patient?

_____

_____

_____

3. What intellectual, technical, interpersonal, and/or ethical/legal competencies are most likely to bring about the desired outcome?

_____

_____

_____

4. What resources might be helpful for Mrs. Ritchie?

_____

_____

_____

Continuity of Care

PRACTICING FOR NCLEX

MULTIPLE CHOICE QUESTIONS

Circle the letter that corresponds to the best answer for each question.

1. Mrs. Rogers is in acute respiratory distress from pneumonia but refuses to stay for treatment. It is the nurse's responsibility to do which of the following?
   a. Restrain the patient until a social worker can talk to her about the possible results of her actions.
   b. Call for a psychological consultation to see if she is mentally stable.
   c. Notify the physician; discuss the outcomes of the patient's decision and have her sign a release form.
   d. Call the patient's family and have them discharge her.

2. Which of the following actions must be performed by the nurse upon discharging a patient from a healthcare agency?
   a. Coordinating future care for the patient
   b. Writing a discharge order for the patient
   c. Writing any orders for future home visits that may be necessary for the patient
   d. Sending the patient's records to the attending physician

3. When patients are transferred within or among healthcare settings, which of the following is most important in ensuring continuity of care?
   a. Notification of all departments of room change
   b. Careful moving of all personal items
   c. Asking family members to take home the patient's jewelry, money, or other valuables
   d. Accurate and complete communication

4. Which of the following healthcare providers is responsible for the comfort and well-being of the patient on arrival to the unit?
   a. Nurse
   b. Physician
   c. Nurse's aide
   d. Admitting office clerk

5. Which of the following statements best describes the use of the word *ambulatory* in ambulatory healthcare facilities?
   a. The patient must be able to walk in.
   b. The patient does not remain overnight.
   c. The patient does not have surgery.
   d. The patient remains overnight but is not bed bound.

6. Which of the following cognitive skills would a nurse need to ensure continuity of care?
   a. The ability to provide the technical nursing assistance to meet the needs of patients and their families
   b. The ability to establish trusting professional relationships with patients, family caregivers, and healthcare professionals in different practice settings
   c. The knowledge of how to communicate patient priorities and the related plan of care as a patient is transferred between different settings

d. Commitment to securing the best setting for care to be provided for patients and the best coordination of resources to support the level of care needed

ALTERNATE-FORMAT QUESTIONS

Multiple Response Questions

Circle the letters that correspond to the best answers for each question.

1. Which of the following pieces of information would be collected during admission to a hospital? *(Select all that apply.)*

    a. Patient's name, address, and date of birth

    b. Names of family members living at home

    c. Occupation and employer of patient

    d. Results of physical assessments

    e. Religious preferences

    f. Nursing diagnoses

2. Which of the following are accurate guidelines for a nurse preparing a room for patient admission? *(Select all that apply.)*

    a. Always open and position the bed in the highest position.

    b. Fold back the top bed linens.

    c. Assemble the necessary equipment and supplies, including a hospital admission pack.

    d. Do not supply pajamas or hospital gowns until it is determined whether the patient will wear his/her own.

    e. Do not assemble special equipment needed by the patient (such as oxygen, cardiac monitors, or suction equipment) because this is the responsibility of the physician.

    f. Adjust the physical environment of the room, including lighting and temperature.

3. Which of the following actions occur initially upon admittance to a hospital? *(Select all that apply.)*

    a. The patient's name and address and the name of his/her closest relative are printed on an identification bracelet that is placed on the patient's wrist.

    b. The patient is told that he/she will be asked to sign consent forms that give consent to treatment and allow the hospital to contact insurance companies as needed.

    c. Information about the patient is printed on an admission sheet, which becomes part of the patient's permanent record.

d. The patient is asked about advance directives that he/she may have already made; if none have been made, an advance directive form is given to the patient to fill out if desired.

e. The patient is given a clear written explanation of how health information will be used and disclosed.

f. The patient is given some form of a patient bill of rights.

4. Which of the following statements describe the procedure for transferring patients from one healthcare facility to another? *(Select all that apply.)*

    a. When a patient is transferred to another room, family members should be called in (if possible) to move the patient's personal belongings to ensure they are not misplaced or lost.

    b. If a patient is moved to an intensive care unit, it may be necessary for family members to take home personal belongings and flowers.

    c. When a patient is transferred from the hospital to a long-term care facility, the patient is not formally discharged from the hospital.

    d. When a patient is transferred to a long-term facility, the original chart goes with him/her to the new facility.

    e. When a patient is transferred to a long-term facility, all personal belongings are carefully packed and sent to the new facility with him/her.

    f. In most cases, a detailed assessment and care plan is sent from the hospital to the long-term facility.

5. Which of the following occur when a patient is discharged from a healthcare setting? *(Select all that apply.)*

    a. Discharge planning is performed to plan for continuity of care.

    b. A hospital administrator coordinates an exchange of information among the patient, caregivers, and those responsible for care while the patient is in the acute care setting and after the patient returns home.

    c. The patient is assessed by the nurse to ensure that the patient does not require any complicated treatment or care performed by family members.

d. The nurse ensures that the family members are taught the knowledge and skills needed to care for the patient.

e. The physician ensures that referrals are made to such agencies as home healthcare or social services to provide support and assistance during the recovery period.

f. Preferably, the nurse who conducts the initial nursing assessment will determine the special needs of the patient being discharged.

DEVELOPING YOUR KNOWLEDGE BASE

FILL-IN-THE-BLANKS

1. _____ care is healthcare provided to people who live within a defined geographic area.

2. New federal mandates that protect patient privacy rights are provided under the _____ Act.

3. A patient who refuses treatment and leaves a hospital must sign a form releasing the physician and institution from legal responsibility for his/her health status. This patient is said to be leaving the hospital _____.

4. _____ is the process of planning for continuity of care as the patient moves from the acute care setting to care at home.

CORRECT THE FALSE STATEMENTS

Circle the word "true" or "false" that follows the statement. If you circled "false," change the underlined word or words to make the statement true. Place your answer in the space provided.

1. The <u>physician</u> is the person who most often is responsible for helping the patient make a smooth transition from one type of care setting to another.

   True   False _____

2. <u>Discharge planning</u> is the coordination of services provided to patients before they enter a healthcare setting, during the time they are in the setting, and after they leave the setting.

   True   False _____

3. People who enter a healthcare setting must take on the role of <u>patient</u>.

   True   False _____

4. <u>Ambulatory facilities</u> are those in which the patient receives healthcare services but does not remain overnight.

   True   False _____

5. The <u>admitting diagnosis</u> is generally included on the identification bracelet that is placed on the patient's wrist during treatment at a healthcare facility.

   True   False _____

6. Hospital admissions and lengths of hospital stay are <u>increasing</u>.

   True   False _____

7. Discharge planning <u>is not indicated</u> when a patient is to be placed in a nursing home or other continuing care setting.

   True   False _____

8. When <u>goals</u> are established with the patient, compliance with the treatment regimen is more likely.

   True   False _____

9. When transferring a patient to a long-term facility for care, the original chart <u>is sent with the patient</u>.

   True   False _____

10. Your patient says, "I'm going home today!" You verify this by checking the <u>nursing care plan</u>.

    True   False _____

SHORT ANSWER

1. Describe how a nurse could help reduce anxiety for a patient who expresses the following concerns on being admitted to a healthcare facility:

   a. "Who will take care of my children when I'm in here?"

   _____

   _____

   b. "Will the procedure be painful?"

   _____

   _____

c. "Will I be able to afford this?"

_____

_____

d. "Who will take care of me after my surgery?"

_____

_____

2. Briefly describe how a nurse should instruct a patient in the following areas of care before discharge:

a. Medications: _____

_____

b. Procedures and treatments: _____

_____

c. Diet: _____

_____

d. Referrals: _____

_____

e. Health promotion: _____

_____

3. Describe how the following methods help provide continuity of care for patients:

a. Discharge planning: _____

_____

b. Collaboration with other members of the healthcare team: _____

_____

c. Involving patient and family in planning: _____

_____

4. List five guidelines that should be followed when admitting and discharging a patient from a hospital, according to the standards established by the Joint Commission on Accreditation of Healthcare Organizations.

a. _____

b. _____

c. _____

d. _____

e. _____

5. List four factors the nurse should assess before discharge planning for a 38-year-old woman hospitalized for a miscarriage in her second month of pregnancy; she has been trying to conceive a child for 2 years.

a. _____

b. _____

c. _____

d. _____

6. Describe the appropriate nursing actions that would be performed during the following patient transfers:

a. Transfer within the hospital setting: ____

_____

_____

b. Transfer to a long-term facility: _____

_____

_____

c. Discharge from a healthcare setting: ____

_____

_____

7. What is the proper procedure for discharging a patient AMA (against medical advice)?

_____

8. Describe how you would prepare a hospital room for a patient who is arriving on a stretcher and is receiving oxygen. _____

_____

_____

APPLYING YOUR KNOWLEDGE

CRITICAL THINKING QUESTIONS

1. More and more hospital services are being performed on an outpatient basis. Although this practice is cost efficient, in many cases, patients are being sent home without the knowledge they need to care for themselves. Think about what can be done to bridge the gap between hospital and home healthcare. How would you use this knowledge to discharge a 59-year-old woman who lives alone and is recovering from back surgery?

2. Imagine that your elderly mother is being discharged from the hospital with a stroke that left her partially paralyzed, and she is no longer able to live alone. Community living options include a life care community, a live-in companion, living with you, or living in a nursing home. Think about the information and support you would need to make this decision. How might this knowledge influence your nursing practice?

REFLECTIVE PRACTICE USING CRITICAL THINKING SKILLS

Use the following expanded scenario from Chapter 9 in your textbook to answer the questions below.

Scenario: Jeff Hart is a 9-year-old with profound mental retardation. He is being transferred from the state home for children to the hospital for respiratory complications associated with pneumonia. His grandmother is present but refuses to sign the consent forms necessary to admit the boy.

1. How might the admitting nurse respond to the grandmother's refusal to sign consent forms?

_____

_____

_____

2. What would be a successful outcome for this patient?

_____

_____

_____

3. What intellectual, technical, interpersonal, and/or ethical/legal competencies are most likely to bring about the desired outcome?

_____

_____

_____

4. What resources might be helpful for the nurse working with this family?

_____

_____

_____

CHAPTER 10

Home Healthcare

PRACTICING FOR NCLEX

MULTIPLE CHOICE QUESTIONS

Circle the letter that corresponds to the best answer for each question.

1. Which of the following statements concerning the characteristics of a home care nurse is accurate?

  a. Clinical skills are less important in a home care setting than in a hospital setting.

  b. The nurse should not make independent decisions about patient care.

  c. The increased autonomy of the nurse reduces the nurse's legal risks.

  d. Physical assessment, nursing diagnoses, and infection control are all part of the nurse's role.

2. Which of the following statements concerning the unique role of the home care nurse is accurate?

  a. Home care is provided to the patient in a setting that is controlled by the nurse.

  b. The nurse should not feel that she is only a "guest" in the patient's home.

  c. The nurse must adapt to the patient's environment instead of the patient adapting to a strange environment.

  d. Home care nurses do not need the patient's permission to adjust furniture or patient belongings to provide a safe environment.

3. Which of the following activities would be performed by a home care nurse in the pre-entry phase of the home visit?

  a. The nurse gathers supplies that may be needed for the patient.

  b. The nurse develops rapport with the patient and family.

  c. The nurse determines desired outcomes, makes assessments, and plans and implements care.

  d. The nurse provides teaching to promote independence in self-care.

4. The 1990s were a time of transition for the home care industry. Which of the following statements accurately describes a probable trend for future home healthcare?

  a. Acuity levels of patients will be lower because of increased care in the hospital setting.

  b. More complex services will be provided in the home setting.

  c. Families will have less responsibility in caring for loved ones at home.

  d. Nursing services will be more generalized to meet the greater demand for home nurses.

ALTERNATE-FORMAT QUESTIONS

Multiple Response Questions

Circle the letters that correspond to the best answers for each question.

1. Which of the following are typical characteristics of a home health nurse? *(Select all that apply.)*

  a. Knowledgeable and skilled

  b. Dependent decision maker

  c. Not accountable for actions made in the home

d. Healthcare coordinator

e. Patient advocate

f. Patient and family educator

2. Which of the following actions take place in the entry phase of the home visit? *(Select all that apply.)*

   a. The nurse reviews the information and calls the patient.

   b. The nurse gathers more information from the patient over the phone.

   c. The nurse gathers the supplies needed for the home visit.

   d. The nurse develops rapport with the patient and family.

   e. The nurse makes assessments and determines nursing diagnoses.

   f. The nurse plans and implements nursing care.

3. Which of the following measures should be followed by the home healthcare nurse to control infection when using a supply bag? *(Select all that apply.)*

   a. Use gloves when reaching into the bag for supplies.

   b. Clean any equipment removed from the bag before returning it to the bag.

   c. Place the bag on a clean hard surface when it is set down in a patient's home.

   d. Wash hands before and after handling equipment in the bag.

   e. Wear gloves when handling blood, body fluids, and contaminated items.

   f. Use strict surgical asepsis when transferring items to and from the bag.

4. Which of the following home healthcare services would be performed by a skilled professional or paraprofessional? *(Select all that apply.)*

   a. Personal care

   b. Physical therapy

   c. Homemaking and housekeeping

   d. Live-in services

   e. Home uterine monitoring

   f. Medical social work

5. Which of the following are eligibility requirements for Medicare-covered home healthcare? *(Select all that apply.)*

   a. A nurse must decide that medical care is needed at home.

   b. A doctor must make a plan of care for the patient at home.

   c. Intermittent skilled nursing care or physical, speech, or occupational therapy must be needed.

   d. The home agency must be Medicare certified.

   e. The patient must have a life-threatening illness.

   f. The patient must be homebound.

DEVELOPING YOUR KNOWLEDGE BASE

FILL-IN-THE-BLANKS

1. _____ is care provided in a patient's place of residence.

2. The _____ provided program coverage for home healthcare to older adults participating in Medicare.

3. The home health nurse who supports a patient's rights is practicing patient _____.

4. In the home setting, the _____ is generally the coordinator of all other healthcare providers visiting the patient.

5. Typically the family members who provide home healthcare for a loved one are _____.

MATCHING EXERCISES

Match the role of the home healthcare nurse in Part A with the appropriate example of that role in Part B. Answers may be used more than once.

PART A

a. Patient advocate

b. Coordinator of services

c. Patient/family educator

PART B

1. ____ The nurse convinces her patient's insurance carrier that there is a need for continued home health services.

2. ____ The nurse provides information on wound care to a patient's family member.

3. ＿＿ The nurse designs a diet for a patient and explains it to the family member who cooks for the household.

4. ＿＿ The nurse arranges for a physical therapist to visit a patient recovering from a broken hip.

5. ＿＿ The nurse calls in a mental health worker to assess the ability of a patient's husband to provide adequate care.

6. ＿＿ The nurse reports the condition of a patient to the physician.

CORRECT THE FALSE STATEMENTS

Circle the word "true" or "false" that follows the statement. If you circled "false," change the underlined word or words to make the statement true. Place your answer in the space provided.

1. One of the changes in the healthcare industry in the past 5 years has been a shift from <u>community-based care to hospital-based care</u>.

   True   False ＿＿＿＿＿＿＿＿＿＿＿＿＿

2. The focus of hospice care is on <u>improving quality of life</u> as opposed to prolonging the length of life.

   True   False ＿＿＿＿＿＿＿＿＿＿＿＿＿

3. The focus of home healthcare is on patients of all ages with <u>acute</u> healthcare needs.

   True   False ＿＿＿＿＿＿＿＿＿＿＿＿＿

4. Once the nurse crosses the threshold of the patient's home, <u>the patient must adapt to the plan of care dictated by the nurse</u>.

   True   False ＿＿＿＿＿＿＿＿＿＿＿＿＿

5. Lillian Wald and <u>William Rathbone</u> opened the Henry Street Settlement House in New York City in 1893.

   True   False ＿＿＿＿＿＿＿＿＿＿＿＿＿

6. The introduction of DRGs in the hospital setting created <u>an earlier</u> discharge from the hospital than patients previously experienced.

   True   False ＿＿＿＿＿＿＿＿＿＿＿＿＿

7. Prior to the late 1980s, home care nurses were considered <u>specialists</u>.

   True   False ＿＿＿＿＿＿＿＿＿＿＿＿＿

8. Nurses providing care in the home <u>are not responsible</u> for independent decision making.

   True   False ＿＿＿＿＿＿＿＿＿＿＿＿＿

9. The <u>home care nurse</u> is responsible for coordinating the community resources needed by the patient.

   True   False ＿＿＿＿＿＿＿＿＿＿＿＿＿

10. During the <u>entry phase</u> of the home visit, the nurse develops rapport with the patient and family, mutually determines desired outcomes, makes assessments, plans and implements prescribed care, and provides teaching.

    True   False ＿＿＿＿＿＿＿＿＿＿＿＿＿

11. Home care is meant to be <u>long term</u>.

    True   False ＿＿＿＿＿＿＿＿＿＿＿＿＿

12. <u>Hospice care</u> provides terminally ill patients a humane option of dying with dignity.

    True   False ＿＿＿＿＿＿＿＿＿＿＿＿＿

13. Home nursing agencies emerged in major cities in the <u>late 1800s</u> to meet the needs of the growing population due to an influx of immigrants.

    True   False ＿＿＿＿＿＿＿＿＿＿＿＿＿

Date	Home Healthcare Provider/Location	Type of Care
1893	Henry Street Settlement House NYC	
Prior to WWII During and Post WWII	Physician Nurses	
Mid 1960s	1965 Social Security Act	
Post 1980	Home care specialists	
2000s	Nurses and families	

SHORT ANSWER

1. Complete the table above describing the history of home care nursing from the 1800s to the present.

2. Give an example of how you have used or witnessed the following characteristics of a home care nurse in your practice.

   a. Knowledge and skills: _____

   _____

   b. Independence: _____

   _____

   c. Accountability: _____

   _____

3. Give a brief definition and example of the following roles of the home health nurse.

   a. Patient advocate: _____

   _____

   b. Coordinator of services: _____

   _____

   c. Educator: _____

   _____

4. List the four basic guidelines for using the bag technique:

   a. _____

   b. _____

   c. _____

   d. _____

5. Describe how teaching is designed and implemented in the home care situation:

   _____

   _____

   _____

   _____

6. Explain why the family is so important to the patient's recovery as healthcare continues to shift from the hospital setting to community-based care:

   _____

   _____

   _____

7. What type of care and skills would a hospice nurse use in caring for a 35-year-old mother, dying of AIDS, who is living at home with her husband and two children, ages 13 and 6?

   _____

   _____

   _____

APPLYING YOUR KNOWLEDGE

CRITICAL THINKING QUESTIONS

1. Identify care priorities for the patients listed below who are being transferred to a home healthcare setting. Be sure to include physical, psychological, socioeconomic, environmental, spiritual, and cultural assessments for each patient. Think about nursing's role in making necessary resources available to the patient and family.

a. A 76-year-old man with advanced cancer is being sent home with a catheter and a patient-controlled analgesic pump. He lives alone, but his son lives 45 minutes away and has promised to check on him once a day. Members of his church have offered to visit him and bring him a meal once a day.

b. A 32-year-old man with advanced AIDS is being sent home to spend his remaining days with his parents. His life partner died of AIDS the previous year, and he is angry about his situation. His parents do not accept his condition and lifestyle, but offer to take care of his healthcare needs.

c. A young single mother who lives with her boyfriend is released from the hospital with an infant who has Down syndrome. Both the mother and her boyfriend work, and two incomes are needed to maintain the household. The mother has expressed concerns about being able to give her infant the proper treatment and attention.

2. Volunteer to help a home healthcare nurse who is practicing in the field. See how this professional bridges the gap between hospital and long-term facility care. Interview some of the patients and ask them if they feel their healthcare needs are being met by home healthcare agencies. Ask the home healthcare nurse if he/she feels the system is working and, if appropriate, what could be done to provide a higher quality of care for these patients.

REFLECTIVE PRACTICE USING CRITICAL THINKING SKILLS

Use the following expanded scenario from Chapter 10 in your textbook to answer the questions below.

Scenario: Alphonse Califano is a 72-year-old widower who lives alone. He was recently discharged from the hospital, where he had been treated for diabetic foot ulcers. He has a history of diabetes, hypertension, and renal disease. A home healthcare nurse is visiting him once a week.

1. What is the role of the home healthcare nurse in providing continuity of care for Mr. Califano?

_____

_____

_____

2. What would be a successful outcome for this patient?

_____

_____

_____

3. What intellectual, technical, interpersonal, and/or ethical/legal competencies are most likely to bring about the desired outcome?

_____

_____

_____

4. What resources might be helpful for Mr. Califano?

_____

_____

_____

CHAPTER 11

Blended Skills and Critical Thinking Throughout the Nursing Process

PRACTICING FOR NCLEX

MULTIPLE CHOICE QUESTIONS

Circle the letter that corresponds to the best answer for each question.

1. Which of the following statements concerning the nursing process is accurate?
   a. The nursing process is nurse oriented.
   b. The steps of the nursing process are separate entities.
   c. The nursing process is nursing practice in action.
   d. The nursing process comprises four steps to promote patient well-being.

2. Which of the following groups legitimized the steps of the nursing process in 1973 by developing standards of practice to guide nursing practice?
   a. American Nurses Association Congress for Nursing Practice
   b. Joint Commission on Accreditation of Healthcare Organizations
   c. National League of Nursing
   d. American Association of Critical Care Nursing

3. Which of the following characteristics of the nursing process could be defined as a great deal of overlapping interaction among the five steps, with each step being fluid and flowing into the next step?
   a. Interpersonal
   b. Dynamic
   c. Systematic
   d. Universally applicable

4. Which of the following statements accurately depicts a step in the critical thinking process?
   a. The first step when thinking critically is to gather as much data related to the question as possible.
   b. Nurses who think critically allow emotions to direct their thinking.
   c. Nurses who use the critical thinking process ultimately must identify alternative decisions and reach a conclusion.
   d. The critical thinking process is based on intuition and excludes the use of outside resources.

5. In which of the following cases is the nursing process applicable?
   a. When nurses work with patients who are able to participate in their care

b. When families are clearly supportive and wish to participate in care

c. When patients are totally dependent on the nurse for care

d. In all the nursing situations listed above

6. Which of the following interpersonal skills is displayed by a nurse who is attentive and responsive to the healthcare needs of individual patients and ensures the continuity of care when leaving the patient?

a. Establishing caring relationships

b. Enjoying the rewards of mutual interchange

c. Developing accountability

d. Developing ethical/legal skills

7. Which of the following traits help nurses develop the attitudes and dispositions to think critically?

a. Thinking independently

b. Being intellectually humble

c. Being curious and persevering

d. All of the above

ALTERNATE-FORMAT QUESTIONS

Multiple Response Questions

Circle the letters that correspond to the best answers for each question.

1. Which of the following statements are key descriptors of the nursing process? *(Select all that apply.)*

a. The nursing process is systematic in that each nursing activity is part of an ordered sequence of activities, depends on the accuracy of the activity that preceded it, and influences the actions that follow it.

b. The nursing process is dynamic, meaning that each step flows into the next step and there is a great deal of interaction and overlapping among the five steps.

c. The nursing process is interpersonal because the human being is always at the heart of nursing.

d. The nursing process is interpersonal in that a patient is viewed as a "problem to be solved" and nurses interact mechanically to provide the solution.

e. The nursing process is outcome oriented in that it is a means to an end, which may not always focus on the outcomes that are patient priorities.

f. The nursing process is universally applicable in nursing situations, meaning that healthcare is provided in an unchanging environment and the nursing process can be used as a tool in any nursing situation.

2. Which of the following statements describe the use of problem solving in the nursing process? *(Select all that apply.)*

a. The trial-and-error problem-solving method is used extensively in the nursing process.

b. The trial-and-error problem-solving method is recommended as a guide for nursing practice.

c. The scientific problem-solving method is closely related to the more general problem-solving process (the nursing process) commonly used by healthcare professionals as they work with patients.

d. Nurse theorists and educators advocate, basing clinical judgments on data alone in an attempt to establish nursing as a science, worthy of the respect of other professions.

e. Today, nurses acknowledge the positive role of intuitive thinking in clinical decision making.

f. Critical thinking in nursing can be intuitive or logical or a combination of both.

3. Which of the following accurately describe the role of documenting in the nursing process? *(Select all that apply.)*

a. The patient record is the chief means of communication among members of the interdisciplinary team.

b. If a nurse is accused of negligent care, a nurse's word that he/she faithfully assessed the patient's needs, diagnosed problems, and implemented and evaluated an effective plan of care is his/her best defense.

c. Legally speaking, a nursing action not documented is a nursing action not performed.

d. It is helpful to practice documentation while learning any given nursing activity.

e. The content of the patient report and nursing documentation helps to establish nursing priorities in a practice setting.

f. Because data collection is ongoing and responsive to changes in the patient's condition, it should be documented in the final step of the nursing process.

4. Which of the following are examples of ethical/legal skills? *(Select all that apply.)*

a. Working collaboratively with the healthcare team as a respected and credible colleague to reach valued goals

b. Being trusted to act in ways that advance the interests of patients

c. Using technical equipment with sufficient competence and ease to achieve goals with minimal distress to patients

d. Selecting nursing interventions that are most likely to yield the desired outcomes

e. Being accountable for practice to oneself, the patient, the caregiving team, and society

f. Acting as an effective patient advocate

5. Which of the following are considered characteristics of a critical thinker? *(Select all that apply.)*

a. Thinking based on the opinions of others

b. Being open to all points of view

c. Acting like a "know-it-all"

d. Resisting "easy answers" to patient problems

e. Thinking "outside the box"

f. Accepting the status quo

Prioritization Questions

1. Place the following nursing activities in the order that they would most likely occur when a healthcare professional uses the nursing process:

a. Modifying the plan of care (if indicated)

b. Carrying out the plan of care

c. Establishing the database

d. Interpreting and analyzing patient data

e. Establishing priorities

f. Measuring how well the patient has achieved desired outcomes

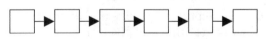

2. Place the following steps of scientific problem solving in the order in which they occur in the process:

a. Hypothesis formulation

b. Plan of action

c. Evaluation

d. Interpretation of results

e. Problem identification

f. Data collection

g. Hypothesis testing

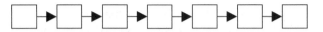

DEVELOPING YOUR KNOWLEDGE BASE

FILL-IN-THE-BLANKS

1. The steps of the nursing process were legitimized in 1973 when the ANA Congress for Nursing Practice developed _____ to guide nursing performance.

2. When a nurse assists a patient to achieve desired goals such as promoting wellness, preventing disease and illness, restoring health, or facilitating coping with altered functioning, he/she is using the _____ step of the nursing process.

3. _____ is an instructional strategy that requires learners to identify, graphically display, and link key concepts.

4. A nurse who reports his/her employer's violation of law to law enforcement agencies outside the employer's facilities is termed a(n) _____.

5. The three important ideas that must be linked together during clinical planning are _____, _____, and _____.

MATCHING EXERCISES

Match the step of the nursing process listed in Part A with the related task listed in Part B. Answers will be used more than once.

PART A

a. Assessing

b. Diagnosing

c. Planning

d. Implementing

e. Evaluating

PART B

1. ____ A nurse performs an initial patient interview.

2. ____ A home care nurse helps the physical therapist exercise the patient's limbs.

3. ____ A nurse sits down with the healthcare team halfway through treatment of a patient to see how effective the treatment has been.

4. ____ A nurse analyzes data to determine what health problems might exist.

5. ____ A nurse sets a goal for an obese teenager to lose 2 pounds a week.

6. ____ A nurse consults with a patient's support people and other healthcare professionals to learn more about a patient's problem.

7. ____ A nurse decides whether to continue, modify, or terminate the healthcare plan.

8. ____ A nurse identifies the strengths a patient with cancer possesses.

9. ____ A home care nurse determines how much nursing care is needed by an elderly stroke patient living with her daughter.

10. ____ A nurse weighs a patient after 3 weeks to determine whether his/her new diet has been effective.

11. ____ A nurse documents respiratory care performed on a patient.

12. ____ A nurse reviews a patient's past medical records.

Match the competencies listed in Part A with the appropriate example of competencies listed in Part B. Answers will be used more than once.

PART A

a. Cognitive competencies
b. Technical competencies
c. Interpersonal competencies
d. Ethical/legal competencies

PART B

13. ____ A nurse conducts a patient interview in such a way that the patient relaxes and "opens up" to her.

14. ____ A nurse skillfully attaches a heart monitor to a patient.

15. ____ A nurse carefully fills out an incident report documenting a fall.

16. ____ A nurse understands the need for palpating the lungs of a patient with pneumonia.

17. ____ A nurse checks the side rails on a bed of an elderly patient with a history of falls.

18. ____ A nurse successfully performs a catheterization of a patient.

19. ____ A nurse is familiar with the various types of medications for high blood pressure and their side effects.

20. ____ A nurse calms the mother of an infant brought to the emergency room with a high fever.

21. ____ A nurse competently starts an IV drip on a patient.

22. ____ A nurse checks a patient's bracelet before administering medications.

SHORT ANSWER

1. List three patient and three nursing benefits of using the nursing process correctly.

   Patient:

   a. _____

   b. _____

   c. _____

   Nursing:

   a. _____

   b. _____

   c. _____

2. Describe how the nurse and patient work together to accomplish the following tasks of the nursing process:

   a. Determining the need for nursing care:

   _____

   _____

   b. Planning and implementing the care:

   _____

   _____

   c. Evaluating the results of the nursing care:

   _____

   _____

3. Define the nursing process:

_____

_____

What are the primary goals of the nursing process?

_____

_____

What skills are necessary to use the nursing process successfully?

_____

_____

Which of these skills do you personally possess and which do you need to develop in your practice?

_____

_____

4. Describe what the following words mean to you and how they apply to your use of the nursing process:

a. Systematic: _____

_____

b. Dynamic: _____

_____

c. Interpersonal: _____

_____

d. Goal oriented: _____

_____

e. Universally applicable: _____

_____

5. Briefly explain how the following considerations are relevant to the successful use of critical thinking competencies:

a. Purpose of thinking: _____

_____

b. Adequacy of knowledge: _____

_____

c. Potential problems: _____

_____

d. Helpful resources: _____

_____

e. Critique of judgment/decision: _____

_____

6. List four good habits nurses should develop to help them master the manual competencies essential to quality nursing process.

a. _____

b. _____

c. _____

d. _____

7. Think of three people you know personally, preferably of different ages, professions, or cultures. What about each of these individuals causes you to respect his/her human dignity? Are some people more deserving of respect than others? How do you show respect for them in your daily contact with them?

_____

_____

_____

_____

8. Follow three different nurses on their daily rounds of patients, noticing how they relate to their patients. Does their attitude say "drop dead," "you mean nothing to me," or "I care about you"? Note what each nurse said or did to display this attitude.

a. Nurse 1: _____

_____

b. Nurse 2: _____

_____

c. Nurse 3: _____

_____

9. Nurses skilled in developing caring relationships often need to direct the conversations with their patients. Develop four opening statements/questions designed to elicit information from a patient that you could use in your own practice.

a. _____

b. _____

c. _____

d. _____

10. List four areas a nurse should consider when seeking to develop a sense of legal and ethical accountability to a patient.

a. _____

b. _____

c. _____

d. _____

APPLYING YOUR KNOWLEDGE

CRITICAL THINKING QUESTIONS

1. Assess your personal blend of the skills nurses need: cognitive, technical, interpersonal, and ethical/legal. Would you want you to be your nurse? What skills do you need to develop to meet the needs of those entrusted to your care?

2. Think about major health problems on campus. How might the school of nursing use the nursing process to address one or more of these problems? Do you as a nursing student have an obligation to address the health problems you encounter?

3. Think about a stressful situation you had to deal with, such as changing a course of study, accepting a job in another city, dealing with a sick relative, deciding on a life partner, and so on. What methods did you use to weigh all your options in making this decision? Where did you turn for information or assistance? How did you reach your final decision? Relate the method you used in your life to the models of problem solving listed in this chapter. Which process most accurately describes your personal process of problem solving? Compare this process to the nursing process.

4. Write down all the qualities you admire in your friends. What is it about them that makes you respect them? What attributes of their personality don't you like? How might this knowledge help you to understand your responses to patients with different personality traits? Are some patients more worthy of your respect than others? Do you feel your attitude toward a patient affects the outcome of treatment?

REFLECTIVE PRACTICE USING CRITICAL THINKING SKILLS

Use the following expanded scenario from Chapter 11 in your textbook to answer the questions below.

Scenario: Charlotte Horvath is a single mother whose 5-year-old daughter is to be discharged soon. Ms. Horvath is scheduled to learn how to perform wound care for her daughter at home but has missed every planned teaching session thus far. When questioned by the nurse, Ms. Horvath says she doesn't have enough time to put a decent meal on the table, let alone learn how to take care of a wound at home. Ms. Horvath works the evening shift and has a babysitter stay with her children from immediately after school until midnight.

1. How might the nurse use blended nursing skills to respond to this patient situation?

_____

_____

_____

2. What would be a successful outcome for this patient and her family?

_____

_____

_____

3. What intellectual, technical, interpersonal, and/or ethical/legal competencies are most likely to bring about the desired outcome?

_____

_____

_____

4. What resources might be helpful for Ms. Horvath?

_____

_____

_____

CHAPTER 12

Assessing

PRACTICING FOR NCLEX

MULTIPLE CHOICE QUESTIONS

Circle the letter that corresponds to the best answer for each question.

1. Data that can be observed by one person and verified by another person observing the same patient are known as:
   a. Subjective data
   b. Covert data
   c. Symptomatic data
   d. Objective data

2. During which of the following phases of the nurse–patient interview does the nurse gather all the information needed to form the subjective database?
   a. Preparatory phase
   b. Introduction
   c. Working phase
   d. Termination

3. Which of the following nurse–patient positioning facilitates an easy exchange of information?
   a. If the patient is in bed, the nurse stands at the foot of the bed.
   b. If both the nurse and patient are seated, their chairs are at right angles to each other, 1 foot apart.
   c. If the patient is in bed, the nurse sits in a chair placed at a 45-degree angle to the bed.
   d. If the patient is in bed, the nurse stands at the side of the bed.

4. Which of the following sources of patient data is usually the primary and best source?
   a. Patient
   b. Support people
   c. Patient records
   d. Reports of diagnostic studies

5. Mrs. Smith is admitted to the hospital with complaints of left-sided weakness and difficulty speaking. Which of the following assessments contains the data that best represent a nursing assessment?
   a. Neurologic examination reveals partial paralysis and aphasic speech.
   b. Brain scan shows evidence of a clot in the middle cerebral artery.
   c. Patient is unable to communicate basic needs and cannot perform hygiene measures with left hand.
   d. Left-sided weakness and speech deficit indicate probable stroke.

6. Mr. Martin is an energetic 80-year-old, admitted to the hospital with complaints of difficulty urinating, bloody urine, and burning on urination. In assessing Mr. Martin, which of the following is a priority?
   a. Assessing only the urinary system
   b. Focusing on altered patterns of elimination common in the elderly
   c. Obtaining a detailed assessment of the patient's sexual history
   d. Conducting a thorough systems review to validate data on the patient's record

7. During the nursing examination, Mrs. Jones becomes very tired, but there are still questions the nurse practitioner would like to address in order to have data for planning care. Which of the following actions would be most appropriate in this situation?
   a. Ask Mrs. Jones to wake up and try to answer your questions.
   b. Ask Mrs. Jones's husband to come in and answer your questions.
   c. Wait until the next day to obtain the answers to your questions.
   d. Ask Mrs. Jones if she objects to your interviewing her husband to obtain the needed data.

8. Mrs. Anderson, age 50, is admitted to your unit with the diagnosis of scleroderma. You are unfamiliar with this condition. Which of the following would be your best source of information?
   a. Consult with the patient.
   b. Consult with the patient's doctor.
   c. Read the patient's chart.
   d. Consult nursing and medical literature.

ALTERNATE-FORMAT QUESTIONS

Multiple Response Questions

Circle the letters that correspond to the best answers for each question.

1. Which of the following nursing actions would occur during the preparatory phase of the nursing interview? *(Select all that apply.)*
   a. The nurse ensures that the interview environment is private and relaxing.
   b. The nurse initiates the interview by stating his or her name and status.
   c. The nurse assesses the patient's comfort and ability to participate in the interview.
   d. The nurse arranges the seating in the interview room to facilitate an easy exchange of information.
   e. The nurse prepares to meet the patient by reading current and past records and reports.
   f. The nurse recapitulates the interview, highlighting key points.

2. Which of the following statements accurately describe the unique focus of nursing assessment? *(Select all that apply.)*
   a. Nursing assessments duplicate medical assessments.
   b. Nursing assessments target data pointing to pathologic conditions.
   c. Nursing assessments focus on the patient's responses to health problems.
   d. The findings from a nursing assessment may contribute to the identification of a medical diagnosis.
   e. The focus of nursing assessment is on actual, not potential, health problems.
   f. An initial assessment establishes a complete database for problem solving and care planning.

3. Which of the following statements reflect the focus of Gordon's functional health patterns model for organizing or clustering data? *(Select all that apply.)*
   a. Data are clustered or organized according to a hierarchy of basic human needs.
   b. Data are collected regarding the health perception/health management of the patient.
   c. The perception of the major roles and responsibilities in the patient's life is explored.
   d. The major body systems are assessed and data are collected.
   e. Data related to human response patterns are collected and organized.
   f. Elimination, activity, sleep, and sexuality are components of the assessment and data collection.

4. Which of the following patient data would be considered subjective data? *(Select all that apply.)*
   a. A nurse observes a patient wringing her hands before signing a consent for surgery.
   b. A nurse observes redness and swelling at an IV site.
   c. A patient describes his pain as an 8 on the pain assessment scale.
   d. A patient feels nauseated after eating his breakfast.
   e. A patient's blood pressure is elevated following physical activity.
   f. A patient complains of being cold and requests an extra blanket.

Prioritization Question

1. Place the following actions performed by a nurse during a patient interview in the order in which they would most likely occur. Keep in mind the four distinct phases of the interview process: preparatory phase, introduction, working phase, and termination.

   a. The nurse gathers all the information needed to form the subjective database.

   b. The nurse prepares to meet the patient by reading current and past records and reports.

   c. The nurse recapitulates the interview, highlighting the key points.

   d. The nurse initiates the interview by stating his or her name, identifying the purpose of the interview, and clarifying the roles of the nurse and patient.

   e. The nurse ensures that the environment in which the interview is to be conducted is private and relaxed.

   f. The nurse assesses the patient's comfort and ability to participate in the interview.

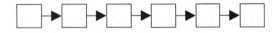

DEVELOPING YOUR KNOWLEDGE BASE

FILL-IN-THE-BLANKS

1. The primary source of patient data is the patient, but two other sources of patient data are _____ and _____.

2. The type of nursing assessment that is performed during the nurse's initial contact with the patient and involves collecting data about all aspects of the patient's health is called the _____.

3. When a nurse confirms or verifies the data collected upon assessment to keep it free of error, bias, or misinterpretation, he/she is performing the act of _____.

4. When a nurse asks a patient how having a newborn at home will affect her lifestyle, she is asking a(n) _____ type of a question.

5. A nurse who gathers data about a newly diagnosed case of hypertension in a 52-year-old African American patient is performing a(n) _____ type of assessment.

6. When the nurse compares the current status of a patient to the initial assessment performed during the admitting process, he/she is performing a(n) _____ type of assessment.

7. Most schools of nursing and healthcare institutions establish the specific information that must be collected from every patient in a structured assessment form. This information is known as a(n) _____.

MATCHING EXERCISES

Match the term in Part A with the definition in Part B.

PART A

a. Database
b. Focused assessment
c. Interview
d. Health assessment
e. Nursing history
f. Objective data
g. Physical assessment
h. Subjective data
i. Validation
j. Observation
k. Time-lapsed assessments

PART B

1. ____ Observable and measurable information that can be seen, heard, or felt by someone other than the person experiencing it

2. ____ The conscious and deliberate use of the five physical senses to gather information

3. ____ Clearly identifies patient strengths and weaknesses, health risks, and potential and existing health problems

4. ____ A planned communication to obtain patient data

5. ____ The examination of a patient for objective data that may better define the patient's condition and help the nurse in planning care

6. ____ The act of confirming or verifying data

7. ____ Compares a patient's current status to baseline data obtained earlier

8. ___ Includes all the pertinent patient information collected by the nurse and other healthcare professionals, enabling a comprehensive and effective plan of care to be designed and implemented for the patient

9. ___ The gathering of data about a specific problem that has already been identified

10. ___ May be used by nurses to help patients identify potential and actual health risks and to explore the habits, behaviors, beliefs, attitudes, and values that influence their health

Match the examples of data in Part B with the type of data in Part A. Answers will be used more than once.

PART A

a. Objective data

b. Subjective data

PART B

11. ___ Redness and swelling are noticed at the site of an incision.

12. ___ A patient complains of pain in his left arm.

13. ___ A patient has a violent spell of coughing.

14. ___ A patient recovering from knee surgery favors his impaired leg when walking.

15. ___ A patient is nauseated at the sight of food.

16. ___ A patient worries about her children during her hospital stay.

SHORT ANSWER

1. List the five functions of the initial comprehensive nursing assessment.

a. _____
b. _____
c. _____
d. _____
e. _____

2. Identify eight sources of patient data, and give an example of each.

a. _____

b. _____
c. _____
d. _____
e. _____
f. _____
g. _____
h. _____

3. Briefly describe why the following characteristics of data are important when collecting and recording patient data.

a. Purposeful: _____

b. Complete: _____

c. Factual and accurate: _____

d. Relevant: _____

4. Give an example of three observations nurses should make each time they encounter a patient.

a. _____
b. _____
c. _____

5. List three patient goals that should be accomplished by the end of the introduction phase of the patient interview.

a. _____
b. _____
c. _____

6. Give two examples of closed questions, open-ended questions, and reflective questions that could be used to elicit information from your patient, a 42-year-old mother of three young children who has recently been diagnosed with diabetes; she is admitted to the hospital overnight for observation.

   a. Closed questions: _____

   _____

   b. Open-ended questions: _____

   _____

   c. Reflective questions: _____

   _____

7. Explain how the following factors affect assessment priorities when collecting patient data.

   a. Patient's health orientation: _____

   _____

   b. Patient's developmental stage: _____

   _____

   c. Patient's need for nursing: _____

   _____

8. Give two examples of when data need to be validated.

   a. _____

   b. _____

9. Explain when the immediate communication of data is indicated.

   _____

   _____

APPLYING YOUR KNOWLEDGE

CRITICAL THINKING QUESTIONS

1. Role-play the following nursing interviews with your classmates:

   a. A 50-year-old woman with diabetes and diabetic foot ulcers is admitted to the emergency room for observation after she experienced a blackout.

   b. An 85-year-old African American man is admitted to the coronary care unit after experiencing a possible stroke.

   c. A teenage boy is admitted to the hospital with severe stomach pains and a possible ruptured appendix.

   Talk about which approaches and types of questions (closed, open-ended, reflective, direct) resulted in the best interviews.

2. Recall the last time you went to a doctor's office for a checkup or medical problem. How were you treated by the doctor's staff? Did they do anything to make you feel comfortable or uncomfortable? What did they do to include you in the process? How did it feel to be a patient at the mercy of others? What would you do to incorporate this learning into your own nursing practice?

REFLECTIVE PRACTICE USING CRITICAL THINKING SKILLS

Use the following expanded scenario from Chapter 12 in your textbook to answer the questions below.

Scenario: Susan Morgan is a 34-year-old woman newly diagnosed with multiple sclerosis. She was recently married to a man she met while hiking the Appalachian Trail. While educating Ms. Morgan about her disease, the nurse notices that she appears distressed and angry. Ms. Morgan says, "How am I going to tell my husband? We were just married last year and planned to do lots of hiking and outdoor sports. It's not fair for him to be tied down to me if I can't be the wife and partner that he thought he married."

1. How might the nurse facilitate Ms. Morgan's ability to cope with disability?

   _____

   _____

   _____

2. What would be a successful outcome for this patient?

   _____

   _____

   _____

3. What intellectual, technical, interpersonal, and/or ethical/legal competencies are most likely to bring about the desired outcome?

_____

_____

_____

4. What resources might be helpful for Ms. Morgan?

_____

_____

_____

CHAPTER 13

Diagnosing

PRACTICING FOR NCLEX

MULTIPLE CHOICE QUESTIONS

Circle the letter that corresponds to the best answer for each question.

1. Which of the following statements regarding nursing diagnoses is accurate?
   a. Nursing diagnoses remain the same for as long as the disease is present.
   b. Nursing diagnoses are written to identify diseases.
   c. Nursing diagnoses are written to describe patient problems that nurses can treat.
   d. Nursing diagnoses focus on identifying healthy responses to health and illness.

2. Which of the following is an actual or potential health problem that can be prevented or resolved by an independent nursing intervention?
   a. Nursing diagnoses
   b. Nursing assessments
   c. Medical diagnoses
   d. Collaborative problems

3. Which of the following would be an appropriate nursing diagnosis for a toddler who has been treated on two different occasions for lacerations and contusions due to the parents' negligence in providing a safe environment?
   a. High Risk for Injury related to abusive parents
   b. High Risk for Injury related to impaired home management
   c. Child Abuse related to unsafe home environment

   d. High Risk for Injury related to unsafe home environment

4. Which of the following nursing diagnoses would be written when the nurse suspects that a health problem exists but needs to gather more data to confirm the diagnosis?
   a. Actual
   b. Potential
   c. Possible
   d. Apparent

5. Which of the following nursing concerns is clearly the responsibility of the nurse?
   a. Monitoring for changes in health status
   b. Promoting safety and preventing harm; detecting and controlling risks
   c. Tailoring treatment and medication regimens for each individual
   d. All of the above

ALTERNATE-FORMAT QUESTIONS

Multiple Response Questions

Circle the letters that correspond to the best answers for each question.

1. Which of the following statements describe the purpose of diagnosing? *(Select all that apply.)*
   a. To identify a disease in an individual, group, or community
   b. To identify how an individual, group, or community responds to actual or potential health and life processes
   c. To identify factors that contribute to, or cause, health problems (etiologies)

d. To provide a legal record for actions performed by the nursing staff

e. To identify resources or strengths the individual, group, or community can draw on to prevent or resolve problems

f. To serve as a basis for the selection of nursing interventions to achieve outcomes for which the nurse is accountable

2. Which of the following statements accurately describe a type of NANDA nursing diagnosis? *(Select all that apply.)*

   a. A wellness diagnosis has four components: label, definition, defining characteristics, and related factor.

   b. A possible diagnosis is a clinical judgment about an individual, group, or community in transition from a specific level of wellness to a higher level of wellness.

   c. A risk nursing diagnosis is a clinical judgment that an individual, family, or community is more likely to develop the problem than others in the same or similar situation.

   d. An actual diagnosis represents a problem that has been validated by the presence of major defining characteristics.

   e. A potential nursing diagnosis is a statement describing a suspected problem for which additional data are needed.

   f. A syndrome nursing diagnosis comprises a cluster of actual or risk nursing diagnoses that are predicted to be present because of certain events or situations.

3. Which of the following nursing diagnoses are written correctly? *(Select all that apply.)*

   a. Deficient Fluid Volume related to abnormal fluid loss

   b. Risk for Impaired Skin Integrity

   c. Grieving related to Body Image Disturbance

   d. Possible Chronic Low Self-Esteem

   e. Nutrition Deficit related to inability to eat a balanced diet

   f. Knowledge Deficit related to noncompliance with physical therapy routine

4. Which of the following are accurate guidelines for writing nursing diagnoses? *(Select all that apply.)*

   a. Phrase the nursing diagnosis as a patient need rather than a patient problem.

   b. Check to make sure that the patient problem follows the etiology.

   c. Make sure the patient problem and etiology are linked by the phrase "related to."

   d. Make sure defining characteristics follow the etiology and are linked by the phrase "as manifested by" or "as evidenced by."

   e. Write nursing diagnoses in legally advisable terms.

   f. Use defining characteristics and medical diagnoses in the problem statement.

5. Which of the following are parts of a nursing diagnosis? *(Select all that apply.)*

   a. Problem

   b. Etiology

   c. Patient needs

   d. Defining characteristics

   e. Medical diagnosis

   f. Legal parameters for nursing actions

DEVELOPING YOUR KNOWLEDGE BASE

FILL-IN-THE-BLANKS

1. When a nurse writes a patient outcome that requires pain medication for goal achievement, the situation is a(n) _____ problem.

2. Patient complaints of chills and nausea are considered significant data or _____.

3. When determining the significance of a patient's urinalysis, the normative values to which the data can be compared are termed a(n) _____.

4. When a nurse groups patient cues that point to the existence of a patient health problem, the cues form what is known as a(n) _____.

5. When a nurse recognizes a cluster of significant patient data indicating that patient teaching and counseling for a colostomy is needed, a(n) _____ should be written.

6. What part of the following nursing diagnosis would be considered the etiology: Spiritual Distress related to inability to accept the death of newborn child? _____

7. What two cues must be present for a valid wellness diagnosis? _____ and _____.

8. _____ nursing diagnoses comprise a cluster of actual or risk nursing diagnoses that are predicted to be present because of a certain event or situation.

MATCHING EXERCISES

Match the examples listed in Part B with the four steps involved in the interpretation and analysis of data listed in Part A. Answers will be used more than once.

PART A

a. Recognizing significant data

b. Recognizing patterns or clusters

c. Identifying strengths and problems

d. Reaching conclusions

PART B

1. ____ A nurse notes that a patient's refusal to stop smoking will adversely affect his recovery from cardiac surgery.

2. ____ A nurse compares a 15-month-old child's motor abilities with the norms for that age group.

3. ____ A nurse recognizes an unhealthy situation developing when her patient, recovering from a mastectomy, cries at night, refuses to eat, and sleeps all day.

4. ____ A nurse decides no further nursing response is indicated for a woman who recovered from gallbladder surgery according to schedule.

5. ____ A maternity nurse notices a newborn's skin tone is markedly different than that of the other babies and checks for jaundice.

6. ____ A nurse determines that a man with a history of diabetes is highly motivated to develop a healthy pattern of nutrition in response to his problem.

7. ____ A nurse notices that a patient with AIDS has an adverse reaction to a drug and consults the prescribing physician.

CORRECT THE FALSE STATEMENTS

Circle the word "true" or "false" that follows the statement. If you circled "false," change the underlined word or words to make the statement true. Place your answers in the space provided.

1. Actual or potential health problems that can be prevented or resolved by independent nursing intervention are termed <u>collaborative problems</u>.

   True False _____

2. <u>Medical diagnoses</u> represent situations that are the primary responsibility of nurses.

   True False _____

3. A <u>cue</u> is a generally accepted rule, measure, pattern, or model that can be used to compare data in the same class or category.

   True False _____

4. A <u>data cluster</u> is a grouping of patient data or cues, which points to the existence of a patient health problem.

   True False _____

5. Nursing diagnoses should be derived from a <u>single cue</u>.

   True False _____

6. The <u>NANDA list</u> is a beginning list of suggested terms for health problems that may be identified and treated by nurses.

   True False _____

7. The <u>problem statement</u> of a nursing diagnosis identifies the physiologic, psychological, sociologic, spiritual, and environmental factors believed to be related to the problem as either a cause or a contributing factor.

   True False _____

8. The <u>etiology</u> of nursing diagnoses directs nursing intervention.

   True False _____

9. A <u>possible</u> nursing diagnosis is written when the nurse suspects that a health problem exists but needs to gather more data to confirm the diagnosis.

   True False _____

10. A <u>wellness diagnosis</u> is a clinical judgment about an individual, family, or community in transition from a specific level of wellness to a higher level of wellness.

    True False _____

11. In the diagnosing step, the nurse <u>collects patient data</u>.

    True False _____

12. A <u>possible nursing diagnosis</u> is a clinical judgment that an individual, family, or community is more likely to develop the problem than others in the same or similar situation.

True   False _____

SHORT ANSWER

1. Place a check next to the nursing diagnoses that are written correctly, and identify the errors in the incorrect diagnoses on the lines that follow.

   a. _____ High Risk for Injury related to absence of restraints and side rails _____

   _____

   b. _____ Impaired Skin Integrity related to mobility deficit _____

   _____

   c. _____ Grieving related to loss of breast ____

   _____

   d. _____ Self-Care Deficit: Bathing related to immobility _____

   _____

   e. _____ Sleep Pattern Disturbance related to insomnia _____

   _____

   f. _____ Alteration in Nutrition: Less Than Body Requirements related to loss of appetite _____

   _____

   g. _____ Powerlessness related to poor family support system _____

   _____

   h. _____ Anxiety: mild, related to changing lifestyle/diet _____

   _____

   i. _____ Ineffective Airway Clearance related to 20-year smoking habit _____

   _____

   j. _____ Alteration in Bowel Elimination: Constipation related to cancer of bowel ____

   _____

   k. _____ Nausea and Vomiting related to medication side effects _____

   _____

   l. _____ Knowledge Deficit related to noncompliance with diet _____

   _____

   m. _____ Alteration in Parenting related to knowledge deficit: child growth and development, discipline _____

   _____

   n. _____ Pain related to discomfort in abdomen _____

   _____

   o. _____ Impaired Physical Mobility: amputation of left leg related to gangrene _____

   _____

   p. _____ Alteration in Nutrition: More Than Body Requirements related to obesity ____

   _____

   q. _____ Noncompliance related to unresolved hostility _____

   _____

   r. _____ Needs assistance walking to bathroom: related to immobility _____

   _____

2. What questions would you ask a patient to validate the following nursing diagnoses?

   a. Altered Urinary Elimination: _____

   _____

   b. Impaired Social Interaction: _____

   _____

   c. Ineffective Individual Coping: _____

   _____

   d. Sleep Pattern Disturbance: _____

   _____

3. Describe the appropriate nursing response to each of the following basic conclusions after interpreting and analyzing patient data.

   a. No problem: _____

   _____

b. Possible problem: _____

_____

c. Actual or potential nursing diagnosis: _____

_____

d. Clinical problem other than nursing diagnosis: _____

_____

4. Give three examples of how standards may be used to identify significant cues.

a. _____

b. _____

c. _____

5. List five questions a nurse should consider when using critical thinking in diagnostic reasoning.

a. _____

b. _____

c. _____

d. _____

e. _____

6. In her book on the nursing process, Alfaro-LeFevre (2006) describes the shift from Diagnose and Treat (DT) to Predict, Prevent, Manage, and Promote (PPMP). The latter approach focuses on early evidence-based intervention to prevent and manage problems and their potential complications. Describe the three activities nurses need to perform to follow this approach in daily nursing care.

a. _____

_____

b. _____

_____

c. _____

_____

7. Read the three mini-cases that follow. In each one, underline the cues that form a data cluster indicating a nursing diagnosis, and write the appropriate nursing diagnosis as a three-part statement.

a. Mr. Klinetob, age 86, has been seriously depressed since the death 6 months ago of his wife of 52 years. Although he suffers

from degenerative joint disease and has talked for years about having "just a touch of arthritis," this never kept him from being up and about. Recently, however, he spends all day sitting in a chair and seems to have no desire to engage in self-care activities. He tells the visiting nurse that he doesn't get washed up anymore because he's "too stiff" in the morning to bathe and "I just don't seem to have the energy." The visiting nurse notices that his hair is matted and uncombed, his face has traces of previous meals, and he has a strong body odor. His children have complained that their normally fastidious father seems not to care about personal hygiene any longer.

Nursing Diagnosis: _____

_____

_____

b. Miss Adams sustained a right-sided cerebral infarct that resulted in left hemiparesis (paralysis on the left side of the body) and left "neglect." She ignores the left side of her body and actually denies its existence. When asked about her left leg, she stated that it belonged to the woman in the next bed—this while she was in a private room. This patient was previously quite active: she walked for 45 to 60 minutes four or five times a week and was an avid swimmer. At present, she cannot move either her left arm or leg.

Nursing Diagnosis: _____

_____

_____

c. After trying to conceive a child for 11 years, Ted and Rosemary Hines sought the assistance of a fertility specialist who was highly recommended by a friend. It was determined that Ted's sperm was inadequate, and Rosemary was inseminated with sperm from an anonymous donor. The couple was told that the donor was healthy and that he was selected because he resembled Ted. Rosemary became pregnant after the second in-vitro fertilization attempt and delivered a healthy baby girl named Sarah.

Sarah is now 7 years old, and Ted and Rosemary have learned from blood tests that their fertility specialist is the biologic father of their child. It seems that he lied to some couples about using sperm from anonymous donors and deceived others into thinking the wives had become pregnant when he had simply injected them with hormones. Ted and Rosemary have joined other couples in pressing charges against this physician.

Rosemary tells the nurse in her pediatrician's office that she is concerned about how all this is affecting her family. "Ted and I both love Sarah and would do nothing to hurt her, but I'm so angry about this whole situation I'm afraid I may be taking it out on her," she says. Questioning reveals that Rosemary has found herself yelling at Sarah for minor disobedience and spanking her, something she rarely did before. Both Ted and Rosemary had commented before about Sarah's striking physical resemblance to the fertility specialist but attributed this to coincidence. Rosemary says, "Whenever I see her now, I can't help but see Dr. Clowser, and everything inside me clenches up and I want to scream." Both Ted and Rosemary express great remorse that Sarah, who is innocent, is bearing the brunt of something that is in no way her fault.

Nursing Diagnosis: _____

_____

_____

APPLYING YOUR KNOWLEDGE

CRITICAL THINKING QUESTIONS

1. With a partner or several classmates, write appropriate nursing diagnoses for the following patient. Be sure to include actual, potential, and possible diagnoses. Compare your diagnoses with your partner's and note similarities and differences. Decide which diagnoses best suit the patient's situation.

A 35-year-old woman presents with chills, fever, and severe vaginal bleeding. She tells you she is 2 months pregnant and has had two previous miscarriages. She is overwrought and says she feels God is punishing her for an abortion she had when she was in college. She and her husband have been trying to have children for years and were counting on this pregnancy to come to term.

2. Interview members of your family or several close friends. Identify wellness diagnoses for each person. What factors contributed to these diagnoses?

REFLECTIVE PRACTICE USING CRITICAL THINKING SKILLS

Use the following expanded scenario from Chapter 13 in your textbook to answer the questions below.

Scenario: Martin Prescott, age 46, comes to the clinic for a routine physical examination. During the assessment, he says, "I've had problems with constipation and I've seen some blood when I wipe myself after a bowel movement. It's just hemorrhoids, right? Nothing to worry about?" Upon further questioning, the nurse discovers that Mr. Prescott's father and an uncle both died in their early 50s from colon cancer.

1. What nursing diagnosis would be appropriate for Mr. Prescott? How might the nurse advocate for Mr. Prescott to ensure that he gets tested for colon cancer?

_____

_____

_____

2. What would be a successful outcome for this patient?

_____

_____

_____

3. What intellectual, technical, interpersonal, and/or ethical/legal competencies are most likely to bring about the desired outcome?

_____

_____

_____

4. What resources might be helpful for Mr. Prescott?

_____

_____

_____

CHAPTER 14

Outcome Identification and Planning

PRACTICING FOR NCLEX

MULTIPLE CHOICE QUESTIONS

Circle the letter that corresponds to the best answer for each question.

1. Which of the following actions would be performed during the planning step of the nursing process?
   a. Interpreting and analyzing patient data
   b. Establishing the database
   c. Identifying factors contributing to patient's success or failure
   d. Selecting nursing measures

2. Which of the following is a correctly written goal for a patient who is scheduled to ambulate following hip surgery?
   a. Over the next 24-hour period, the patient will walk the length of the hallway assisted by the nurse.
   b. The nurse will help the patient ambulate the length of the hallway once a day.
   c. Offer to help the patient walk the length of the hallway each day.
   d. Patient will become mobile within a 24-hour period.

3. Mr. Conner is a 48-year-old patient with a new colostomy. Which of the following patient goals for Mr. Conner is written correctly?
   a. Explain to Mr. Conner the proper care of the stoma by 3/29/12.

   b. Mr. Conner will know how to care for his stoma by 3/29/12.
   c. Mr. Conner will demonstrate proper care of stoma by 3/29/12.
   d. Mr. Conner will be able to care for stoma and cope with psychological loss by 3/29/12.

4. The etiology of the nursing diagnosis contains which of the following factors?
   a. Identification of the unhealthy response preventing desired change
   b. Identification of factors causing undesirable response and preventing desired change
   c. Suggestion of patient goals to promote desired change
   d. Identification of patient strengths

5. Mr. Rose, an overweight, highly stressed 50-year-old executive, is being discharged from the hospital after undergoing coronary bypass surgery. Which of the following demonstrates an affective goal for this patient?
   a. By 6/30/12, the patient will list three benefits of daily exercise.
   b. By 6/30/12, the patient will correctly demonstrate breathing techniques to reduce stress.
   c. By 6/30/12, the patient will value his health sufficiently to reduce the cholesterol in his diet.
   d. By 6/30/12, the patient will be able to plan healthy weekly menus.

6. Which of the following statements concerning nursing interventions is accurate?
   a. Nursing interventions are a separate entity from the original goal/outcome.
   b. Nursing interventions are dated when written and when the plan of care is reviewed.
   c. Nursing interventions are signed by the attending physician.
   d. Nursing interventions do not describe the nursing action to be performed.

7. According to Maslow's hierarchy of human needs, which of the following examples would be the highest priority for a patient?
   a. Self-actualization needs
   b. Love and belonging needs
   c. Physiologic needs
   d. Safety needs

ALTERNATE-FORMAT QUESTIONS

Multiple Response Questions

Circle the letters that correspond to the best answers for each question.

1. Which of the following actions are performed by the nurse in the planning step of the nursing process? *(Select all that apply.)*
   a. Establishing priorities
   b. Collecting and interpreting patient data
   c. Identifying expected patient outcomes
   d. Selecting evidence-based nursing interventions
   e. Recording patient outcomes
   f. Communicating the plan of nursing care

2. Which of the following actions occur during the initial planning of patient care? *(Select all that apply.)*
   a. The initial plan is developed by the nurse who performs the admission nursing history and the physical assessment.
   b. After the initial plan is developed, nursing diagnoses are prioritized.
   c. Patient goals and the related nursing care are identified in the initial plan.
   d. Standardized care plans should not be used as a basis for the initial plan.
   e. New data are collected and analyzed to make the plan more specific and effective.

   f. The focus of initial planning is using teaching and counseling skills to help the patient carry out necessary self-care behaviors at home.

3. According to Maslow, which of the following needs rank first, second, and third in the hierarchy of human needs? *(Select all that apply.)*
   a. Self-esteem needs
   b. Self-actualization needs
   c. Physiologic needs
   d. Safety needs
   e. Love and belonging needs
   f. Spiritual needs

4. Which of the following are guidelines that nurses should consider when writing outcomes? *(Select all that apply.)*
   a. Each set of outcomes should be derived from a combination of nursing diagnoses.
   b. At least one of the outcomes should show a direct resolution of the problem statement in the nursing diagnosis.
   c. The patient and family need not value the outcomes as long as they support the plan of care.
   d. Each outcome should be brief and specific.
   e. The outcomes should be supportive of the total treatment plan.
   f. Not all outcomes need to specify a time line.

5. Which of the following would be considered a cognitive outcome? *(Select all that apply.)*
   a. Within 1 week after teaching, the patient will list three benefits of quitting smoking.
   b. By 6/8/12, the patient will correctly demonstrate injecting himself with insulin.
   c. Before discharge, the patient will verbalize valuing health sufficiently to follow a healthy diet.
   d. By 6/8/12, the patient will describe a meal plan that is high in fiber.
   e. By 6/8/12, the patient will correctly demonstrate ambulating with a walker.
   f. After viewing the film, the patient will verbalize four benefits of daily exercise.

6. Which of the following are components of a measurable outcome? *(Select all that apply.)*
   a. Object
   b. Modifiers

  c. Performance criteria

  d. Conditions

  e. Subject

  f. Target time

7. Which of the following goals are written correctly? *(Select all that apply.)*

  a. Demonstrate the correct use of crutches to the patient prior to discharge.

  b. The patient will know how to dress her wound after receiving a demonstration.

  c. After attending an infant care class, the patient will correctly demonstrate the procedure for bathing her newborn.

  d. By 4/5/12, the patient will demonstrate how to care for a colostomy.

  e. The patient will list the dangers of smoking and quit.

  f. After counseling, the patient will describe two coping measures to deal with stress.

8. Which of the following accurately describe the purposes of a plan of nursing care? *(Select all that apply.)*

  a. It represents an effective philosophy of nursing and is intended to advance only the nursing aim of promoting recovery.

  b. It is prepared by the nurse who knows the patient best and is recorded on the day the patient presents for treatment and care, according to agency policy.

  c. It is a general guideline for care that is not always a response to the individual characteristics and needs of the patient.

  d. It clearly identifies the nursing assistance the patient needs and nursing's collaborative responsibilities for fulfilling the medical and interdisciplinary plan of care.

  e. It is separate from the discharge plan and does not deal with teaching and counseling.

  f. When appropriate, it is compatible with the medical plan of care and that of the disciplinary team.

DEVELOPING YOUR KNOWLEDGE BASE

FILL-IN-THE-BLANKS

1. A(n) _____ is an expected conclusion to a patient health problem.

2. When a nurse contemplates, while driving to a restaurant for lunch, how to help a young cancer patient accept the loss of a limb, he/she is using the process of _____.

3. In acute care settings, the three basic stages of planning that are critical to comprehensive nursing care are _____, _____, and _____.

4. From what part of the nursing diagnosis "Pain related to delayed healing of surgical incision" would outcomes be derived?

   _____

5. The _____, developed by the Iowa Outcomes Project, presents the first comprehensive standardized language used to describe the patient outcomes that are responsive to nursing intervention.

6. When a nurse writes a statement regarding a patient's achievement of the desired outcome and lists actual patient behavior as evidence supporting the statement, he/she is writing a(n) _____ statement.

7. A(n) _____ is any treatment based on clinical judgment and knowledge that a nurse performs to enhance patient outcomes.

8. When a nurse supplies education to an obese teenager regarding the fat content in food and helps him choose a nutritious diet, he/she is performing a(n) _____ intervention.

9. When a nurse administers physician-prescribed pain medication to a patient after surgery, he/she is performing a(n) _____ intervention.

10. A(n) _____ is a set of steps (typically embedded in a branching flowchart) that approximates the decision process of an expert clinician and is used to make a decision.

11. The _____ is the written guide that directs the efforts of the nursing team as the nurses work with patients to meet health goals.

MATCHING EXERCISES

Match the definition in Part B with the type of care plan listed in Part A. Answers may be used more than once.

PART A

  a. Initial care plan

  b. Ongoing, problem-solving care plan

c. Discharge care plan

d. Standardized care plan

e. Kardex care plan

f. Computerized care plan

g. Case management care plan

h. Critical care plan

i. Concept map care plan

PART B

1. ____ A care plan developed by the nurse who performs the admission nursing history and physical assessment

2. ____ A care plan that is concisely recorded on a card and filed in a central file

3. ____ Benefits of this type of care plan include ready access to an expanded knowledge base, improved record keeping and documentation, and decreased paperwork.

4. ____ The chief purpose of this type of planning is to keep the plan up to date.

5. ____ Prepared plans of care that identify the nursing diagnoses

6. ____ This type of plan for leaving the institution is best prepared by the nurse who has worked most closely with the patient, in conjunction with a social worker familiar with the patient's community.

7. ____ The emphasis of this care plan is to clearly state expected patient outcomes and the specific times by which it is reasonable to achieve these outcomes.

8. ____ The emphasis of this type of care plan is to individualize the plan to meet unique patient needs.

9. ____ This diagram of patient problems and interventions is used to organize data, analyze data, and take a holistic view of the patient situation.

Match the patient goals in Part B with the type of goal listed in Part A. Answers may be used more than once.

PART A

a. Cognitive goals

b. Psychomotor goals

c. Affective goals

PART B

10. ____ By 3/30/12, patient will successfully navigate length of hallway with walker.

11. ____ By 3/30/12, patient will list five low-fat snacks to replace high-fat foods.

12. ____ By 3/30/12, patient will bathe infant on her own.

13. ____ By 3/30/12, patient will value her health sufficiently to stop smoking.

14. ____ By 3/30/12, patient will list three reasons to continue taking blood pressure medication.

15. ____ By 3/30/12, patient will show concern for his well-being and participate in AA meetings.

Match the descriptions in Part B with the type of planning being performed in Part A. Answers may be used more than once.

PART A

a. Initial planning

b. Ongoing planning

c. Discharge planning

PART B

16. ____ Used to keep the nursing plan up to date

17. ____ Addresses each problem listed in the prioritized nursing diagnoses and identifies appropriate patient goals and related nursing care

18. ____ States nursing diagnoses more clearly and develops new diagnoses

19. ____ Should be carried out by the nurse who has worked most closely with the patient and family

20. ____ Involves teaching and counseling skills to help the patient and family carry out self-care behaviors at home

21. ____ Standardized care plans provide an excellent basis for this type of planning if the nurse individualizes them.

SHORT ANSWER

1. Give an example of an appropriate nursing order for the following patients:

   a. A child with asthma who must be taught to use an inhaler: _____

   _____

   b. An elderly woman recovering from hip surgery who must learn to ambulate with a walker: _____

   _____

   c. An obese teenager who needs weight counseling: _____

   _____

   d. A new mother who must ambulate after undergoing a cesarean section: _____

   _____

2. Briefly define the following elements of planning. Explain why they are necessary to the planning step of the nursing process.

   a. Setting priorities: _____

   _____

   b. Writing goals/outcomes that determine the evaluative strategy: _____

   _____

   c. Selecting appropriate evidence-based nursing interventions: _____

   _____

   d. Communicating the plan of nursing care: _____

   _____

3. List two examples of informal planning.

   _____

   _____

   _____

   _____

4. Explain how a formal plan of care benefits the nurse and patient.

   _____

   _____

   _____

5. Individualize the following standard plans to meet the patient's specific goals.

   a. Manage pain for a terminally ill patient:

   _____

   _____

   b. Explore support people for a patient with AIDS: _____

   _____

   c. Provide sensory stimulation for an elderly man in a nursing home: _____

   _____

   d. Teach self-help to a stroke patient in the home care setting: _____

   _____

   _____

6. Describe the following types of nursing care and give an example of each type.

   a. Nursing care related to basic human needs:

   _____

   Example: _____

   b. Nursing care related to nursing diagnoses:

   _____

   Example: _____

   c. Nursing care related to the medical and interdisciplinary plan of care: _____

   _____

   Example: _____

7. List four considerations a nurse should employ when planning nursing care for each day.

   a. _____

   b. _____

   c. _____

   d. _____

8. Place a check mark next to the patient goals that are written correctly, and on the line below, rewrite those that are written incorrectly:

   a. _____ Teach Mrs. Myers one lesson per day on the nutritional value of foods.

   _____

b. _____ Mrs. Gray will know the dangers of smoking after viewing a film on smoking.

_____

c. _____ By end of shift, patient ambulates in hallway using crutches. _____

_____

d. _____ By 2/7/12, patient correctly demonstrates subcutaneous injections using normal saline.

_____

e. _____ By next visit, the patient will understand the benefits of psychotherapy.

_____

f. _____ By 6/12/12, patient correctly demonstrates application of wet-to-dry dressing on leg ulcer. _____

_____

9. Identify a patient goal that shows a direct resolution of the health problem expressed in the nursing diagnoses below.

a. Nursing diagnosis: Fluid Volume Deficit related to decreased fluid intake during fever

Patient goal: _____

_____

b. Nursing diagnosis: Altered Sexual Patterns: Loss of Desire related to change in body image and feelings of unattractiveness following mastectomy

Patient goal: _____

_____

c. Nursing diagnosis: Stress Incontinence related to age-related degenerative changes and weak pelvic muscles and structural supports

Patient goal: _____

_____

d. Nursing Diagnosis: Activity Intolerance related to decreased amount of oxygenated blood available to tissues

Patient goal: _____

_____

e. Nursing Diagnosis: Acute Postoperative Pain related to fear of taking prescribed analgesics

Patient goal: _____

_____

10. List six measures nurses should consider to correctly plan healthcare for a patient.

a. _____

b. _____

c. _____

d. _____

e. _____

f. _____

11. Give four examples of questions a nurse should ask when thinking critically about setting priorities for a patient plan of care.

a. _____

b. _____

c. _____

d. _____

APPLYING YOUR KNOWLEDGE

CRITICAL THINKING QUESTIONS

1. Think about what type of goals would be appropriate in each of the three stages of planning (initial planning, ongoing planning, discharge planning) using the following patient data.

a. A mother brings her 5-year-old son to the emergency room. She says he has been running a low fever and complaining of abdominal pain and headache. You notice his skin is pale and there are several bruises on his arms and legs. On examination, you notice his spleen is enlarged and the abdominal area is tender. A medical diagnosis confirms the child has acute leukemia.

b. A 45-year-old man presents with low fever, weight loss, chronic fatigue, and heavy sweating at night. He has a productive cough with yellowish mucus and chest pain. A TB skin test comes back positive.

c. A 12-year-old girl presents with fatigue, weight loss, excessive thirst, and frequent urination. Laboratory tests confirm a diagnosis of diabetes mellitus.

Why is the identification of goals in each stage necessary for optimal care and outcomes?

2. Some nurses may tell you that care plans are a waste of time. Think about what knowledge and experience you need to respond to this comment. If possible, interview nurses or search through the literature to discover how plans can make a difference.

REFLECTIVE PRACTICE USING CRITICAL THINKING SKILLS

Use the following expanded scenario from Chapter 14 in your textbook to answer the questions below.

Scenario: Glenda Kronk, age 35, comes to the health center for a routine checkup. Upon assessment, the nurse notes that she is 25 pounds overweight and has high-normal blood pressure. During the visit, she verbalizes a strong motivation and desire to become physically fit, lose weight, increase her muscle tone, and improve her cardiorespiratory capacity. She says, "I know it'll involve some major lifestyle changes, including diet and exercise. What's with all these diets and diet supplements now?"

1. How might the nurse respond to Ms. Kronk's questions regarding fitness?

_____

_____

_____

2. What would be a successful outcome for this patient?

_____

_____

_____

3. What intellectual, technical, interpersonal, and/or ethical/legal competencies are most likely to bring about the desired outcome?

_____

_____

_____

4. What resources might be helpful for Ms. Kronk?

_____

_____

_____

CHAPTER 15

Implementing

PRACTICING FOR NCLEX

MULTIPLE CHOICE QUESTIONS

Circle the letter that corresponds to the best answer for each question.

1. Which of the following phrases best describes the unique focus of nursing implementation?
   a. The selected aspects of the patient's treatment regimen
   b. The response of the patient to the plan of care in general
   c. The response of the patient to the illness
   d. The patient's ability to work with support people to promote wellness

2. Which of the following nursing actions is considered an independent (nurse-initiated) action?
   a. Executing physician orders for a catheter
   b. Meeting with other healthcare professionals to discuss a patient
   c. Helping to allay a patient's fears about surgery
   d. Administering medication to a patient

3. Which of the following terms denotes a nurse's authority to initiate actions that normally require the order or supervision of a physician?
   a. Protocols
   b. Nursing interventions
   c. Collaborative orders
   d. Standing orders

4. As the nurse bathes a patient, she notes his skin color and integrity, his ability to respond to simple directions, and his muscle tone.

Which of the following statements best explains why such continuing data collection is so important?
   a. It is difficult to collect complete data in the initial assessment.
   b. It is the most efficient use of the nurse's time.
   c. It enables the nurse to revise the care plan appropriately.
   d. It meets current standards of care.

5. Your patient, who presented with high blood pressure, is put on a low-salt diet and instructed to quit smoking. You find him in the cafeteria eating a cheeseburger and french fries. He also tells you there is no way he can quit smoking. What is your first objective when implementing care for this patient?
   a. Explain to the patient the effects of a high-salt diet and smoking on blood pressure.
   b. Identify why the patient is not following the therapy.
   c. Collaborate with other healthcare professionals about the patient's treatment.
   d. Change the nursing care plan.

ALTERNATE-FORMAT QUESTIONS

Multiple Response Questions

Circle the letters that correspond to the best answers for each question.

1. Which of the following activities would be carried out during the implementation step of the nursing process? *(Select all that apply.)*
   a. Collecting additional patient data
   b. Modifying the patient plan of care

c. Performing an initial assessment of the patient

d. Developing patient outcomes and goals

e. Measuring how well the patient has achieved patient goals

f. Collecting a database to enable an effective plan of care

2. Which of the following are goals of the research behind the Nursing Outcomes Classifications (NOCs)? *(Select all that apply.)*

a. To identify, label, and validate nursing-sensitive patient outcomes and indicators

b. To teach decision making

c. To ensure appropriate reimbursement for nursing services

d. To communicate nursing to non-nurses

e. To evaluate the validity and usefulness of the classification in clinical field testing

f. To define and test measurement procedures for the outcomes and indicators

3. Which of the following are advantages of having standard Nursing Interventions Classifications (NIC)? *(Select all that apply.)*

a. Limiting the amount of reimbursement allowed for nursing services.

b. Teaching decision making

c. Allocating nursing resources

d. Allowing the use of multiple systems of nomenclature

e. Developing information systems

f. Communicating nursing to non-nurses

4. Which of the following are listed in the ANA's *Nursing: Scope and Standards of Practice* for Standard 5: Implementation? *(Select all that apply.)*

a. The nurse demonstrates quality by documenting the application of the nursing process in a responsible, accountable, and ethical manner.

b. The nurse incorporates new knowledge to initiate changes in nursing practice if the desired outcomes are not achieved.

c. The nurse develops expected outcomes that provide direction for the continuity of care.

d. The nurse documents implementation and any modifications, including changes or omissions, of the identified plan.

e. The nurse utilizes community resources and systems to implement the plan.

f. The nurse utilizes evidence-based interventions and treatments specific to the diagnosis or problem.

DEVELOPING YOUR KNOWLEDGE BASE

FILL-IN-THE-BLANKS

1. When a nurse administers medications that were prescribed by the patient's doctor, he/she is carrying out a(n) _____ intervention.

2. _____ are written plans that detail the nursing activities to be executed in specific situations.

3. _____ are interventions targeted to promote and preserve the health of populations.

4. A(n)_____ intervention is a treatment performed away from the patient but on behalf of a patient or group of patients.

5. McCloskey and Bulechek published a report of research to construct a taxonomy of nursing interventions known as _____

6. Interventions that are performed jointly by nurses and other members of the healthcare team are known as _____

MATCHING EXERCISES

Match the examples in Part B with the types of nursing interventions listed in Part A. Answers may be used more than once.

PART A

a. Nurse-initiated independent intervention

b. Physician-initiated dependent intervention

c. Collaborative interdependent intervention

PART B

1. ____ A nurse notices that her patient is extremely anxious before surgery and recommends psychiatric evaluation by the psychiatric nurse specialist.

2. ____ A nurse administers the prescribed dosage of pain medication for a patient recovering from knee surgery.

3. ____ A nurse teaches the daughter of a patient who has leg ulcers how to apply the dressings.

4. ____ A nurse meets with a patient's physician to describe what she feels is the patient's lack of response to prescribed therapy.

5. ____ A nurse prepares a patient for surgery by performing a bowel cleansing.

6. ____ A nurse meets in conference with a patient's physician, social worker, and psychiatrist to discuss the patient's failure to progress.

CORRECT THE FALSE STATEMENTS

Circle the word "true" or "false" that follows the statement. If you circled "false," change the underlined word or words to make the statement true. Place your answer in the space provided.

1. The <u>physician</u> is legally responsible for the assessments nurses make and for their nursing responses.

   True   False _____

2. <u>Nurse-initiated interventions</u> involve carrying out nurse-prescribed orders written on the nursing plan of care.

   True   False _____

3. <u>Standing orders</u> are written plans that detail the nursing activities to be executed in specific situations.

   True   False _____

4. The <u>physician</u> plays the role of coordinator within the healthcare team.

   True   False _____

5. The <u>nursing team</u> carries out the nursing orders detailed in the nursing plan of care.

   True   False _____

6. When working with patients to achieve the goals/outcomes specified in the plan of care, it is important to remember that <u>everything about the plan of care is fixed</u>.

   True   False _____

7. When choosing nursing interventions, it is important to consider the <u>patient's</u> <u>background</u>.

   True   False _____

8. Sincere motivation to benefit the patient and conscientious attempts to implement nursing orders are <u>sufficient</u> to protect a nurse from legal action due to negligence.

   True   False _____

9. When a patient fails to follow the plan of care despite the nurse's best efforts, it is time to <u>change the patient's attitude toward his care</u>.

   True   False _____

10. If a plan of care is well written, <u>carrying out its orders</u> is the nurse's most important task and should receive top priority.

    True   False _____

11. <u>All nursing actions for implementing the plan of care</u> must be consistent with standards for practice.

    True   False _____

SHORT ANSWER

1. List three duties nurses perform when acting as coordinator for the healthcare team.

   a. _____

   b. _____

   c. _____

2. Give an example of a nurse variable, a patient variable, and a healthcare variable that might influence the implementation of the plan of care.

   a. Nurse variable: _____

   b. Patient variable: _____

   c. Healthcare variable: _____

3. Explain why the following nursing actions are important to the continuity of nursing care.

   a. Promoting self-care: teaching, counseling, and advocacy _____

   _____

   _____

   b. Assisting patients to meet health goals _____

   _____

   _____

4. Mr. Franks, a new resident in a nursing home, is recovering from minor surgery. He shows no interest in his condition and refuses to participate in self-care. You suspect an underlying problem of loneliness and boredom stemming from his admittance to the home, which was not mentioned in his original plan of care. How would you reevaluate the nursing care

plan and incorporate self-care for Mr. Franks, taking into consideration his mental state?

_____

_____

_____

5. Your patient is a pregnant woman, living in a subsidized housing development. You believe she is not receiving proper nutrition. She has two other children and complains that there is not enough money to put three square meals a day on the table. When evaluating her plan of care, you notice there is no mention of providing counseling in this area. How would you reevaluate the nursing care plan for this patient to include options for proper nutrition?

_____

_____

_____

6. Give an example of the following types of interventions defined by the Nursing Intervention Classification (NIC).

   a. Direct care intervention: _____

   _____

   b. Indirect care intervention: _____

   _____

   c. Community (or public health) intervention:

   _____

APPLYING YOUR KNOWLEDGE

CRITICAL THINKING QUESTIONS

1. Work with your classmates to list all the factors (nurse, healthcare team, patient/family, healthcare setting, resources, and so on) that might interfere with the nurse's ability to implement a plan of care for the following patients. Then identify facilitating factors. Think about how you can use this knowledge.

   a. A 5-year-old girl with cystic fibrosis is being discharged into the care of her family, which consists of a single working mother and two older brothers.

   b. A 17-year-old single mother who is living with her parents is being sent home with her newborn son. She is having difficulty nursing the baby, and the baby is being treated for jaundice.

2. Spend some time observing nurses as they care for patients. List all the nursing actions you observe. Determine whether these actions involved the use of the nurse's cognitive skills, interpersonal skills, technical skills, ethical/legal skills, or a blend of these skills. Rate your own skills in these areas and note in which areas you feel confident and in which areas you need improvement. Write a plan of action to help you improve these skills.

REFLECTIVE PRACTICE USING CRITICAL THINKING SKILLS

Use the following expanded scenario from Chapter 15 in your textbook to answer the questions below.

Scenario: Antoinette Browne, a toddler, is brought to the well-child community clinic by her grandmother, who lives with the child and her mother. Physical examination reveals a negligible gain in height and weight, lethargy, and a delay in achieving developmental milestones. The grandmother says, "The baby keeps me awake all night with her crying. I can't take it anymore." Further questioning reveals that the mother is a single woman who works nights and sleeps most of the day, leaving the bulk of the childcare to the grandmother.

1. What might be the nurse's response when advocating for Antoinette and her family?

_____

_____

_____

2. What would be a successful outcome for this patient?

_____

_____

_____

3. What intellectual, technical, interpersonal, and/or ethical/legal competencies are most likely to bring about the desired outcome?

_____

_____

_____

4. What resources might be helpful for this family?

_____

_____

_____

CHAPTER 16

Evaluating

PRACTICING FOR NCLEX

MULTIPLE CHOICE QUESTIONS

Circle the letter that corresponds to the best answer for each question.

1. Which of the following actions is the most important act of evaluation performed by the nurse?
   a. Evaluating the patient's goal/outcome achievement
   b. Evaluating the plan of care
   c. Evaluating the competence of nurse practitioners
   d. Evaluating the types of healthcare services available to the patient

2. The nurse collects data in the evaluation step to determine which of the following?
   a. Patient health problems
   b. Assessment of the patient's underlying health problems
   c. Solution of health problems through goal achievement
   d. The effect of medical diagnosis

3. Which of the following patient goals would be considered a psychomotor goal?
   a. By 8/18/12, patient will value his health sufficiently to quit smoking.
   b. By 8/18/12, patient will have full motion in left arm.
   c. By 8/18/12, patient will list three foods that are low in salt.
   d. By 8/18/12, patient will learn three exercises designed to strengthen leg muscles.

4. Which of the following statements concerning quality improvement is accurate?
   a. Quality improvement is externally driven.
   b. Quality improvement follows organizational structure rather than patient care.
   c. Quality improvement focuses on individuals rather than processes.
   d. Quality improvement has no endpoints.

5. Which of the following actions should the nurse take when patient data indicate that the stated goals have not been achieved?
   a. Collect more data for the database.
   b. Review each preceding step of the nursing process.
   c. Implement a standardized plan of care.
   d. Change the nursing orders.

6. For a patient with self-care deficit, the long-term goal is that the patient will be able to dress himself by the end of the 6-week therapy. For best results, the nurse should evaluate the patient's progress toward this goal at which of the following times?
   a. When the patient is discharged
   b. At the end of the 6-week therapy
   c. Only when the patient shows some progress
   d. As soon as possible

7. The quality assurance model of the ANA identifies three essential components of quality care. Which one of these components does the nurse use when determining whether a patient has met the goals stated on the care plan?
   a. Structure
   b. Process

c. Retrospect

d. Outcome

8. Which of the following actions would be an appropriate nursing action when evaluating a patient's responses to a plan of care?

a. Reinforce the plan of care when each expected outcome is achieved.

b. Terminate the plan if there are difficulties achieving the goals/outcomes.

c. Terminate the plan of care upon patient discharge.

d. Continue the plan of care if more time is needed to achieve the goals/outcomes.

ALTERNATE-FORMAT QUESTIONS

Multiple Response Questions

Circle the letters that correspond to the best answers for each question.

1. Which of the following are physiologic goals? *(Select all that apply.)*

a. By 4/6/12, the baby will demonstrate adequate sleep–wakefulness patterns.

b. Before discharge, the parents of the baby will verbalize decreased anxiety about taking care of a newborn.

c. By 4/6/12, the parents will list appropriate resources in case questions arise after discharge.

d. By 4/6/12, the baby will show an adequate comfort level indicating satisfactory parenting.

e. Before discharge, the baby will have reached a target weight gain of 8 lb (birthweight: 7 lb, 6 oz).

f. Before discharge, the parents will demonstrate confidence in bathing and feeding their baby.

2. Which of the following statements accurately describe the appropriate documentation of the evaluation process? *(Select all that apply.)*

a. After the data have been collected to determine patient outcome achievement, the nurse writes an evaluative statement to summarize the findings.

b. The nurse writes a two-part evaluative statement that includes a decision about how well the outcome was met, along with patient data that support the decision.

c. The nurse has three decision options for how goals have been met.

d. The nurse determines whether a patient goal has been met or not met. In each case, the goal is discontinued.

e. The nurse does not increase the complexity of a goal after it has been achieved to prevent patient anxiety and distrust.

f. If a nurse writes a properly written goal, it is not affected by patient, nurse, or healthcare variables.

3. Which of the following rules are recommended by the Institute of Medicine's Committee on Quality of Health Care in America to redesign and improve care? *(Select all that apply.)*

a. Care should be based on nursing needs and values.

b. The nurse should be the source of control for patient care.

c. Care should include evidence-based decision making.

d. Customization of care should be based on availability of resources.

e. Care should include shared knowledge and the free flow of information.

f. The need for transparency and decrease in waste affects patient care.

4. Which of the following are recommended steps in performance improvement? *(Select all that apply.)*

a. Discover a problem.

b. Plan a strategy using indicators.

c. Organize a task force to implement the change.

d. Assess the change.

e. If the goal is not met, discontinue efforts to force change.

f. Use management to reduce resistance to change.

5. Which of the following statements accurately describe the process of quality assurance in nursing practice? *(Select all that apply.)*

a. Quality assurance programs are primarily small programs conducted by nurses on nursing units to improve nursing care.

b. Quality assurance programs enable the nursing profession to be accountable to society for the quality of nursing care.

c. Quality assurance programs ensure survival of the profession.

d. Quality as opportunity focuses on finding deficient workers and removing them.

e. In the quality-by-inspection system, mistakes are viewed not as being caused by a lack of motivation or effort, but rather as a result of a problem in the system.

f. The ANA model of quality assurance directs attention to three essential components of quality care: structure, process, and outcome.

6. Which of the following are major premises of quality improvement? *(Select all that apply.)*

a. Focus on organizational mission

b. Sporadic improvement

c. Healthcare worker orientation

d. Leadership commitment

e. Not crossing boundaries

f. Focus on process

DEVELOPING YOUR KNOWLEDGE BASE

FILL-IN-THE-BLANKS

1. During the evaluation step of the nursing process, based on the patient's responses to the plan of care, the nurse decides to _____, _____, or _____ the plan of care.

2. Nurses are involved in many types of evaluations, but the _____ is always the nurse's primary concern.

3. The most important act of evaluation performed by nurses is evaluating _____ with the patient.

4. _____ are measurable qualities, attributes, or characteristics that specify skills, knowledge, or health states.

5. _____ are the levels of performance accepted and expected by the nursing staff or other healthcare team members established by authority, custom, or consent.

6. _____ are recommendations for how care should be managed in specific diseases, problems, or situations.

7. Specially designed programs that promote excellence in nursing are called _____.

8. _____ evaluation or audit focuses on the environment in which care is provided.

9. When a healthcare worker evaluates nursing care by reviewing patient records to assess the outcomes of nursing care or the process by which these outcomes were achieved, he/she is conducting a(n) _____.

MATCHING EXERCISES

Match the term in Part A with the correct definition listed in Part B.

PART A

a. Concurrent evaluation

b. Retrospective evaluation

c. Outcome evaluation

d. Process evaluation

e. Structure evaluation

f. Introspective evaluation

PART B

1. ___ An evaluation that focuses on the environment in which care is provided

2. ___ An evaluation that focuses on measurable changes in the health status of the patient

3. ___ An evaluation of nursing care and patient goals while the patient is receiving the care

4. ___ An evaluation that focuses on the nature and sequence of activities carried out by the nurse implementing the nursing process

5. ___ An evaluation to collect data after discharge

Match the measurement tool in Part A with its appropriate example in Part B. Answers may be used more than once.

PART A

a. Criteria

b. Standard

PART B

6. ___ Patient will be able to walk the length of the hall by 5/15/12.

7. ___ The admission database will be completed on all patients within 24 hours of admission to the unit.

8. ___ All patients in active labor will have continuous external fetal heart monitoring.

9. ___ Upon completion of an ECG course, the nurse will be able to recognize common arrhythmias when they appear on a heart monitor.

10. ___ The student will be able to name and describe steps of the nursing procedure by the end of the semester.

SHORT ANSWER

1. Explain how you would evaluate whether a patient has achieved the following goals.

   a. Cognitive goals: _____
   _____

   b. Psychomotor goals: _____
   _____

   c. Affective goals: _____
   _____

2. Explain how the following elements of evaluation help to determine whether goals/outcomes have been met.

   a. Identifying evaluative criteria: _____
   _____

   b. Determining whether these criteria and standards are met: _____
   _____

   c. Terminating, continuing, or modifying the plan: _____
   _____

3. Give an example of a variable that may influence goal/outcome achievement in the following areas.

   a. Patient: _____

   b. Nurse: _____

   c. Healthcare system: _____

4. Mr. Bogash, a 28-year-old man with leukemia, recently had a bone marrow transplantation. His medical condition has improved, but he is unable to meet his goal of being up and alert during the daytime hours. What would be the appropriate step to take after evaluating Mr. Bogash? How would you document Mr. Bogash's failure to progress? How would you revise his plan of care?

   _____
   _____
   _____

5. Explain the following three essential components of quality care and how nursing care is evaluated in each area.

   a. Structure: _____
   _____

   b. Process: _____
   _____

   c. Outcome: _____
   _____

6. Explain why the following revisions may be made to a plan of care.

   a. Delete or modify the nursing diagnosis: ___
   _____

   b. Make the goal statement more realistic: ___
   _____

   c. Adjust the time criteria in the goal statement:
   _____

   d. Change nursing interventions: _____
   _____

7. Would you rather work in an environment that ensures the quality of the profession using quality by inspection or quality as opportunity? Explain your answer. _____
   _____

8. Give four examples of the type of evaluations nurses are involved in as members of the healthcare team.

   a. _____

   b. _____

   c. _____

   d. _____

APPLYING YOUR KNOWLEDGE

CRITICAL THINKING QUESTIONS

1. Interview friends and family members who have experienced a stay in the hospital. Ask them if they were aware of specific nursing plans geared to their recovery. See if they were given goals and taught behaviors to accomplish them. Was goal attainment evaluated before they were discharged? Were further goals incorporated into their discharge plan? What do they feel could have been done to help them attain their health goals? How can you use this knowledge to help you develop the blended skills necessary to help patients achieve goals?

2. Reflect on the role that evaluation plays in promoting your scholastic achievement. Has it been positive or negative? Think of specific ways nurses can use evaluation to motivate patients to achieve healthy goals.

3. Give an example of each of the following "Seven Crucial Conversations in Health Care" and brainstorm with a friend or the class to provide a recommendation for solving the problems.
   a. Broken rules
   b. Mistakes
   c. Lack of support
   d. Incompetence
   e. Poor teamwork
   f. Disrespect
   g. Micromanagement

REFLECTIVE PRACTICE USING CRITICAL THINKING SKILLS

Use the following expanded scenario from Chapter 16 in your textbook to answer the questions below.

Scenario: Mrs. Mioshi Otsuki, an elderly woman with a history of heart failure being treated with diuretics, is receiving home care. Mrs. Otsuki lives alone and has a daughter nearby who checks on her once a day. Questioned about her prescribed drug therapy regimen, the patient says, "I take this one labeled 'furosemide' every day in the morning, along with this other one labeled 'Lasix.'"

1. What should be the focus of an evaluation of Mrs. Otsuki's nursing care plan conducted by the home healthcare nurse?

   _____

   _____

   _____

2. What would be a successful outcome for this patient?

   _____

   _____

   _____

3. What intellectual, technical, interpersonal, and/or ethical/legal competencies are most likely to bring about the desired outcome?

   _____

   _____

   _____

4. What resources might be helpful for Mrs. Otsuki?

   _____

   _____

   _____

CHAPTER 17

Documenting, Reporting, Conferring, and Using Informatics

PRACTICING FOR NCLEX

MULTIPLE CHOICE QUESTIONS

Circle the letter that corresponds to the best answer for each question.

1. Which of the following is a nurse's best defense against allegations of negligence by a patient or patient's surrogate?

 a. Nursing team

 b. Flow sheet

 c. Medication record

 d. Patient record

2. Which of the following statements regarding the patient record is accurate?

 a. A patient's chart may be shared only with close family members.

 b. Student nurses are not granted access to patient records.

 c. The patient record is generally the responsibility of one caregiver.

 d. Most patient records are microfilmed and stored in computers.

3. In which of the following systems would a nurse organize data according to the SOAP format?

 a. Source-oriented method

 b. PIE charting method

 c. Problem-oriented method

 d. Focus charting method

4. Abnormal status can be seen immediately with narrative easily retrieved in which of the following documentation formats?

 a. Charting by exception

 b. PIE

 c. Narrative notes

 d. SOAP notes

5. Which of the following is a key component to facilitate data and outcome comparisons by using uniform definitions to create a common language among multiple healthcare data users?

 a. Kardex care plan

 b. Minimum data sets

 c. Computer-based records

 d. Critical/collaborative pathways

6. You are finding it difficult to plan and implement care for Mr. Rivers and decide to have a nursing care conference. Which of the following best defines this action?

   a. You consult with someone in order to exchange ideas or seek information, advice, or instructions.

   b. You meet with nurses or other healthcare professionals to discuss some aspect of patient care.

   c. You and other nurses visit similar patients individually at each patient's bedside in order to plan nursing care.

   d. You send or direct someone for action in a specific nursing care problem.

7. Which of the following is an accurately written documentation of the effectiveness of a patient's pain management?

   a. Mr. Gray is receiving sufficient relief from pain medication.

   b. Mr. Gray appears comfortable and is resting adequately.

   c. Mr. Gray reports that on a scale of 1 to 10, the pain he is experiencing is a 3.

   d. Mr. Gray appears to have a low tolerance for pain and complains frequently about the intensity of his pain.

8. Which of the following guidelines for charting patient information is accurate?

   a. Nursing interventions should be charted chronologically on consecutive lines.

   b. If a mistake is made on a chart, correcting fluid should be used to change the mistake.

   c. Charting should be done in pencil to facilitate correction of mistakes.

   d. If a procedure is repeated frequently, it is proper to use dittos to decrease recording time.

9. Which of the following is a form used to record specific patient variables such as pulse, respiratory rate, blood pressure, and body temperature?

   a. Progress notes

   b. Flow sheets

   c. Graphic sheets

   d. Medical records

ALTERNATE-FORMAT QUESTIONS

Multiple Response Questions

Circle the letters that correspond to the best answers for each question.

1. Which of the following statements are accurate guidelines for communicating and documenting patient information? *(Select all that apply.)*

   a. The patient record is the only permanent legal document that details the nurse's interactions with the patient.

   b. The patient record should not be relied on as a defense against nursing negligence charges.

   c. Omissions and errors in the nursing documentation always affect patient care.

   d. Documentation should be accurate, concise, legally prudent, and confidential.

   e. Only information regarding the patient that pertains to patient care is considered confidential.

   f. Personal codes of ethics, agency policies, and state and federal privacy legislation dictate how patient information can be communicated.

2. According to HIPAA, patients have the right to do which of the following with their health record? *(Select all that apply.)*

   a. See their health record.

   b. Copy their health record.

   c. Destroy their health record.

   d. Change their health record.

   e. Update their health record.

   f. Request a restriction on all uses and disclosures.

3. Which of the following are potential documentation errors that increase the risk for legal problems? *(Select all that apply.)*

   a. The content reflects patient needs.

   b. The content includes descriptions of situations that are out of the ordinary.

   c. The content is not in accordance with professional or healthcare organization standards.

   d. There are lines between the entries.

   e. The documentation is not countersigned.

   f. Dates and times of entries are omitted.

4. Which of the following are incidental disclosures of patient health information that are permitted by HIPAA? *(Select all that apply.)*

   a. The use of sign-in sheets that contain information about the reason for the patient visit

   b. The possibility of a confidential conversation being overheard, provided that the surroundings are appropriate and voices are kept down

   c. The unlimited use of white boards

   d. X-ray light boards that can be seen by passersby, provided that patient x-rays are not left unattended on them

   e. Calling out names in the waiting room, provided that the reason for the patient visit is not mentioned

   f. Leaving detailed appointment reminder messages on a patient's voice mail

5. Which of the following statements accurately describe a method of documentation? *(Select all that apply.)*

   a. In a source-oriented record, each healthcare group keeps data on its own separate form.

   b. In a problem-oriented record, the entire healthcare team works together in identifying a master list of patient problems and contributes collaboratively to the plan of care.

   c. In the PIE charting system, a separate plan of care is developed.

   d. In focus charting, a problem list of nursing or medical diagnoses is used that incorporates many aspects of a patient and patient care.

   e. In charting by exception, only significant findings or "exceptions" to these standards are documented.

   f. In the case management model, a collaborative pathway is part of a computerized documentation system that integrates the collaborative pathway and documentation flow sheets designed to match each day's expected outcomes.

6. Which of the following are basic components of the Resident Assessment Instrument (RAI)? *(Select all that apply.)*

   a. Patient record

   b. Maximum data set

   c. Triggers

   d. Resident assessment protocols

   e. Utilization guidelines

   f. Resident nurse practice acts

Hot Spot Question

1. Place an X on the clock below that shows the military time of 2230.

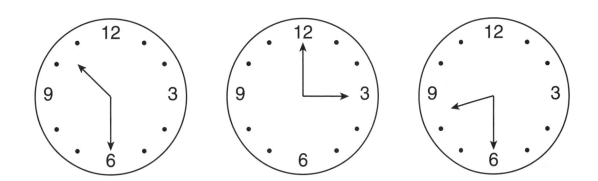

DEVELOPING YOUR KNOWLEDGE BASE

FILL-IN-THE-BLANKS

1. A(n) _____ is a compilation of a patient's health information.

2. The usual format for _____ charting is the unexpected event, the cause of the event, actions taken in response to the event, and discharge planning if appropriate.

3. _____ are a key component to facilitate data and outcome comparisons. They are specific categories of information that use uniform definitions to create a common language among multiple healthcare data users.

4. The _____ is a group of data elements that represent core items of a comprehensive assessment for an adult home care patient and form the basis for measuring patient outcomes for purposes of outcome-based quality improvement.

5. Documentation in long-term care settings is specified by the _____, which helps the staff gather definitive information on a resident's strengths and needs and address these in an individualized plan of care.

6. A nurse who communicates oral, written, or audiotaped patient data to the nurse replacing him/her on the next shift is giving a(n) _____ report.

7. A(n) _____ is a tool used by healthcare agencies to document the occurrence of anything out of the ordinary that results in, or has the potential to result in, harm to a patient, employee, or visitor.

8. A(n) _____ is a meeting of nurses to discuss some aspect of a patient's care.

MATCHING EXERCISES

Match the formats of nursing documentation listed in Part A with their appropriate example listed in Part B.

PART A

a. Initial nursing assessment
b. Plan of nursing care
c. Critical/collaborative pathways
d. Progress notes
e. Graphic record
f. 24-hour fluid balance record
g. Medication record
h. 24-hour nursing care record
i. Discharge and transfer summary
j. Home care documentation
k. Long-term care documentation

PART B

1. ____ The nurse documents the case management plan for a patient population with a designated diagnosis, which includes expected outcomes, interventions to be performed, and the sequence and timing of these interventions.

2. ____ The nurse documents a diabetic patient's intake and output of fluids.

3. ____ The nurse summarizes a patient's reason for treatment, significant findings, procedures performed and treatment rendered, and any specific instructions for the patient/family.

4. ____ The nurse uses this form to record a patient's pulse, respiratory rate, blood pressure, body temperature, weight, and bowel movements.

5. ____ The nurse documents routine aspects of care that promote goal achievement, safety, and well-being.

6. ____ The nurse records the database obtained from the nursing history and physical assessment.

7. ____ The nurse documents the administration of Cipro IV, 400 mg every 12 hours.

8. ____ The nurse documents a patient's diagnosis of AIDS, expected outcomes, and specific nursing interventions.

9. ___ A nurse documents that a patient is homebound and still needs nursing care.

10. ___ A nurse uses RAI to document care.

SHORT ANSWER

1. List four areas of nursing care data that, according to the Joint Commission, must be permanently integrated into the patient record.

   a. _____

   b. _____

   c. _____

   d. _____

2. Briefly describe the following methods of reporting patient data.

   a. Change-of-shift reports: _____

   b. Telephone reports: _____

   c. Telephone orders: _____

   d. Transfer and discharge reports: _____

   e. Reports to family members and significant others: _____

   f. Incident reports: _____

   g. Conferring about care: _____

   h. Consultations and referrals: _____

   i. Nursing care conference: _____

   j. Nursing care rounds: _____

3. Briefly explain the following purposes of the patient record.

   a. Communication: _____

   b. Care planning: _____

   c. Quality review: _____

   d. Research: _____

   e. Decision analysis: _____

   f. Education: _____

   g. Legal documentation: _____

   h. Reimbursement: _____

   i. Historical document: _____

4. List five guidelines nurses should follow when reporting a significant change in a patient's condition to other healthcare professionals by telephone.

   a. _____

   b. _____

   c. _____

   d. _____

   e. _____

5. List four benefits of using the Resident Assessment Instrument (RAI).

   a. _____

   b. _____

   c. _____

   d. _____

6. Complete the chart below listing the purpose, advantages, and disadvantages of the various methods of documentation.

Documentation Method	Description/Advantages/Disadvantages
SOURCE-ORIENTED RECORD	Description: Advantages: Disadvantages:
PROBLEM-ORIENTED MEDICAL RECORDS	Description: Advantages: Disadvantages:
PIE–PROBLEM, INTERVENTION, EVALUATION	Description: Advantages: Disadvantages:
FOCUS CHARTING	Description: Advantages: Disadvantages:
CHARTING BY EXCEPTION	Description: Advantages: Disadvantages:
CASE MANAGEMENT MODEL	Description: Advantages: Disadvantages:
VARIANCE CHARTING	Description: Advantages: Disadvantages:
COMPUTERIZED RECORDS	Description: Advantages: Disadvantages:

APPLYING YOUR KNOWLEDGE

CRITICAL THINKING QUESTIONS

1. Consider the following patient: A 79-year-old woman with Alzheimer's disease is admitted to a long-term care unit. She has a history of falls and has fractured her left hip in the past. She no longer recognizes her daughter, who was taking care of her. The daughter states she can no longer handle her mother's condition. The daughter insists that the nurses restrain her mother physically to prevent falls.

   Think about the information the team will need to provide safe, quality care for this patient. What types of data should the admitting nurse record, and what system of documentation is most likely to bring the information to the attention of everyone who needs it?

2. How would you go about scheduling a consultation for a male amputee who needs physical therapy? Write a brief summary of the patient's condition and how you would present his case to the referred agency.

3. Make an appointment to interview the risk manager of a healthcare system. Find out how important the documentation of patient care is to the patient, nurse, and health agency when legal questions arise. How can this knowledge help to safeguard your practice?

REFLECTIVE PRACTICE USING CRITICAL THINKING SKILLS

Use the following expanded scenario from Chapter 17 in your textbook to answer the questions below.

   Scenario: Philippe Baron, age 52, is being discharged from the outpatient surgery department after undergoing a colonoscopy for removal of three polyps. Upon admittance, Mr. Baron stated that he was allergic to a pain medication but couldn't remember the name of it. The RN phoned the doctor's office to check his medical record. His attending gave an order via phone for a PRN analgesic that worked in the past. He will be going home with his wife, who is a nurse, and they require discharge teaching.

1. What should be the focus of discharge teaching for Mr. Baron and his wife?

2. What would be a successful outcome for this patient?

3. What intellectual, technical, interpersonal, and/or ethical/legal competencies are most likely to bring about the desired outcome?

4. What resources might be helpful for Ms. Baron?

CHAPTER 18

Developmental Concepts

PRACTICING FOR NCLEX

MULTIPLE CHOICE QUESTIONS

Circle the letter that corresponds to the best answer for each question.

1. The human process of growth and development is the result of which two interrelated factors?
   a. Heredity and environment
   b. Heredity and religion
   c. Faith and culture
   d. Physical and psychosocial skills

2. Which of the following theorists listed the unconscious mind, the id, the ego, and the superego as the primary aspects of the psycho-analytic theory?
   a. Erik Erikson
   b. Robert Havighurst
   c. Jean Piaget
   d. Sigmund Freud

3. Which of Freud's stages of development marks the transition to adult sexuality during adolescence?
   a. Latency stage
   b. Anal stage
   c. Phallic stage
   d. Genital stage

4. The expansion of Freud's theory to include cultural and social influences in addition to biologic processes is credited to which of the following theorists?
   a. Erik Erikson
   b. Robert Havighurst
   c. Jean Piaget
   d. Lawrence Kohlberg

5. Which of the following theorists believed that living and growing are based on learning, and that a person must continuously learn to adjust to changing societal conditions?
   a. Erik Erikson
   b. Robert Havighurst
   c. Jean Piaget
   d. Sigmund Freud

6. A child who learns that he must sit quietly during story hour in kindergarten, thereby integrating this new experience into his exist-ing schemata, is applying the process of:
   a. Accommodation
   b. Dissemination
   c. Assimilation
   d. Orientation

7. In which stage of Piaget's cognitive develop-ment theory is logical thinking developed with an understanding of reversibility, relations between numbers, and loss of egocentricity?
   a. Sensorimotor stage
   b. Preoperational stage
   c. Concrete operational stage
   d. Formal operational stage

8. According to Piaget, the use of abstract thinking and deductive reasoning occurs during which of the following stages of development?
   a. Sensorimotor stage
   b. Preoperational stage
   c. Concrete operational stage
   d. Formal operational stage

9. Which of the following theorists developed the theory that males and females have different ways of dealing with moral issues?
   a. Lawrence Kohlberg
   b. Jean Piaget
   c. James Fowler
   d. Carol Gilligan

ALTERNATE-FORMAT QUESTIONS

Multiple Response Questions

Circle the letters that correspond to the best answers for each question.

1. Which of the following generalizations about growth and development are accurate? *(Select all that apply.)*
   a. Growth and development do not occur in a specific order or sequence.
   b. Growth and development follow irregular and unpredictable trends.
   c. Growth and development are differentiated and integrated.
   d. Different aspects of growth and development cannot be modified.
   e. Within each developmental level, certain milestones can be identified.
   f. Cephalocaudal development is the first trend in growth and development.

2. Which of the following statements regarding the effects of environment and nutrition development are accurate? *(Select all that apply.)*
   a. Infants who are malnourished in utero develop the same amount of brain cells as infants who had adequate prenatal nutrition.
   b. Substance abuse by a pregnant woman increases the risk for congenital anomalies in her developing fetus.
   c. Failure to thrive cannot be linked to emotional deprivation.
   d. Abuse of alcohol and drugs is more prevalent in teenagers who have poor family relationships.

   e. An increased incidence of teenage pregnancy can be linked to substance abuse by adolescents.
   f. Child abuse can lead to deficits in physical development, but psychosocial development is not affected.

3. Which of the following are components of Freud's theory of psychoanalytic development? *(Select all that apply.)*
   a. Ego
   b. Id
   c. Yin and yang
   d. Altered consciousness
   e. Superego
   f. Conscious mind

4. Which of the following concepts are components of Erikson's theory of psychosocial development? *(Select all that apply.)*
   a. Cognitive development
   b. Psychosexual stages
   c. Developmental goals or tasks
   d. Psychosocial crises
   e. The process of coping
   f. Spiritual growth

5. Which of the following concepts accurately describe the developmental stages and concepts of Kohlberg's theory of moral development? *(Select all that apply.)*
   a. The preconventional level is based on external control as the child learns to conform to rules imposed by authority figures.
   b. The postconventional level involves identifying with significant others and conforming to their expectations.
   c. Few adults ever reach stage 6 of the postconventional level.
   d. Males and females have different ways of looking at the world.
   e. In the preconventional level, moral judgment is based on shared norms and expectations, and societal values are adopted.
   f. In stage 1 of the preconventional level, punishment and obedience orientation, the motivation for choices of action is fear or physical consequences of authority's disapproval.

Prioritization Questions

1. Place the following stages of Sigmund Freud's theory of psychoanalytic development in the order in which they occur:

   a. Phallic stage

   b. Latency stage

   c. Oral stage

   d. Genital stage

   e. Anal stage

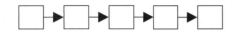

2. Place the following stages of Havighurst's theory of development (developmental tasks) in the order in which they occur:

   a. Achieving gender-specific social role; achieving independence; acquiring a set of values and ethical system to guide behavior

   b. Learning sex differences; forming concepts; getting ready to read

   c. Learning to walk; learning to talk; learning to control body waste elimination

   d. Achieving social and civic responsibility; accepting and adjusting to physical changes

   e. Learning physical skills; learning to get along with others; developing conscience and morality

   f. Adjusting to decreasing physical status and health; adjusting to retirement

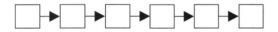

DEVELOPING YOUR KNOWLEDGE BASE

FILL-IN-THE-BLANKS

1. The second trend in growth and development is _____, meaning that growth progresses from gross motor movements to fine motor movements.

2. According to developmental theorist Sigmund Freud, the period from adolescence to adulthood is known as the _____ stage.

3. According to the developmental theorist _____, during the preschool to early school years, a child imitates the religious behavior of others.

4. According to Jean Piaget, during the _____ years, an individual integrates others' viewpoints into his/her own understanding of truth.

5. Freud identified the underlying stimulus for human behavior as sexuality, which he called _____.

6. _____ is the process of integrating new experiences into existing schemata.

7. The _____ stage of Piaget's theory of cognitive development is characterized by the use of abstract thinking and deductive reasoning.

8. Levinson and associates based their theory of human development on the organizing concept of _____.

MATCHING EXERCISES

Match Erikson's stages of development listed in Part A with the appropriate example listed in Part B. Some answers will be used more than once.

PART A

a. Trust versus mistrust

b. Autonomy versus shame and doubt

c. Initiative versus guilt

d. Industry versus inferiority

e. Identity versus role confusion

f. Intimacy versus isolation

g. Generativity versus stagnation

h. Ego integrity versus despair

PART B

1. ___ A 10-year-old boy proudly displays his principal's award certificate.

2. ___ An infant believes that his parents will feed him.

3. ___ A 22-year-old woman picks a circle of friends with whom she spends her free time.

4. ___ A 13-year-old girl fights with her mother about appropriate dress.

5. ___ A nursing home resident reflects positively on her past life experiences.

6. ___ A 15-year-old boy worries about how his classmates treat him.

7. ____ A 45-year-old man meets a goal of guiding his two children into rewarding careers.

8. ____ A kindergarten student learns the alphabet.

9. ____ A 2-year-old boy expresses interest in dressing himself.

10. ____ A 35-year-old woman volunteers Saturday mornings to work with the homeless.

Match the stages of faith development listed in Part A with the appropriate definition listed in Part B. Note which of the following stages you have personally experienced in your lifetime. Give an example from your past that illustrates your passage through each stage on the lines provided at the end of the definitions.

PART A

a. Stage 1: Intuitive–projective faith
b. Stage 2: Mythical–literal faith
c. Stage 3: Synthetic–conventional faith
d. Stage 4: Individuative–reflective faith
e. Stage 5: Conjunctive faith
f. Stage 6: Universalizing faith

PART B

11. _____ This stage integrates other viewpoints about faith into one's understanding of truth. One is able to see the paradoxical nature of the reality of one's own beliefs. Personal example: _____

_____

12. _____ This is the characteristic stage for many adolescents. An ideology has emerged, but it has not been closely examined until now; attempts to stabilize own identity. Personal example: _____

_____

13. _____ This stage involves making tangible the values of absolute love and justice for humankind; total trust in principle of being and existence of future. Personal example: _____

_____

14. _____ In this stage, children imitate religious gestures and behaviors of others; they follow parental attitudes toward religious or moral beliefs without a thorough understanding of them. Personal example: _____

_____

15. _____ This stage is critical for older adolescents and young adults because the responsibility for their commitments, beliefs, and attitudes becomes their own. Personal example: _____

_____

16. _____ This stage predominates in the school-aged child with increased social interaction. Stories represent religious and moral beliefs, and the existence of a deity is accepted. Personal example: _____

_____

CORRECT THE FALSE STATEMENTS

Circle the word "true" or "false" that follows the statement. If you circled "false," change the underlined word or words to make the statement true. Place your answer in the space provided.

1. The human processes of growth and development result from two interrelated factors: <u>heredity and environment</u>.

   True False _____

2. Growth and development follow <u>irregular and unpredictable</u> trends.

   True False _____

3. Different aspects of growth and development occur at <u>the same</u> stages and rates.

   True False _____

4. Freud identified the underlying stimulus for human behavior as <u>faith</u>.

   True False _____

5. According to Freud, the <u>ego</u> is the part of the psyche concerned with self-gratification by the easiest and quickest available means.

   True False _____

6. In Freud's <u>phallic</u> stage, the child has increased interest in gender differences, and curiosity about the genitals and masturbation increases.

   True False _____

7. According to Havighurst, developing a conscience, morality, and a scale of values should occur in <u>middle childhood</u>.

   True False _____

8. In Kohlberg's <u>preconventional level, stage 2, instrumental relativist orientation</u>, the motivation for choices of action is fear of physical consequences or authority's disapproval.

True   False _____

9. According to Gould, between the ages of <u>22 and 28</u>, self-acceptance increases as the need to prove oneself disappears.

True   False _____

SHORT ANSWER

1. Complete the following chart, using the first theorist (Sigmund Freud) as an example.

Theorist and Theory	Basic Concepts of Theory	Stages of Development
Sigmund Freud Psychoanalytic theory	Stressed the impact of instinctual human drives on determining behavior: Unconscious mind, the id, the ego, the superego, stages of development based on sexual motivation	Oral stage Anal stage Phallic stage Latent stage Genital stage
Erik Erikson		
Robert J. Havighurst		
Jean Piaget		
Lawrence Kohlberg		
Carol Gilligan		
James Fowler		

2. Describe Lawrence Kohlberg's three levels of moral development, and give an example of behavior that would typify each level.

   a. Preconventional level: _____

      _____

     Example: _____

      _____

   b. Conventional level: _____

      _____

     Example: _____

      _____

   c. Postconventional level: _____

      _____

     Example: _____

      _____

3. A 6-year-old girl with leukemia is admitted to the hospital for her first session of chemotherapy. What insight into this patient's needs could be gained from the following theorists?

   a. Freud: _____

   b. Erikson: _____

   c. Havighurst: _____

   d. Piaget: _____

   e. Kohlberg: _____

   f. Gilligan: _____

   g. Fowler: _____

4. Identify the stage of the theorists noted below that the nurse could use in responding to the following statements made by a 15-year-old boy who has been admitted to the hospital following an ATV accident. He has multiple fractures and several deep cuts in his face that require stitches.

   a. Freud: _____ "My dad told me not to ride that thing. I should have listened to him, and this never would have happened."

   b. Erikson: _____ "I'm going to be so ugly with these scars on my face. No girl will ever look at me again."

   c. Piaget: _____ "What's the best way to be sure I don't lose strength in my muscles? If I do those exercises you taught me, I'll be able to go back to school and play basketball next year."

   d. Fowler: _____ "I don't believe in God. If there were a God, He never would have let this happen to me."

5. What role does the family play in health promotion and illness prevention? How has your family affected your attitudes toward health and illness? _____

APPLYING YOUR KNOWLEDGE

CRITICAL THINKING QUESTIONS

1. Reflect on the nursing plan you would develop for a 3-year-old, a 10-year-old, and a 16-year-old undergoing heart surgery. How would your plan differ to take into consideration the age differences of the patients? How would you explain the procedure to each child? Give a rationale for each nursing intervention planned. Support your rationale by using a different developmental theory for each age group's nursing plan.

3-year-old:

10-year-old:

16-year-old:

2. Make a chart listing Freud's stages of psychosexual development, Piaget's psychosocial development of different ages, and Havighurst's developmental tasks. Observe children in different settings and find an example of each stage of development. Talk with classmates about how these findings would influence your nursing practice.

REFLECTIVE PRACTICE USING CRITICAL THINKING SKILLS

Use the following expanded scenario from Chapter 18 in your textbook to answer the questions below.

Scenario: Joseph Logan, age 70, fell and fractured his hip while repairing the exterior of his home. He has a wife and two grown children. His son, age 42, is mentally challenged and lives at home with the couple. His wife tells you she is apprehensive about having to care for two people now. When the nurse comes into Mr. Logan's room to perform AM care, he says, "Go away and leave me alone. I'm a grown man; I can take care of myself. And get rid of this tray. I'm not hungry!" Further investigation reveals that Mr. Logan has been the traditional head of his household and is now troubled by needing others, including his wife, to care for him.

1. What developmental considerations may affect care planning for Mr. Logan?

_____

_____

_____

2. What would be a successful outcome for this patient?

_____

_____

_____

3. What intellectual, technical, interpersonal, and/or ethical/legal competencies are most likely to bring about the desired outcome?

_____

_____

_____

4. What resources might be helpful for Mr. Logan and his family?

_____

_____

_____

Conception Through Young Adult

PRACTICING FOR NCLEX

MULTIPLE CHOICE QUESTIONS

Circle the letter that corresponds to the best answer for each question.

1. Which of the following numbers is a normal score on the Apgar rating scale for newborns taken 1 and 5 minutes after birth?
   a. 1 to 3
   b. 4 to 6
   c. 7 to 10
   d. 11 to 15

2. Which of the following statements concerning neonates is accurate?
   a. A neonate can see color and forms.
   b. A neonate cannot hear sounds.
   c. A neonate is insensitive to touch and pain.
   d. A neonate has no labile temperature control.

3. A preschooler who clings excessively to his mother and uses infantile speech patterns is exhibiting which of the following behaviors?
   a. Separation anxiety
   b. Regression
   c. Negativism
   d. Self-expression

4. In which of the following stages of puberty do ova and sperm begin to be produced by the reproductive organs?
   a. Prepubescence
   b. Pubescence
   c. Postpubescence
   d. None of the above

5. In which of the following stages of development would a person be most likely to think in the abstract and question beliefs and practices that no longer serve to stabilize identity or purpose?
   a. Toddler
   b. School-aged
   c. Adolescent
   d. Older adult

6. In which of the following stages of development of a fetus have all the basic organs been developed?
   a. Preembryonic stage
   b. Embryonic stage
   c. Fetal stage
   d. Neonatal stage

7. A child would be most likely to develop separation anxiety in which of the following stages of development?
   a. Infant
   b. Toddler
   c. Preschooler
   d. School-aged

8. You have been asked to implement a sex education program in the public schools. With which grade level would you begin the program?
   a. Kindergarten
   b. Elementary
   c. Middle school/junior high
   d. High school

9. Which of the following toys would be most appropriate for the toddler?
   a. Tricycle
   b. Basketball
   c. Building blocks
   d. Stuffed animal

10. The most influential group in stabilizing self-concept in the adolescent is his or her:
    a. Parents
    b. Siblings
    c. Peers
    d. Teachers

11. Which of the following cell layers of the fetus become the skeleton, connective tissue, cartilage, and muscles, as well as the circulatory, lymphoid, reproductive, and urinary systems?
    a. Ectoderm
    b. Endoderm
    c. Mesoderm
    d. None of the above

12. During which stage of development would the fetus be most susceptible to maternal use of alcohol?
    a. Preembryonic stage
    b. Embryonic stage
    c. Fetal stage

13. When assessing the health of a neonate, the nurse should be aware of which of the following accurate statements?
    a. The neonate has not yet developed reflexes that allow sucking, swallowing, or blinking.
    b. The neonate has labile temperature control that responds slowly to environmental temperatures.
    c. The neonate is alert to the environment but cannot distinguish color and form.
    d. The neonate hears and turns toward sound and can smell and taste.

ALTERNATE-FORMAT QUESTIONS

Multiple Response Questions

Circle the letters that correspond to the best answers for each question.

1. Which of the following are physical characteristics of the normal neonate? *(Select all that apply.)*
   a. Reflexes include the Moro reflex and the stepping reflex.
   b. Body temperature responds slowly to the environmental temperature, necessitating the use of warming devices.
   c. Senses are not developed enough to feel pain.
   d. Stool and urine are eliminated.
   e. Both an active crying state and a quiet alert state are exhibited.
   f. The neonate inherits a transient immunity from infections as a result of immunoglobulins that cross the placenta.

2. Which of the following are physical characteristics of an infant? *(Select all that apply.)*
   a. Brain grows to about one third the adult size.
   b. Body temperature stabilizes.
   c. Eyes begin to focus and fixate.
   d. Heart triples in weight.
   e. Heart rate slows and blood pressure rises.
   f. Birth weight usually doubles by 1 year.

3. Which of the following are considered growth and development characteristics of the toddler? *(Select all that apply.)*
   a. Brain growth slows.
   b. The long bones of the arms and legs increase in length.
   c. The toddler does not achieve bladder control during this stage.
   d. At 2 years of age, a toddler is typically four times the birthweight.
   e. The toddler turns pages in a book and draws stick people.
   f. The toddler walks forward and backward but cannot run or climb stairs.

4. Which of the following statements describing the psychosocial development of the preschooler are accurate? *(Select all that apply.)*

a. The preschooler is in Piaget's preoperational stage of development.

b. The preschooler is in Freud's phallic stage.

c. The preschooler is in Erickson's stage of industry versus inferiority.

d. According to Havighurst, the preschooler has the developmental task of developing conscience and morality.

e. According to Fowler, the preschooler imitates the religious behaviors of others.

f. According to Kohlberg, the preschooler is aware of the need to respect authority.

5. Which of the following statements accurately describe the physiologic development of the school-aged child? *(Select all that apply.)*

a. The brain reaches 90% to 95% of adult size.

b. The nervous system is 50% matured, resulting in coordinated body movements.

c. Sexual organs grow but are dormant until late in this period.

d. All permanent teeth are present.

e. Height increases 2 to 3 inches a year.

f. Weight increases 3 to 6 pounds a year.

6. Which of the following accurately describe the cognitive and psychosocial development of the adolescent? *(Select all that apply.)*

a. The concept of time and its passage enables the adolescent to set long-term goals.

b. According to Piaget, adolescence is the stage when the cognitive development of formal operations is developed.

c. In the adolescent, egocentrism diminishes and is replaced by an awareness of the needs of others.

d. Based on Erikson's theory, the adolescent tries out different roles and personal choices and beliefs in the stage called generativity versus stagnation.

e. The parents act as the greatest influence on the adolescent.

f. According to Havighurst, more mature relationships with boys and girls are achieved by the adolescent.

Chart/Exhibit Question

Use the chart below to determine the 5-minute Apgar score of the following neonates:

1. A neonate has a pink skin tone on the body with blue extremities, displays minimum resistance to having extremities extended, has a hearty cry, and has a heart rate of 105 beats per minute. Score _____

2. A neonate has a pale skin tone, heart rate of 96 beats per minute, respiratory rate of 20 breaths per minute, a weak cry, and no response to being slapped on the sole. Score _____

3. A neonate has a pink skin color, cries vigorously, clenches fists and flexes knees, and has a heart rate of 130 beats per minute. Score _____

Apgar Scoring Chart			
Category*	0	1	2
Heart rate	Absent	Slow (less than 100 beats/min)	More than 100 beats/min
Respiratory effort	Absent	Slow, irregular	Good, crying
Muscle tone	Flaccid	Some flexion of extremities	Active motion
Reflex irritability	No response	Weak cry or grimace	Vigorous cry
Color	Blue, pale	Body pink, extremities blue	Completely pink

*Each category is rated as 0, 1, or 2. The rating for each category is then totaled to a maximum score of 10. Normal neonates score between 7 and 10. Neonates who score between 4 and 6 require special assistance; those who score below 4 are in need of immediate life-saving support.

DEVELOPING YOUR KNOWLEDGE BASE

FILL-IN-THE-BLANKS

1. The three distinct cell layers of the zygote are the _____, _____, and _____.

2. The _____ stage of the development of the fetus occurs from the fourth through the eighth week, initiating rapid growth and differentiation of the cell layers.

3. The most commonly used measurement scale to assess the neonate at birth is the _____.

4. _____ occurs when a mother forms an emotional link to her newborn.

5. _____ is a condition of inadequate growth in height and weight resulting from the infant's inability to obtain or use calories needed for growth.

6. The unexpected death of an infant under the age of 1 year in which postmortem examination fails to reveal a cause of death is known as _____.

7. A test that is commonly used to determine quickly and inexpensively atypical developmental patterns in infants and children is the _____.

MATCHING EXERCISES

Match the stage of development listed in Part A with the risk factor associated with that age listed in Part B.

PART A

a. Neonate

b. Infant

c. Toddler

d. Preschooler

e. School-aged

f. Adolescent and young adult

PART B

1. ___ Hormonal changes cause physical symptoms.

2. ___ Communicable diseases and respiratory tract infections begin to develop in this stage.

3. ___ Congenital disorders, such as hypospadias, inguinal hernias, and cardiac anomalies, require surgery at this stage.

4. ___ The suicide rate is highest for this group.

5. ___ A mother who smokes cigarettes, drinks alcohol, or uses drugs may cause developmental deficits in this stage.

6. ___ Accidents, poisonings, burns, drowning, aspiration, and falls remain the major causes of death in this stage.

7. ___ Gastroenteritis, food allergies, and skin disorders are common in this stage of development.

8. ___ Scabies, impetigo, and head lice are more prevalent in this stage.

SHORT ANSWER

1. Write down the age group in which the following physiologic characteristics and behaviors are commonly developed. Use *N* for neonate, *I* for infant, *T* for toddler, *P* for preschooler, *S* for school-aged, and *A* for adolescent/young adult.

_____ Motor abilities include skipping, throwing and catching, copying figures, and printing letters and numbers.

_____ Puberty begins.

_____ Brain grows to about half the adult size.

_____ Reflexes include sucking, swallowing, blinking, sneezing, and yawning.

_____ Temperature control responds quickly to environmental temperatures.

_____ Walks forward and backward, runs, kicks, climbs, and rides tricycle

_____ Drinks from a cup and uses a spoon

_____ Sebaceous and axillary sweat glands become active.

_____ Height increases 2 to 3 inches and weight increases 3 to 6 pounds a year.

_____ The feet, hands, and long bones grow rapidly, and muscle mass increases.

_____ Alert to environment, sees color and form, hears and turns to sound

_____ Birthweight usually triples.

_____ Full set of 20 deciduous teeth; baby teeth fall out and are replaced.

_____ Body is less chubby and becomes leaner and more coordinated.

_____ Primary and secondary development occurs with maturation of genitals.

_____ Typically four times the birthweight and 23 to 37 inches in height

_____ Body temperature stabilizes.

_____ Average weight is 45 pounds.

_____ Brain reaches 90% to 95% of adult size; nervous system is almost mature.

_____ Head is close to adult size.

_____ Motor abilities develop, allowing feeding self, crawling, and walking.

_____ Can smell and taste and is sensitive to touch and pain

_____ Begins to eliminate stool and urine

_____ Deciduous teeth begin to erupt.

_____ All permanent teeth are present except for second and third molars.

_____ Attains bladder control during the day and sometimes during the night

_____ Holds a pencil and eventually writes in script and sentences

_____ Full adult size is reached.

_____ Drinks breast milk, glucose water, and plain water

_____ Eyes begin to focus and fixate.

_____ Turns pages in a book and by age 3 draws stick people

_____ Heart doubles in weight, heart rate slows, blood pressure rises.

_____ Rapid brain growth; increase in length of long bones of the arms and legs

_____ Uses fingers to pick up small objects

_____ Sexual organs grow but are dormant until late in this period.

2. Write down the age group in which the following psychosocial characteristics and behaviors are commonly developed. Use *N* for neonate, *I* for infant, *T* for toddler, *P* for preschooler, *S* for school-aged, and *A* for adolescent/young adult.

_____ Is in oral stage (Freud); strives for immediate gratification of needs; strong sucking need

_____ Developmental task of learning appropriate sex's social role

_____ In Freud's genital stage, libido reemerges in mature form.

_____ Is in anal stage (Freud); focus on pleasure of sphincter control

_____ Self-concept is being stabilized, with peer group as greatest influence.

_____ Develops trust (Erikson) if caregiver is dependable to meet needs

_____ Achieves personal independence; develops conscience, morality, and scale of values

_____ Tries out different roles, personal choices, and beliefs (identity versus role confusion)

_____ Meets developmental tasks (Havighurst) by learning to eat, walk, and talk

_____ Develops skill in reading, writing, and calculating, as well as concepts for everyday living

_____ More mature relationships with both males and females of same age

_____ Enters Erikson's stage of autonomy versus shame and doubt

_____ Is in Erikson's stage of initiative versus guilt

_____ Inner turmoil/examination of propriety of actions by rigid conscience

_____ Getting ready to read and learning to distinguish right from wrong

_____ One's personal appearance accepted; set of values internalized

_____ Freud's latency stage; strong identification with own sex

_____ Developmental tasks of learning to control elimination; begins to learn sex differences, concepts, language, and right from wrong

_____ Focuses on learning useful skills with an emphasis on doing, succeeding, and accomplishing

_____ Developmental tasks of describing social and physical reality through concept formation and language development

_____ Is in phallic stage (Freud) with biologic focus on genitals

_____ Superego and conscience begin to develop

_____ Developmental tasks of learning sex differences and modesty

_____ Developmental task of learning physical game skills

_____ Is in Erikson's industry versus inferiority stage

3. Briefly describe the growth and development of the fetus in the following three stages of fetal growth.

a. Preembryonic stage: _____

_____

b. Embryonic stage: _____

_____

c. Fetal stage: _____

_____

4. List four critical areas of development that are assessed by the Denver Developmental Screening test.

a. _____

b. _____

c. _____

d. _____

5. After observing infants in a neonatal unit, describe the physical symptoms of the following temperaments:

a. "Easy": _____

b. "Slow to warm": _____

c. "Difficult": _____

6. Define the following infant health problems and the role of the nurse in treating/preventing them.

a. Colic: _____

_____

b. Failure to thrive: _____

_____

c. Sudden infant death syndrome: _____

_____

d. Child abuse: _____

_____

7. Describe age-appropriate methods for preparing the following age groups for eye surgery; explain why you have chosen this method.

a. Toddler: _____

_____

_____

b. Preschooler: _____

_____

_____

c. School-aged child: _____

_____

_____

d. Adolescent and young adult: _____

_____

8. The nurse plays an important role in healthcare for each stage of development. Explain how you would tailor your care plan for the various age groups listed below.

a. Infant: _____

_____

b. Toddler: _____

_____

c. Preschooler: _____

_____

d. School-aged child: _____

_____

e. Adolescent and young adult: _____

_____

9. Briefly describe the following stages of puberty.

a. Prepubescence: _____

_____

b. Pubescence: _____

_____

c. Postpubescence: _____

_____

APPLYING YOUR KNOWLEDGE

CRITICAL THINKING QUESTIONS

1. A child is admitted to the intensive care unit with third-degree burns. How would your nursing care plan differ for a child in each of the stages listed below? Be sure to include the type of dialog you would use to explain painful procedures to each age group.

   a. Toddler: _____

   _____

   _____

   b. Preschooler: _____

   _____

   _____

   c. School-aged child: _____

   _____

   _____

   d. Adolescent: _____

   _____

   _____

2. No two parents are the same in their methods of raising children. Although there aren't always clear-cut right or wrong ways to raise children, some parents just seem to do a better job of it than others. Interview some of your friends to find out how successful they feel their parents were in raising them. Ask them about their parents' methods of discipline, motivation, and encouragement. Compare their answers with your own thoughts about how you were raised by your parents. What is nursing's role in promoting good parenting?

REFLECTIVE PRACTICE USING CRITICAL THINKING SKILLS

Use the following expanded scenario from Chapter 19 in your textbook to answer the questions below.

Scenario: Patricia Leming, age 26, is in the first trimester of pregnancy. At a clinic visit, she says, "I've been trying to cut back on smoking and drinking alcohol, but I haven't had much success." Upon assessment, the nurse notes that Ms. Leming appears nervous and slightly underweight. Ms. Leming also states that she hasn't had much of an appetite since she's been pregnant. She tells the nurse, "My boyfriend was furious when he found out I was pregnant, and he wants nothing to do with the baby."

1. What should be the focus of the nursing care plan developed for Ms. Leming?

   _____

   _____

   _____

2. What would be a successful outcome for this patient?

   _____

   _____

   _____

3. What intellectual, technical, interpersonal, and/or ethical/legal competencies are most likely to bring about the desired outcome?

   _____

   _____

   _____

4. What resources might be helpful for Ms. Leming?

   _____

   _____

   _____

CHAPTER 20

The Aging Adult

PRACTICING FOR NCLEX

MULTIPLE CHOICE QUESTIONS

Circle the letter that corresponds to the best answer for each question.

1. Which of the following accurately describes the behavior of the middle adult?
   a. Believes in establishment of self but fears being pulled back into the family
   b. Usually substitutes new roles for old roles and perhaps continues formal roles in a new context
   c. Looks inward, accepts life span as having definite boundaries, and has special interest in spouse, friends, and community
   d. Looks forward but also looks back and begins to reflect on his/her life

2. Which of the following aging theories assumes that healthy aging is related to the ability of the older adult to continue similar patterns of behavior that existed in young to middle adulthood?
   a. Identity-continuity theory
   b. Disengagement theory
   c. Activity theory
   d. Life review theory

3. Based on an understanding of the cognitive changes that normally occur with aging, what would you expect a newly hospitalized older adult to do?
   a. Talk rapidly but be confused
   b. Withdraw from strangers
   c. Interrupt with frequent questions
   d. Take longer to respond and react

4. Which of the following nursing actions would help maintain safety in the older adult?
   a. Treat each patient as a unique individual.
   b. Orient the patient to new surroundings.
   c. Encourage independence.
   d. Provide planned rest and activity times.

5. As defined by Erickson, in what stage of human development is the older adult?
   a. Intimacy versus isolation
   b. Identity versus role diffusion
   c. Ego-integrity versus despair
   d. Generativity versus stagnation

6. According to Havighurst, which of the following is a developmental task of older adulthood?
   a. Adjusting to declining physical strength and health
   b. Moving from one's own home to the home of others
   c. Learning to live by oneself after losing a spouse
   d. Establishing oneself in the community

7. Which of the following adult developmental theorists viewed the middle years as a time when adults increase their feelings of self-satisfaction, value their spouse as a companion, and become more concerned with health?
   a. Erickson
   b. Levinson
   c. Piaget
   d. Gould

8. Which of the following is a developmental task of the middle adult?

a. Selecting a life partner

b. Establishing and guiding the next generation

c. Establishing a social network

d. Forming a personal philosophical and ethical structure

9. Which of the following statements about the older adult is accurate?

a. Old age begins at age 65.

b. Personality is not changed by chronologic aging.

c. Most older adults are ill and institutionalized.

d. Intelligence declines with age.

ALTERNATE-FORMAT QUESTIONS

Multiple Response Questions

Circle the letters that correspond to the best answers for each question.

1. Which of the following are considered to be normal physical changes in the middle adult? *(Select all that apply.)*

a. Skin moisture increases.

b. Hormone production increases.

c. Hearing acuity diminishes.

d. Cognitive ability diminishes.

e. Cardiac output begins to decrease.

f. There is a loss of calcium from bones.

2. Which of the following statements accurately describe the role of the middle adult? *(Select all that apply.)*

a. A task of the middle adult is to guide the next generation.

b. A task of the middle adult is to prepare for separation from family and friends.

c. One role of the middle adult is to adjust to the needs of aging parents.

d. According to Levinson, middle adults may choose either to continue an established lifestyle or reorganize their life in a period of midlife transition.

e. Gould viewed the middle years as a time when adults look inward and accept their life span as having definite boundaries.

f. Persons in the middle adult years must adjust to decreased personal freedom and economic instability.

3. Which of the following statements concerning the physical condition of older adults are accurate? *(Select all that apply.)*

a. In older adults, all organs undergo some degree of decline in overall functioning.

b. Body functions that require integrated activity of several organ systems are affected the most in older adults.

c. Most older adults experience severe limitations in activities.

d. Statistically, one out of every five older adults suffers from at least one chronic illness.

e. An older adult who lives alone is at greatest risk for loss of independence.

f. An older adult's ability to adapt determines whether he/she is ill or healthy.

4. Which of the following facts regarding Alzheimer's disease (AD) are accurate? *(Select all that apply.)*

a. AD accounts for about one third of the cases of dementia in the United States.

b. AD primarily affects young to middle adults.

c. Scientists estimate that more than 5 million people have AD.

d. The number of people with AD doubles every 20 years.

e. AD affects brain cells and is characterized by patchy areas of the brain that degenerate.

f. AD is a progressively serious but not a life-threatening disease.

5. Which of the following accurately describe conditions found in older adulthood? *(Select all that apply.)*

a. Sundowning syndrome is a condition in which an older adult habitually becomes confused, restless, and agitated after dark.

b. Delirium is a permanent state of confusion occurring in older adulthood.

c. Depression is a prolonged or extreme state of sadness occurring in many older adults.

d. As many as 50% of adults 65 years and older experience an episode of delirium during a hospitalization.

e. Polypharmacy is a term that is used to describe the habit of older adults to use many pharmacies to obtain their prescription drugs.

f. A significant percentage of older adults limit their activities because of fear of falling that might result in serious health consequences.

DEVELOPING YOUR KNOWLEDGE BASE

FILL-IN-THE-BLANKS

1. _____ is a chemical reaction that produces damage to the DNA and cell death.

2. A middle adult is considered to be in the age range of _____.

3. The term _____ describes the middle adult who is involved in relationships with his/her own children and aging family members.

4. The older adult period is often further divided into the young-old, ages _____; the middle-old, ages _____; and the old-old, ages _____.

5. A nurse who believes that all older adults take more time to answer interview questions due to slowed mental processes is guilty of a form of stereotyping known as _____.

6. The _____ theory of aging assumes that healthy aging is related to the older adult's ability to continue similar patterns of behavior from young and middle adulthood.

7. When an older adult tells the nurse about his successes on the golf course, he is engaging in what is termed _____ or _____.

8. _____ is the most common degenerative neurologic illness and the most common cause of cognitive impairment.

9. A nurse who shows a patient with dementia a calendar and points to the present date and the date of a visit from her family is practicing what is commonly known as _____.

10. _____ is the scientific and behavioral study of all aspects of aging and its consequences.

SHORT ANSWER

1. Briefly describe the following characteristics of middle and older adulthood.

   a. Middle adulthood

   Physiologic development: _____

   _____

   Psychosocial development: _____

   _____

   Cognitive, moral, and spiritual development:

   _____

   b. Older adulthood

   Physiologic development: _____

   _____

   Psychosocial development: _____

   _____

   Cognitive, moral, and spiritual development:

   _____

2. List five health-promotion activities recommended for all middle adults.

   a. _____

   b. _____

   c. _____

   d. _____

   e. _____

3. Briefly describe the following theories on aging.

   a. Genetic theory: _____

   _____

   b. Immunity theory: _____

   _____

   c. Cross-linkage theory: _____

   _____

   d. Free radical theory: _____

   _____

   e. Disengagement theory: _____

   _____

   f. Activity theory: _____

   _____

   g. Identity-continuity theory: _____

   _____

4. You are a visiting nurse for a patient with Alzheimer's disease. Describe what physical and psychological changes you would expect to occur in this patient over time. _____

   _____

   _____

5. Give an example of how older adulthood may affect the following body systems.

   a. Integumentary: _____

   _____

   b. Musculoskeletal: _____

   _____

   c. Neurologic: _____

   _____

   d. Cardiopulmonary: _____

   _____

   e. Gastrointestinal: _____

   _____

   f. Genitourinary: _____

   _____

APPLYING YOUR KNOWLEDGE

CRITICAL THINKING QUESTIONS

1. Because of advances in medical technology and the increased awareness of the need to eat right and exercise, there has been a dramatic increase in the number of active older adults. Although adults in this age group as a whole are healthier than the generations that preceded them, they still have specific health risks and needs that must be identified by the nursing process. Consider the older adults you know personally and identify nursing strategies that would enhance their cognitive development and overall functioning (physiologic, social, emotional, spiritual).

2. Identify healthy middle-age adults and older adults among your family and friends. Interview them to learn about their physical, emotional, and spiritual selves. Compare their long- and short-range goals, life stressors, physical ability, and emotional stability. How have age factors affected their life experiences? What can you learn from this healthy group that will enable you to help others?

3. Take a look at the way older adults are portrayed on TV dramas. Are these dramas a realistic representation of this age group? Identify several health risks for older adults and preventive methods to promote health and safety.

REFLECTIVE PRACTICE USING CRITICAL THINKING SKILLS

Use the following expanded scenario from Chapter 20 in your textbook to answer the questions below.

Scenario: Larry Jenkins is a 67-year-old man with diabetes who lives with his wife, Mary. Mrs. Jenkins brings her husband to the clinic for a checkup and says she is worried about her husband's physical and emotional health. She reports that their three children live in different states and don't visit often. Mr. and Mrs. Jenkins moved to Florida 5 months ago when Mr. Jenkins retired, and Mrs. Jenkins says they have had trouble finding friends "as good as the ones we had at home." During the nursing interview, Mr. Jenkins says, "Everything's gone downhill since I retired." He reports that he is "bored out of my mind" and is drinking more alcohol, "simply because there's nothing else to do!"

1. How might the nurse use blended nursing skills to provide holistic, developmentally sensitive care for Mr. and Mrs. Jenkins?

   _____
   _____
   _____

2. What would be a successful outcome for this patient?

   _____
   _____
   _____

3. What intellectual, technical, interpersonal, and/or ethical/legal competencies are most likely to bring about the desired outcome?

   _____
   _____
   _____

4. What resources might be helpful for Mr. and Mrs. Jenkins?

   _____
   _____
   _____

CHAPTER 21

Communicator

PRACTICING FOR NCLEX

MULTIPLE CHOICE QUESTIONS

Circle the letter that corresponds to the best answer for each question.

1. Which of the following statements about the communication process is accurate?

   a. Communication is a reciprocal process in which both the sender and receiver of messages take turns participating.

   b. One-to-one communication occurs when three or more people are involved in the communication process.

   c. Nursing instructors and students seldom experience the communication process in large groups.

   d. Communicating people receive and send messages through verbal and nonverbal means, which occur simultaneously.

2. In which of the following phases of the helping relationship is an agreement or contract about the relationship established?

   a. Orientation phase

   b. Working phase

   c. Termination phase

   d. All of the above

3. An active listener in a group is performing which of the following group roles?

   a. Task roles

   b. Maintenance roles

   c. Self-serving roles

   d. Administrative roles

4. A group member who delegates responsibilities to other members is performing which of the following group roles?

   a. Task roles

   b. Maintenance roles

   c. Self-serving roles

   d. Administrative roles

5. In a helping relationship, the nurse would most likely perform which of the following activities?

   a. Encourage the patient to independently explore goals that allow his/her human needs to be satisfied

   b. Set up a reciprocal relationship in which patient and nurse are both helper and person being helped

   c. Establish communication that is continuous and reciprocal

   d. Establish goals for the patient that are not set in a specific time frame

6. Which of the following techniques would a nurse employ when using listening skills appropriately?

   a. The nurse would try to avoid body gestures when listening to the patient.

   b. The nurse would not allow conversation to lapse into periods of silence.

   c. The nurse would listen to the themes in the patient's comments.

   d. The nurse would stand close to the patient and maintain eye contact.

7. Which of the following senses is most highly developed at birth?

a. Hearing

b. Taste

c. Sight

d. Touch

8. A nurse who "unblocks" and "clears" congested areas of energy in a patient's body is applying the phenomenon known as:

a. "Unruffling" touch

b. Interpersonal touch

c. Tactile manipulation

d. Therapeutic Touch

9. A 36-year-old patient who underwent a hysterectomy 4 days ago says to the nurse, "I wonder if I'll still feel like a woman." Which of the following responses would most likely encourage the patient to expand on this and express her concerns in more specific terms?

a. "When did you begin to wonder about this?"

b. "Do you want more children?"

c. "Feel like a woman . . ."

d. Remaining silent

10. When attending a staff meeting, a nurse is participating in which of the following types of communication?

a. Intrapersonal communication

b. Interpersonal communication

c. Small-group communication

d. Organizational communication

ALTERNATE-FORMAT QUESTIONS

Multiple Response Questions

Circle the letters that correspond to the best answers for each question.

1. Which of the following are parts of the communication model identified by Berlo (1960)? *(Select all that apply.)*

a. Stimulus

b. Encoder

c. Subscriber

d. Medium

e. Component

f. Process

2. Which of the following are levels of communication that the nurse engages in during nursing practice? *(Select all that apply.)*

a. Personal communication

b. Small-group communication

c. Organizational communication

d. Observational communication

e. Large-group communication

f. Interpersonal communication

3. Which of the following statements accurately describe the functions of group dynamics? *(Select all that apply.)*

a. Ideally, a group leader is selected, who alone uses his or her talents and interpersonal strengths to assist the group to accomplish goals.

b. Effective groups possess members who elicit mutually respectful relationships.

c. The group's ability to function at a high level depends on only the group leader's sensitivity to the needs of the group and its individual members.

d. If a group member dominates or thwarts the group process, the leader or other group members must confront him or her to promote the needed collegial relationship.

e. In an effective group, power is used to "fix" immediate problems without considering the needs of the powerless.

f. In an effective group, members support, praise, and critique one another.

4. Which of the following statements accurately describe the roles of group members? *(Select all that apply.)*

a. Task-oriented roles focus on the other members of the group.

b. An information giver or seeker is taking on a maintenance role.

c. Group-building roles focus on the well-being of people doing the work.

d. A person who uses humor to relieve tension in a group meeting is performing a self-serving role.

e. Self-serving roles advance the needs of individual members at the group's expense.

f. A group member who pleads with other members to lighten the workload on his unit is performing a self-serving role.

5. Which of the following statements accurately describe how various factors influence communication? *(Select all that apply.)*

a. The rate of language development is directly correlated with the patient's neurologic competence and cognitive development.

b. Men and women possess similar communication styles.

c. Culture influences a person's worldview and relationships with the surrounding environment, religion, time, and others.

d. Stereotypical perceptions of the patient, derived from the patient's occupation, help the nurse understand the patient's manner of communicating.

e. A nurse performing a patient interview should sit as close to the patient as possible in order to obtain accurate information, regardless of the patient's sense of "private space."

f. Communication is influenced by the way people value themselves, one another, and the purpose of any human interaction.

6. Which of the following are qualities of a helping relationship? *(Select all that apply.)*

a. The helping relationship occurs spontaneously.

b. The helping relationship is characterized by an equal sharing of information.

c. The helping relationship is built on the patient's needs, not on those of the helping person.

d. A friendship must develop from an effective helping relationship.

e. A helping relationship is dynamic.

f. A helping relationship is purposeful and time limited.

7. Which of the following guidelines would most likely help nurses improve their communications with patients and achieve a more effective helping relationship? *(Select all that apply.)*

a. The nurse should control the tone of his/her voice so that it conveys exactly what is meant.

b. The nurse should remain focused on the topic at hand and not allow the patient to diverge to another topic.

c. The nurse should make statements that are as simple as possible, gearing conversation to the patient's level.

d. The nurse should feel free to use words that might have different interpretations when using the same language as the patient.

e. The nurse should never admit a lack of knowledge to the patient to avoid undermining the patient's confidence in the helping relationship.

f. The nurse should take advantage of any available opportunities to communicate information to patients in routine caregiving situations.

8. Which of the following are recommended techniques to help improve listening skills? *(Select all that apply.)*

a. Sit with the patient in a comfortable environment with arms and legs crossed in a relaxed position.

b. Always maintain eye contact with the patient in a face-to-face pose.

c. Use appropriate facial expressions and body gestures to indicate that you are paying attention to what the patient is saying.

d. Think before responding to the patient, even if this creates a lull in the conversation.

e. Listen for themes in the patient's comments.

f. If an action being performed does not allow for conversation, pretend to listen to the patient rather than interrupting the patient's conversation.

DEVELOPING YOUR KNOWLEDGE BASE

FILL-IN-THE-BLANKS

1. The communication process is initiated based on a(n) _____.

2. When a doctor communicates with a nurse by telephone to prescribe pain medication for a patient, the telephone is considered to be the _____ of this communication.

3. A patient who verbally acknowledges understanding of discharge instructions is providing _____ to the caregiver.

4. A patient who expresses anger at a diagnosis by slamming a food tray on the table is using _____ communication.

5. When a nurse helps a patient achieve goals that allow his/her human needs to be satisfied, the nurse and patient are involved in a(n) _____ relationship.

6. When a nurse and patient meet and learn to identify each other by name and clarify their roles, they are in the _____ phase of the helping relationship.

7. A nurse is using a(n) _____ comment/question when she says to her patient, "You have been following a diet high in fiber at home. Are you continuing to get enough fiber in the foods you've been eating since you've been here?"

8. Anger and aggressive behavior between nurses, or nurse-to-nurse hostility, has been labeled _____.

MATCHING EXERCISES

Match the elements of the communication process in Part A with the appropriate definition in Part B.

PART A

a. Source

b. Message

c. Channel

d. Receiver

e. Noise

f. Communication

g. Feedback

PART B

1. ___ The actual product of the encoder

2. ___ He/she must translate and make a decision about the product.

3. ___ Verbal and nonverbal evidence that the patient received and understood the product

4. ___ He/she prepares and sends the product.

5. ___ The medium selected to convey the product

6. ___ Factors that distort the quality of the product

Match the examples of patient goals in Part B with the appropriate phase in which they should occur listed in Part A. Answers may be used more than once.

PART A

a. Orientation phase

b. Working phase

c. Termination

PART B

7. ___ The patient will demonstrate ability to maneuver on crutches.

8. ___ The patient will acknowledge the goals he has accomplished in physical therapy.

9. ___ The patient will learn the name of the physical therapist and address him by his name.

10. ___ An anorexic patient will establish an agreement with her healthcare professional to return gradually to a normal eating pattern.

11. ___ The patient will express his desire to go home despite the excellent care he received at the agency.

12. ___ The patient will attend a counseling session dealing with smoking.

13. ___ The patient will verbalize the goals set forth in his transition to a home health-care setting.

14. ___ The patient will establish an agreement with the home healthcare worker about the frequency and length of contacts.

15. ___ The patient will express his concerns about pending surgery to the nurse.

Match the interviewing questions in Part B with the interviewing techniques useful in nurse–patient interactions listed in Part A. Answers may be used more than once.

PART A

a. Validating question/comment

b. Clarifying question/comment

c. Reflective question/comment

d. Sequencing question/comment

e. Directing question/comment

PART B

16. ___ "You say you've always been healthy and active; is this the first time you've been hospitalized?"

17. ___ "You expressed concern about your children at home . . ."

18. ___ "At home you've been treating your ulcer with an antacid. Did you take any today?"

19. ___ "You've been on your present medication for 3 years. Did you experience any side effects?"

20. ___ "Your chest pain began after exercising on a lifecycle?"

21. ___ "You've been upset about taking medication . . ."

SHORT ANSWER

1. Give an example of the following nonverbal forms of communication and explain how they can provide clues to the patient's health status.

   a. Touch: _____

   _____

   b. Eye contact: _____

   _____

   c. Facial expressions: _____

   _____

   d. Posture: _____

   _____

   e. Gait: _____

   _____

   f. Gestures: _____

   _____

   g. General physical appearance: _____

   _____

   h. Mode of dress and grooming: _____

   _____

   i. Sounds: _____

   _____

   j. Silence: _____

   _____

2. Briefly describe how you would alter your explanation of a surgical procedure to take into account the developmental considerations of the following patients:

   a. An 8-year-old boy: _____

   _____

   b. A 16-year-old girl: _____

   _____

   c. A 65-year-old man with a hearing impairment: _____

   _____

3. What clues to a person's identity can sometimes be determined by knowing that person's occupation? _____

   _____

4. Briefly explain the role that communication plays in the following steps of the nursing process.

   a. Assessing: _____

   _____

   b. Diagnosing: _____

   _____

   c. Planning: _____

   _____

   d. Implementing: _____

   _____

   e. Evaluating: _____

   _____

   f. Documenting: _____

   _____

5. Explain why the following variables must be considered when establishing rapport between a nurse and patient.

   a. Having specific objectives: _____

   _____

   b. Providing a comfortable environment: ___

   _____

   c. Providing privacy: _____

   _____

   d. Maintaining confidentiality: _____

   _____

   e. Maintaining patient focus: _____

   _____

   f. Using nursing observations: _____

   _____

   g. Using optimal pacing: _____

   _____

   h. Providing personal space: _____

   _____

   i. Developing therapeutic communication skills: _____

   _____

j. Developing listening skills: _____

_____

k. Using silence as a tool: _____

_____

6. Rewrite the following questions/statements to promote more effective communication with the patient.

a. "Did you have a good night?" _____

_____

b. "Are you ready to try walking on that foot?" _____

_____

c. "I can't believe you stopped taking your insulin!" _____

_____

d. "You aren't afraid of taking that test, are you?" _____

_____

e. "No one should be afraid of that procedure; it's been done a million times!" _____

_____

f. "Don't worry; everything will be all right." _____

_____

7. Underline the nonverbal communication in the following paragraph:

Mrs. Clarke, age 42, underwent a mastectomy. She has a husband and two children, ages 10 and 5. When the nurse enters Mrs. Clarke's room, she finds her patient's eyes are teary and there is a worried expression on her face. When asked how she is feeling, Mrs. Clarke replies "fine," although her face is rigid and her mouth is drawn in a firm line. She is moving her foot back and forth under the covers. On further investigation, the nurse finds that Mrs. Clarke is worried about her children and her own ability to be a healthy, functioning wife and mother again. After prompting, Mrs. Clarke says, "I don't know if my husband will still love me like this." She sighs and falls silent, reflecting upon her recovery. The nurse tries to make Mrs. Clarke comfortable and puts her hand over Mrs. Clarke's hand. She establishes eye contact with Mrs. Clarke and

reassures her that things have a way of working out and suggests that she give her situation some time.

8. Mr. Uhl is a 72-year-old man with early signs of Alzheimer's disease. He is living with his daughter and son-in-law in a large city, where he is functioning well under supervision. His doctor suggests a daycare center to fill in the gaps when the daughter is away at her part-time job. Nurse Parish, employed by the daycare center, enters into a helping relationship with Mr. Uhl, even though she knows she will be starting a new job at the end of the month that will force them to terminate their relationship. Write two patient goals the nurse may prepare for Mr. Uhl in the following phases of their short helping relationship.

a. Orientation phase:

(1) _____

(2) _____

b. Working phase:

(1) _____

(2) _____

c. Termination phase:

(1) _____

(2) _____

9. Give an example of the following interpersonal skills necessary for the promotion of a healthy nurse–patient relationship. Rate your own skills in these areas on a scale of 1 to 10.

a. Warmth and friendliness: _____

b. Openness: _____

c. Empathy: _____

d. Competence: _____

e. Consideration of patient variables: _____

_____

10. Mr. Johnson, age 69, has been diagnosed with prostate cancer. He is despondent and refuses to participate in his own care. Give an example of a nurse's dialog with Mr. Johnson that shows each component of the assertive response:

a. Empathic component: _____

_____

b. Description: _____

_____

c. Expectation: _____

_____

d. Consequence: _____

_____

11. List five common blocks to communication and describe nursing's role in overcoming these obstacles.

a. _____

_____

b. _____

_____

c. _____

_____

d. _____

_____

e. _____

_____

APPLYING YOUR KNOWLEDGE

CRITICAL THINKING QUESTIONS

1. Write a general script for communicating with patients beginning with, "Hello, my name is . . ." to the end of the conversation. Make your script specific to the needs of the following patients:

a. A 4-year-old boy is admitted to the hospital with multiple fractures following a car accident.

b. A teenage girl is admitted to the burn unit with third-degree burns following a fire in her home.

c. A 29-year-old rape victim is brought to the emergency room for treatment and testing.

d. A 60-year-old man with a history of strokes is brought to the emergency room with left-sided paralysis.

How competent and comfortable are you in each situation? What skills do you need to develop?

2. Pick a partner and try to communicate the following messages using only nonverbal communication:

a. I'm thirsty.

b. I have a pain in my stomach.

c. It's too hot in here.

d. I'd like you to read me a story.

e. I'd like to go home now.

f. Where is the bathroom?

g. Can I have another pain reliever?

h. I'd like to go to sleep now.

i. It's too noisy in here.

j. I can't fall asleep.

Reflect on the importance of nonverbal communication.

3. Observe and interpret a patient's nonverbal communication, and then ask the patient if your interpretation was correct; for example, "You seem to be in a lot of pain; is that correct?"

4. Ask a friend who has been a close confidant of yours to rate you on the following attributes that stimulate a healthy nurse–patient relationship: warmth and friendliness, openness, empathy, competence, and consideration of patient variables. See if this evaluation is consistent with your own feelings when practicing patient care. Work on the areas on which you had a lower score the next time you are with patients.

REFLECTIVE PRACTICE USING CRITICAL THINKING SKILLS

Use the following expanded scenario from Chapter 21 in your textbook to answer the questions below.

Scenario: Mrs. Irwina Russellinski is a 75-year-old woman transferred from the emergency department, diagnosed with pneumonia. Her chart reveals that she is hard of hearing, "slightly confused" at times, and speaks "broken English." Mrs. Russellinski has a daughter living nearby who is listed as a contact person. Mrs. Russellinski tells the nurse not to call her daughter because "she is too busy with her own family and shouldn't have to bother with a sick mother." A nursing assessment is needed.

1. What communication skills might the nurse use to complete an assessment of Mrs. Russellinski?

   _____

   _____

   _____

2. What would be a successful outcome for this patient?

   _____

   _____

   _____

3. What intellectual, technical, interpersonal, and/or ethical/legal competencies are most likely to bring about the desired outcome?

   _____

   _____

   _____

4. What resources might be helpful for Mrs. Russellinski?

   _____

   _____

   _____

Teacher and Counselor

PRACTICING FOR NCLEX

MULTIPLE CHOICE QUESTIONS

Circle the letter that corresponds to the best answer for each question.

1. Which of the following developmental considerations is a nurse assessing when he/she determines that an 8-year-old boy is not equipped to understand the scientific explanation of his disease?

   a. Intellectual development

   b. Motor development

   c. Emotional maturity

   d. Psychosocial development

2. Which of the following is the best source of assessment information for the nurse?

   a. Nursing plan of care

   b. Physician

   c. Patient

   d. Family and friends

3. Which of the following diagnoses would best describe a situation in which a woman has a knowledge deficit concerning child safety for her toddler, who is currently being treated for burns and was previously treated for a fracture from a fall?

   a. Knowledge Deficit: child safety, related to inexperience with the active developmental stage of a toddler

   b. Toddler at High Risk for Injury, related to mother's lack of knowledge about child safety

   c. Potential for Enhanced Parenting, related to child safety knowledge deficit

   d. Knowledge Deficit: child safety, related to mother's lack of experience and socioeconomic level

4. When writing learner objectives for a patient, the nurse should consider which of the following statements?

   a. It is better to use one or two broad objectives than several specific objectives.

   b. The objectives written in the "learner objectives" column of the sample teaching plan are general statements that could be accomplished in any amount of time.

   c. Planning of learner objectives should be done by the nurse or another healthcare professional before obtaining input from the patient/family.

   d. One long-term objective could be stated for each diagnosis, followed by several specific objectives.

5. When deciding what information the patient needs to meet the learner objectives successfully, the nurse is planning which part of the teaching plan?

   a. Content

   b. Teaching strategies

   c. Learning activities

   d. Learning domains

6. A nurse could attempt to help a patient solve a situational crisis during which of the following types of counseling sessions?

   a. Long-term counseling

   b. Motivational counseling

c. Short-term counseling

d. Professional counseling

7. When a patient says, "I don't care if I get better; I have nothing to live for, anyway," which type of counseling would be appropriate?

a. Long-term counseling

b. Motivational counseling

c. Short-term counseling

d. Professional counseling

8. When teaching an adult patient how to control stress through relaxation techniques, the nurse should consider which of the following assumptions concerning adult learners?

a. As an adult matures, his/her self-concept becomes more dependent; therefore, this patient must be made aware of the importance of reducing stress.

b. The adult learner is not as concerned with the immediate usefulness of the material being taught as he/she is with the quality of the material.

c. As patients, adults are the least likely to resist learning because of preconceived ideas about the teaching/learning process.

d. The nurse should be able to draw from the previous experience of the patient to emphasize the importance of stress reduction.

9. Which of the following principles of teaching–learning is an accurate guideline for the nurse/teacher?

a. Patient teaching should occur independent of the nursing process.

b. Past life experience should not be a factor when helping patients assimilate new knowledge.

c. The teaching–learning process can be facilitated by a helping relationship.

d. Planning learner objectives should be done by the teacher alone.

10. When planning for learning, who must decide who should be included in the learning sessions?

a. The healthcare team

b. The doctor and nurse

c. The nurse and the patient

d. The patient and the patient's family

ALTERNATE-FORMAT QUESTIONS

Multiple Response Questions

Circle the letters that correspond to the best answers for each question.

1. Which of the following is a Joint Commission standard for patient and family education? *(Select all that apply.)*

a. The patient and family are provided with education that can enhance knowledge, skills, and behaviors that are necessary to benefit fully from the healthcare interventions provided by the organization.

b. The organization recognizes the nurse and other healthcare staff as the sole authority on planning patient education.

c. The patient and family educational process is interdisciplinary as appropriate to the plan of care.

d. The organization plans and supports the provision and coordination of patient and family education activities and resources.

e. The patient and family receive standard education regardless of the patient's needs, capabilities, and readiness.

f. Information about discharge instructions is given to the patient, who in turn is responsible for providing the information to the organization or individual responsible for the continuing care of the patient.

2. Which of the following statements accurately reflect the aims of patient teaching and counseling? *(Select all that apply.)*

a. Patient education influences patient behavior while facilitating changes in the knowledge, attitudes, and skills needed to maintain and improve health.

b. Patient education is ongoing and interactive.

c. Patient education is standardized for each knowledge deficit and can be used interchangeably from patient to patient.

d. Patient education plans should be developed to include only the nursing staff and patient.

e. The basic purpose of teaching is to help patients and families accept minimal functioning and diminished quality of life.

f. Counseling provides the resources and support patients need to participate actively in self-care.

3. Which of the following topics would most likely be taught to a patient with the aim of restoring health? *(Select all that apply.)*
   a. Stress management
   b. Patient and nurse's expectations of one another
   c. Community resources
   d. Hygiene
   e. Orientation to treatment center and staff
   f. The medical and nursing regimens and how the patient can participate in care

4. Which of the following is an accurate description of the acronym TEACH? *(Select all that apply.)*
   a. Turn to the doctor for support.
   b. Educate the patient before treatment.
   c. Act on every teaching moment.
   d. Clarify often.
   e. Help the patient cope when education fails.
   f. Honor the patient as a partner in the education process.

5. Which of the following statements accurately reflect recommended steps of the teaching–learning process? *(Select all that apply.)*
   a. Use anticipatory guidance when assessing learning needs and learning readiness.
   b. Identify general, attainable, measurable, and long-term goals for patient learning when developing learning objectives.
   c. Include group teaching and formal teaching in every teaching plan.
   d. Do not allow time constraints, schedules, and the physical environment to influence the choice of teaching strategies when developing a teaching plan.
   e. Formulate a verbal or written contract with the patient.
   f. Relate new learning material to the patient's past life experiences to help him/her to assimilate new knowledge.

6. Which of the following statements accurately describe the way developmental factors affect patient learning? *(Select all that apply.)*
   a. What people learn and how learning occurs change according to developmental stages.
   b. Emotional maturity and moral and spiritual development do not affect a person's learning processes.
   c. School-aged children are capable of logical reasoning and should be included in the teaching–learning process whenever possible.
   d. The cognitive processes of adolescents are different from those of adults, so they require different content and teaching strategies for patient teaching.
   e. As a person matures, his/her self-concept is likely to move from independence to dependence.
   f. Most adults' orientation to learning is that material should be useful immediately rather than at some time in the future.

7. According to the health belief model, which of the following are health beliefs that are critical for enhanced patient motivation? *(Select all that apply.)*
   a. Patients do not view themselves as susceptible to the disease in question.
   b. Patients view the disease as a serious threat.
   c. Patients believe there are actions that will help reduce the probability of contracting the disease.
   d. Patients believe that the threat of taking actions against a disease is not as great as the disease itself.
   e. Patients believe that noncompliance is not an option.
   f. Patients believe that doing nothing is preferable to painful treatments.

DEVELOPING YOUR KNOWLEDGE BASE

FILL-IN-THE-BLANKS

1. A nurse who counsels an overweight teenager to eat a healthy diet and exercise daily is practicing the aim of patient education of _____.

2. When a nurse and patient establish a relationship in which mutual respect and trust are established, they have developed a(n) _____ relationship.

3. A patient who describes how insulin injections control diabetes has experienced learning by using the _____ domain of learning.

4. A patient who expresses a desire to control binge eating and to return to eating a healthy

diet has experienced the _____ domain of learning.

5. Generally, _____ are considered the best source of assessment information.

6. _____ is an internal impulse (such as emotion or physical pain) that encourages the patient to take action or change behavior.

7. Content that is supported by nursing research and reflects the most accurate and clinically supported information is called _____.

8. When a nurse assists a patient to decide to quit smoking, the nurse is fulfilling the role of _____.

MATCHING EXERCISES

Match the examples in Part B with the appropriate teaching strategy listed in Part A. Answers may be used more than once.

PART A

a. Role modeling
b. Lecture
c. Discussion
d. Demonstration
e. Discovery
f. Role-playing
g. AV materials
h. Printed material
i. Computer-assisted instruction programs

PART B

1. ____ A nurse speaks to a group of patients about the dangers of smoking.

2. ____ A nurse chooses a low-calorie meal for herself when having lunch with an obese patient.

3. ____ A nurse performs a bathing procedure on a newborn in front of several new mothers.

4. ____ A nurse obtains pamphlets for a 16-year-old that describe how STIs are transmitted.

5. ____ One student pretends to be a patient while another student conducts a nursing interview.

6. ____ A nurse uses a videotape to teach a patient about heart disease.

7. ____ A nurse describes the symptoms of an anxiety attack to a patient with panic disorder and lets him choose measures to take during and after the attack.

8. ____ A nurse shows a film on relaxation techniques to a cardiac patient.

9. ____ A nurse shows a diabetic patient how to give herself insulin by injecting an orange.

10. ____ A nurse talks to a patient about the patient's feelings of powerlessness following a transient ischemic attack.

Match the examples of teaching strategies in Part B with the aims of nursing listed in Part A. Answers may be used more than once.

PART A

a. Promoting health
b. Preventing illness
c. Restoring health
d. Facilitating coping

PART B

11. ____ A nurse demonstrates to a postoperative patient the proper way to bandage his incision.

12. ____ A nurse explains to a new mother the importance and availability of immunizations for her baby.

13. ____ A nurse counsels a woman in her first trimester on proper nutrition.

14. ____ A nurse refers a recovering alcoholic to a local group meeting.

15. ____ A nurse presents a lecture on baby-proofing a home to a group of parents.

16. ____ A nurse teaches a young athlete stretching exercises to be used before running track.

17. ____ A nurse refers the daughter of a terminally ill patient to a counseling session on coping with death and dying.

18. ____ A nurse introduces a patient recovering from a broken hip to the physical therapy staff.

19. ____ A nurse refers a 42-year-old woman to a clinic providing free mammograms.

20. ____ A nurse teaches relaxation techniques to a patient recovering from coronary bypass surgery.

Match the learning domain listed in Part A with the example of the domain listed in Part B. Answers may be used more than once.

PART A

a. Cognitive learning

b. Psychomotor learning

c. Affective learning

PART B

21. ____ A patient learns how to care for his surgical wound.

22. ____ A patient explains how eating a proper diet will lower his cholesterol level.

23. ____ A patient learns how to perform range-of-motion exercises after surgery.

24. ____ A patient expresses self-confidence after she completes a class to stop smoking.

25. ____ A patient decides to get dressed in the morning following treatment for depression.

26. ____ A patient reiterates the need for prenatal and infant care to her social worker.

SHORT ANSWER

1. Briefly explain how teaching and counseling patients can facilitate the following nursing aims.

   a. Promoting health: _____

   _____

   b. Preventing illness: _____

   _____

   c. Restoring health: _____

   _____

   d. Facilitating coping: _____

   _____

2. How would you modify your teaching plan to motivate the following patients to learn a new skill?

   a. An adult who has a fear of failure: _____

   _____

   b. An adult who resists learning because of preconceived ideas about the process and your expectations of him/her: _____

   _____

c. An older adult who is afraid to learn something new: _____

_____

3. Mr. Lang is a 75-year-old man recovering from a stroke in a home care setting. He has partial paralysis of his left side and must be taught exercises for rehabilitation. List three teaching strategies you would use in treating this patient, and give an example of each.

   a. _____

   _____

   b. _____

   _____

   c. _____

   _____

4. List two solutions to the problem that time constraints place on the nurse when planning patient learning.

   a. _____

   _____

   b. _____

   _____

5. Briefly describe the following types of teaching, and give an example of each:

   a. Formal: _____

   _____

   b. Informal: _____

   _____

6. Give an example of a method that could be used to evaluate the following types of learning.

   a. Cognitive domain: _____

   b. Affective domain: _____

   c. Psychomotor domain: _____

7. How would you document successfully teaching a new mother how to bathe her infant? _____

   _____

   _____

8. Define the following types of counseling, and give an example of a case in which each type would be used by the nurse.

a. Short-term counseling: _____

_____

b. Long-term counseling: _____

_____

c. Motivational counseling: _____

_____

9. List four elements that should be considered in each assessment of patient learning needs.

a. _____

b. _____

c. _____

d. _____

10. Give an example of the following teaching strategies that you have experienced in your personal/student life. Which of these strategies do you feel were most effective for you?

a. Role modeling: _____

_____

b. Lecture: _____

_____

c. Discussion: _____

_____

d. Panel discussion: _____

_____

e. Demonstration: _____

_____

f. Discovery: _____

_____

g. Role-playing: _____

_____

h. AV materials: _____

_____

i. Programmed instruction: _____

_____

j. Computer-assisted instruction: _____

_____

11. List four measures that promote patient and family compliance.

a. _____

b. _____

c. _____

d. _____

12. List five common mistakes that hinder patient teaching.

a. _____

b. _____

c. _____

d. _____

e. _____

APPLYING YOUR KNOWLEDGE

CRITICAL THINKING QUESTIONS

1. As a child, you learned many things from your parents. Consider the types of teaching that you experienced, and think about how you could use both formal and informal teaching to help children accomplish the following goals:

   a. Avoiding drugs and alcohol

   b. Learning how to cook a healthy meal

   c. Dealing with peer pressure

2. Observe nurses teaching and counseling patients and family members to promote health, prevent illness, restore health, or facilitate coping. What methods did the nurse use to identify each patient's learning needs? Was the nurse successful in teaching this patient? How would you have handled the teaching process differently? Assess each patient's knowledge, attitudes, and skills needed to independently manage his/her own healthcare.

3. Devise a plan to teach a woman how to lose weight by reducing the fat content in her diet and developing an exercise routine using the following methods:

   a. Lecture

   b. Discussion

   c. Demonstration

   d. Role-playing

What was the advantage/disadvantage of each method?

REFLECTIVE PRACTICE USING CRITICAL THINKING SKILLS

Use the following expanded scenario from Chapter 22 in your textbook to answer the questions below.

Scenario: Marco García Ramírez accompanies his wife, Claudia, to the antepartal clinic for a routine visit. They are expecting their first child in 5 months. He reports that they are happy and excited but also scared and very nervous. They are planning for a home birth and ask the nurse what she thinks of this method of childbirth. They are also asking lots of questions about childbirth and their new responsibilities as parents. Mr. Ramírez says, "We're both wondering if we'll be good parents." They also ponder whether they will have the resources to provide for a new child.

1. What should be the focus of patient teaching for this couple?

   _____

   _____

   _____

2. What would be a successful outcome for Mr. and Mrs. Ramirez?

   _____

   _____

   _____

3. What intellectual, technical, interpersonal, and/or ethical/legal competencies are most likely to bring about the desired outcome?

   _____

   _____

   _____

4. What resources might be helpful for this couple?

   _____

   _____

   _____

CHAPTER 23

Nurse Leader and Manager

PRACTICING FOR NCLEX

MULTIPLE CHOICE QUESTIONS

Circle the letter that corresponds to the best answer for each question.

1. In which of the following styles of leadership are group satisfaction and motivation primary benefits?
   a. Democratic
   b. Autocratic
   c. Laissez-faire
   d. Transformational

2. Which of the following styles of leadership is rarely used in a hospital setting because of the difficulty of task achievement by independent nurses?
   a. Democratic
   b. Autocratic
   c. Laissez-faire
   d. Transformational

3. When a nurse arranges all the resources available to teach a teenage girl how to manage her asthma, he/she is performing which of the following roles of a nurse manager?
   a. Planning role
   b. Organizing role
   c. Directing role
   d. Controlling role

4. Which of the following is a characteristic of a decentralized management system?
   a. Decisions are generally made by senior managers.
   b. Nurses further down the hierarchy of an organization are often responsible for implementing decisions into which they had little input.
   c. Decisions are made by those who are most knowledgeable about the issues being decided.
   d. Nurse managers are not accountable for patient census, staffing, supplies, or budgets.

5. In which of the following nursing care delivery models is one nurse responsible for overseeing the quality and financial outcomes of patient care while working collegially with physicians and other caregivers as well as with payers to manage patients along an agreed-on clinical pathway?
   a. Functional nursing
   b. Case management
   c. Primary nursing
   d. Collaborative practice model

6. According to Lewin, in which of the following stages of change is change initiated after a careful process of planning?
   a. Moving
   b. Freezing
   c. Unfreezing
   d. Transforming

ALTERNATE-FORMAT QUESTIONS

Multiple Response Questions

Circle the letters that correspond to the best answers for each question.

1. Which of the following are examples of individuals with implied power? *(Select all that apply.)*

   a. A class president

   b. A nurse manager

   c. A teen idol

   d. An editor of a major newspaper

   e. A class clown

   f. A folk hero

2. Which of the following is a characteristic of a magnet hospital? *(Select all that apply.)*

   a. Self-scheduling

   b. Centralized decision making

   c. Autonomous, accountable professional nursing practice

   d. Higher staff turnover

   e. Higher levels of staff burnout and exodus from the bedside

   f. Supportive nurse managers

3. Which of the following is a characteristic of laissez-faire leadership? *(Select all that apply.)*

   a. The leader is the authority on all issues.

   b. The leader relinquishes power to the group.

   c. The leader depends on the strengths of followers to direct the group activities.

   d. The leader and nurses work independently, making task accomplishment difficult.

   e. There is a sense of equality among the leader and other participants.

   f. The leader is able to inspire and motivate others.

4. In which of the following models of nursing care delivery do the nurse and other team members care for a group of patients? *(Select all that apply.)*

   a. Functional nursing

   b. Team nursing

   c. Primary nursing

   d. Total care nursing

   e. Case management

   f. Patient-centered care

5. Which of the following activities could be delegated to a UAP? *(Select all that apply.)*

   a. The determination of a nursing diagnosis for a patient with breast cancer

   b. Giving a bed bath to a patient

   c. Planning patient education for a patient with a colostomy

   d. Taking routine vital signs

   e. Administering medications to patients

   f. Transferring a patient to another floor

6. Which of the following principles regarding the regulation, education, and use of the UAP are recommended by the American Nurses Association? *(Select all that apply.)*

   a. It is the healthcare institution that determines the scope of nursing practice.

   b. It is the LPN who supervises any assistant involved in providing direct patient care.

   c. It is the purpose of assistive personnel to work in a supportive role to the registered nurse.

   d. It is the role of the assistive personnel to carry out tasks to enable the professional nurse to concentrate on nursing care for the patient.

   e. It is the role of the LPN to assign nursing duties to the UAP.

   f. It is the registered nurse who is responsible and accountable for nursing practice.

DEVELOPING YOUR KNOWLEDGE BASE

FILL-IN-THE-BLANKS

1. Power that is attained by virtue of a position is known as _____ power.

2. A charge nurse who makes all the decisions for the nursing team without considering their feelings or ideas is using the _____ style of leadership.

3. In hospitals, the autocratic style of leadership is gradually being replaced by the _____ style of leadership.

4. In the _____ leadership style, healthcare leaders must be able to communicate to others their vision of the future and bring energy and commitment to the reformation of the system.

5. _____ is the ability to influence others to achieve a desired effect.

6. When an experienced nurse advises a less experienced nurse regarding patient care, their relationship is known as a(n) _____.

MATCHING EXERCISES

Match the examples of leadership in Part B with the types of leadership they imply listed in Part A. Some answers may be used more than once.

PART A

a. Autocratic leadership

b. Democratic leadership

c. Laissez-faire leadership

d. Transformational leadership

e. Situational leadership

f. Quantum leadership

PART B

1. ____ A nurse unites with other nurses to create a shelter for battered women in their neighborhood.

2. ____ A nurse opens a discussion among healthcare team members to determine the best care plan for a patient.

3. ____ A nurse takes control during a "code blue" and directs all activities to resuscitate the patient.

4. ____ A nurse leads other nurses in developing a schedule to cook meals for the homeless.

5. ____ A nurse manager adjusts the work schedule of the unit each week to accommodate the current caseload.

6. ____ A nurse in charge of scheduling suggests that the nurses meet and work out the schedule on their own.

7. ____ A nurse seeks input from coworkers to solve a problem of understaffing.

8. ____ A head nurse makes schedules of ANA meetings available to any staff members who are interested.

9. ____ A head nurse directs the triage unit after several earthquake victims arrive at the emergency room.

10. ____ A head nurse issues a memo describing step-by-step documentation procedures that she wants initiated in the emergency room.

11. ____ A head nurse openly seeks critiques of his work.

SHORT ANSWER

1. Describe what the following leadership qualities mean to you and how they would help motivate patients in your practice to achieve their goals.

   Leaders should:

   a. Be dynamic: _____
   _____

   b. Be enthusiastic: _____
   _____

   c. Be self-directed: _____
   _____

   d. Have a positive self-image: _____
   _____

   e. Be a role model: _____
   _____

   f. Have vision: _____
   _____

2. Mr. Eng is a 75-year-old man dying of lung cancer in a hospice. Give an example of how a nurse could use each of the following leadership skills to help relieve his suffering.

   a. Communication skills: _____
   _____

   b. Problem-solving skills: _____
   _____

   c. Management skills: _____
   _____

   d. Self-evaluation skills: _____
   _____

3. List the steps you would employ to change a nursing unit from paper records to a computerized method of record keeping. How would you handle people who resist the change?

_____

_____

_____

_____

4. Briefly describe the following reasons why people resist change, and state how you would confront the problem in your own practice.

a. Threat to self: _____

_____

_____

b. Lack of understanding: _____

_____

_____

c. Limited tolerance to change: _____

_____

_____

d. Disagreements about the benefits of change: _____

_____

_____

e. Fear of increased responsibility: _____

_____

_____

5. Explain how you, as a nurse leader, can help change the negative portrayals of nursing in the media. _____

_____

_____

6. Describe how you would use the following management functions to organize fellow students to form a group to help control binge drinking on campus.

a. Planning: _____

_____

b. Organizing: _____

_____

c. Motivating: _____

_____

d. Controlling: _____

_____

7. Give an example from your present situation (home, school, work) where you feel that you may have the power to influence change. Explain what steps you would take to overcome resistance to this change.

_____

_____

_____

8. Explain how a nurse manager might accomplish the following leadership goals.

a. Identifying strengths: _____

_____

b. Evaluating work accomplishment: _____

_____

c. Clarifying values: _____

_____

d. Determining where he/she belongs and what he/she can contribute: _____

_____

e. Assuming responsibility for relationships: _____

_____

9. Briefly describe four factors a nurse should consider before planning to make a change:

a. _____

b. _____

c. _____

d. _____

10. List seven factors a nurse should consider before delegating a nursing intervention.

a. _____

b. _____

c. _____

d. _____

e. _____

f. _____

g. _____

11. Explain why the following rights of delegation are important when deciding whether or not to delegate a nursing intervention.

   a. The right task: _____

   _____

   b. The right circumstance: _____

   _____

   c. The right person: _____

   _____

   d. The right direction/communication: _____

   _____

   e. The right supervision: _____

   _____

APPLYING YOUR KNOWLEDGE

CRITICAL THINKING QUESTIONS

1. Imagine you are the team leader on a busy intensive care unit. After giving the team members their patient assignments for the day, you notice that several RNs and float nurses are upset with their assignments. The unit is currently understaffed, and all team members are required to take on more responsibility than usual in order to keep the unit running efficiently. You overhear one RN say she'd rather quit than start taking on additional duties.

   a. As a leader, how would you handle this situation?

   b. What type of leadership style would you feel most comfortable using?

   c. How might your response to this situation be different depending on whether you were working in a magnet hospital or a nonmagnet hospital?

2. Review the leadership styles of the people who have been authority figures in your life. What makes them effective or ineffective leaders? Which leadership styles have you tried? Which do you feel will be most helpful to you as you try to help patients/families and health-care teams achieve health goals?

REFLECTIVE PRACTICE USING CRITICAL THINKING SKILLS

Use the following scenario from Chapter 23 in your textbook to answer the questions below.

Scenario: Rehema Kohls is a college sophomore who comes to the healthcare center requesting information about sexually transmitted infections (STIs). She says, "So many of my friends are concerned about STIs. They all say we should start a group on campus to discuss this problem, and they want me to set it up and be the leader. But I wouldn't know where to start or what to do!"

1. How might the nurse empower Ms. Kohls with the knowledge and ability to be a leader of her peers?

   _____

   _____

   _____

2. What would be a successful outcome for Ms. Kohls?

   _____

   _____

   _____

3. What intellectual, technical, interpersonal, and/or ethical/legal competencies are most likely to bring about the desired outcome?

   _____

   _____

   _____

4. What resources might be helpful for Ms. Kohls?

   _____

   _____

   _____

Vital Signs

PRACTICING FOR NCLEX

MULTIPLE CHOICE QUESTIONS

Circle the letter that corresponds to the best answer for each question.

1. Which of the following is the primary source of heat in the human body?
   a. Metabolism
   b. Hormones
   c. Sympathetic neurotransmitters
   d. Hypothalamus

2. Which of the following is the primary mechanism or site of heat loss?
   a. Contraction of pilomotor muscles of the skin
   b. Warming and humidifying of inspired air
   c. Skin surface
   d. Urine and feces

3. What would be the cardiac output of an adult with a stroke volume of 75 mL and a pulse of 78 beats/minute?
   a. 5,000 mL
   b. 5,550 mL
   c. 5,850 mL
   d. 6,000 mL

4. Which of the following conditions occurs when an adult has a pulse rate of 100 to 180 beats/minute?
   a. Bradycardia
   b. Arrhythmia
   c. Pulse amplitude
   d. Tachycardia

5. Which of the following statements concerning respiratory rates is accurate?
   a. Infants and young children have a lower respiratory rate than adults.
   b. Healthy adults breathe about 12 to 20 times per minute.
   c. The respiratory rate decreases in response to the increased metabolic rate during pyrexia.
   d. An increase in intracranial pressures stimulates the respiratory center and increases the respiration rate.

6. Which of the following statistics regarding blood pressure is accurate?
   a. Blood pressure tends to be lower in a prone or supine position than in a seated or standing position.
   b. Men usually have a lower blood pressure than women of the same age.
   c. Blood pressure decreases after eating.
   d. Blood pressure is usually highest on arising in the morning.

7. The average normal temperature in degrees Fahrenheit for well adults in the rectal site is which of the following?
   a. 94.0
   b. 97.6
   c. 98.6
   d. 99.5

8. Which of the following conditions tends to lower blood pressure?
   a. High viscosity of the blood
   b. Low blood volume
   c. Decreased elasticity of walls of arterioles
   d. Strong pumping action of blood into the arteries

9. After taking vital signs, you write down your findings as T = 98.6, P = 66, R = 18, BP = 124/82. Which of these numbers represents the systolic blood pressure?
   a. 98.6
   b. 124
   c. 82
   d. 66

ALTERNATE-FORMAT QUESTIONS

Multiple Response Questions

Circle the letters that correspond to the best answers for each question.

1. Which of the following are normal variations in vital signs that occur at various ages? *(Select all that apply.)*
   a. The normal blood pressure for a newborn is 73/55.
   b. Normal respirations for a 6- to 8-year-old are 15 to 25.
   c. Normal blood pressure for a teenager is 120/85.
   d. Normal pulse for a person older than 70 years is 80 to 180.
   e. Normal oral temperature for an adult is 37°C.
   f. Normal respirations for a 10-year-old are 20 to 40.

2. Which of the following statements regarding heat production in the body and body temperature are accurate? *(Select all that apply.)*
   a. Heat is produced as a byproduct of metabolic activities that generate energy for cellular functions.
   b. Thyroid hormone, produced by the thyroid gland, decreases metabolism and heat production.

c. Exercise decreases heat production through muscular activity.
d. Body temperature is usually about 1°F to 2°F higher in the early morning than in the late afternoon and early evening.
e. Women tend to have more fluctuation in body temperatures than men.
f. When a set temperature point in the body is increased, the hypothalamus initiates shivering and vasoconstriction.

3. Which of the following are accurate steps when assessing body temperature by various methods? *(Select all that apply.)*
   a. When assessing tympanic membrane temperature, wipe the tympanic probe cover with alcohol before inserting it snugly into the ear.
   b. When assessing an oral temperature with an electronic thermometer, place the probe beneath the patient's tongue in the posterior sublingual pocket.
   c. When assessing rectal temperature with an electronic thermometer, lubricate about 1" of the probe with a water-soluble lubricant.
   d. When assessing axillary temperature using a glass thermometer, place the bulb in the center of the axilla and bring the patient's arm down close to the body. Leave the thermometer in place for 3 minutes.
   e. When assessing temperature with an electronic thermometer, hold the thermometer in place in the assessment site until you hear a beep.
   f. Note the assessment site used because axillary temperatures are generally about 1° more than oral temperatures and rectal temperatures are generally about 1° less than oral temperatures.

4. Which of the following statements correctly describe pulse physiology? *(Select all that apply.)*
   a. The pulse is regulated by the autonomic nervous system; parasympathetic stimulation by the vagus nerve increases the heart rate, and sympathetic stimulation decreases the heart rate.

b. The pulse rate is the number of pulsations felt over a peripheral artery or heard over the apex of the heart in 30 seconds.

c. When stroke volume decreases, such as when blood volume is decreased due to hemorrhage, the heart rate increases in an attempt to maintain the same cardiac output.

d. The normal pulse rate ranges from 60 to 100 beats/minute.

e. A rapid heart rate (tachycardia) increases cardiac filling time, which in turn increases stroke volume and cardiac output.

f. Pulse rate is normally slower in men, in thin people, and in sleep.

5. Which of the following statements accurately describe the factors controlling respirations? *(Select all that apply.)*

a. Under normal conditions, healthy adults breathe about 12 to 20 times each minute.

b. Tachypnea occurs in response to a decreased metabolic rate during pyrexia.

c. During bradypnea, a decrease in intracranial pressure depresses the respiratory center, resulting in irregular or shallow breathing, slow breathing, or both.

d. Apnea refers to periods during which there is no breathing.

e. Dyspnea is difficult or labored breathing. A dyspneic patient usually has rapid, shallow respirations and appears anxious.

f. Dyspneic people can often breathe more easily in a prone position, a condition known as orthopnea.

6. Which of the following statements regarding blood pressure are accurate? *(Select all that apply.)*

a. Maximum blood pressure is exerted on the walls of arteries when the right ventricle of the heart pushes blood through the aortic valve into the aorta at the beginning of systole.

b. Blood pressure rises as the ventricle contracts and falls as the heart relaxes.

c. The continuous contraction and relaxation of the left ventricle creates a pressure wave that is transmitted through the arterial system.

d. The highest pressure is the systolic pressure; the lowest pressure is the diastolic pressure.

e. The difference between the systolic pressure and diastolic pressure is known as the pulse amplitude.

f. When the radial pulse is irregular, counting at the apex of the heart and at the radial artery simultaneously may assess the apical-radial pulse rate.

7. Which of the following guidelines would be implemented when properly assessing a patient's blood pressure? *(Select all that apply.)*

a. Have the patient assume a comfortable lying or sitting position.

b. Have the forearm supported below the level of the heart and the palm of the hand downward.

c. Center the bladder of the cuff over the brachial artery, about midway on the arm, so that the lower edge of the cuff is about 2.5 to 5 cm above the inner aspect of the elbow.

d. Check that a mercury manometer is in the horizontal position and the mercury is in the zero area with the gauge at eye level.

e. Inflate the cuff while continuing to palpate the artery. Pump the pressure 30 mm Hg above the point at which the systolic pressure was palpated and estimated.

f. Note the point on the gauge at which there is appearance of the first faint but clear sound that slowly increases in intensity; note this number as the diastolic pressure.

Fill-in-the-Blank Questions

1. The cardiac output (in liters per minute) of a patient with a stroke volume of 75 mL and a heart rate of 70 beats/minute would be _____.

2. The bladder width and length (in centimeters) that would typically be used on a child with an arm circumference of 20 cm would be _____ and _____.

3. A number that would describe the pulse amplitude for a weak pulse would be _____.

4. If a patient's oral temperature is 101°F, the axillary temperature would most likely be _____ .

5. A patient's temperature of 39°C would be _____ Fahrenheit.

6. A patient's temperature of 99.5°F would be _____ Celsius.

DEVELOPING YOUR KNOWLEDGE BASE

IDENTIFICATION

1. Identify the pulse assessment sites on the figure below by placing your answers on the lines provided.

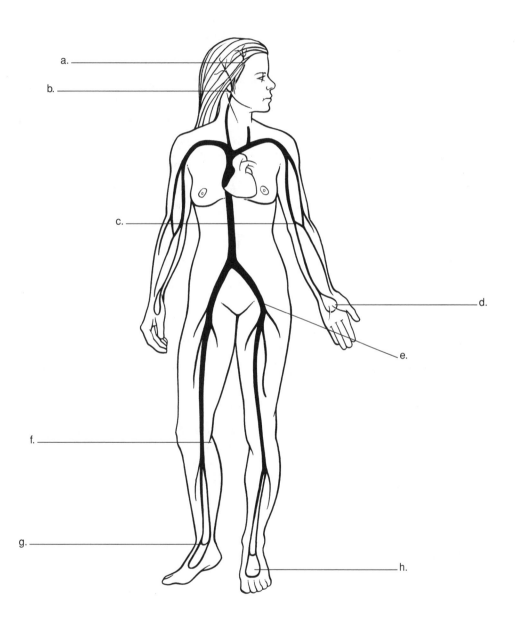

MATCHING EXERCISES

Match the following definitions related to pulse in Part B with the appropriate term listed in Part A.

PART A

a. Pulse

b. Pulse rate

c. Tachycardia

d. Palpitation

e. Bradycardia

f. Pulse rhythm

g. Pulse amplitude

h. Arrhythmia

i. Stroke volume

j. Cardiac output

k. Ventricular contraction

l. Pulse deficit

PART B

1. ___ Number of pulsations felt in a minute

2. ___ Quantity of blood forced out of the left ventricle with each contraction

3. ___ Person is aware of own heartbeat without having to feel for it

4. ___ Quality of the pulse in terms of fullness; reflects strength of left ventricular contraction

5. ___ Light tap caused by expansion of the aorta sending a wave through the walls of the arterial system

6. ___ Irregular pattern of heartbeats

7. ___ Heart rate below 60 beats/minute in an adult

8. ___ The amount of blood pumped per minute

9. ___ A rapid heart rate

10. ___ The pattern of pulsations and pauses between them

11. ___ The difference between the apical and radial pulse rates

Match the term in Part A with the correct definition in Part B.

PART A

a. Inspiration

b. Expiration

c. Apnea

d. Dyspnea

e. Orthopnea

f. Internal respiration

g. External respiration

h. Eupnea

i. Tachypnea

j. Pulmonary ventilation

k. Bradypnea

PART B

12. ___ A fast respiratory rate

13. ___ The exchange of oxygen and carbon dioxide between the alveoli of the lungs and the circulating blood

14. ___ Difficult or labored breathing

15. ___ The act of breathing in

16. ___ The exchange of oxygen and carbon dioxide between the circulating blood and tissue cells

17. ___ Movement of air in and out of the lungs

18. ___ Normal respirations with equal rate and depth

19. ___ Being able to breathe more easily in an upright position

20. ___ Periods during which there is no breathing

21. ___ Slow breathing

Match the definitions of body temperatures and variations in Part B with the appropriate term listed in Part A.

PART A

a. Pyrexia

b. Febrile

c. Afebrile

d. Hyperpyrexia

e. Hypothermia

f. Hyperthermia

g. Ineffective thermoregulation

PART B

22. ___ Body temperature below limit of normal

23. ____ State in which temperature fluctuates between above-normal and below-normal ranges

24. ____ Body temperature elevated above normal range

25. ____ Body temperature above normal

26. ____ Person with normal body temperature

27. ____ High fever, usually above 105.8°F

b. Age: _____

c. Gender: _____

d. Stress: _____

e. Environmental temperature: _____

SHORT ANSWER

1. Briefly describe how the following factors affect body temperature.

   a. Circadian rhythms: _____

2. Complete the table below describing the types of thermometers used to assess body temperature.

Type of Thermometer	Brief Description	Contraindication	Normal Reading
A. GLASS oral rectal			
B. ELECTRONIC			
C. TYMPANIC MEMBRANE			
D. TEMPERATURE SENSITIVE PATCH			
E. AUTOMATED MONITORING DEVICE			

3. List three methods that can be used to assess the pulse by palpating or auscultating.

a. _____

b. _____

c. _____

4. Briefly describe how the following variables may affect a patient's blood pressure.

a. Pumping action of the heart: _____

_____

b. Blood volume: _____

_____

c. Viscosity of blood: _____

_____

d. Elasticity of vessel walls: _____

_____

5. Briefly define the following NANDA nursing diagnoses for altered respirations.

a. Impaired Gas Exchange: _____

_____

b. Ineffective Airway Clearance: _____

_____

c. Ineffective Breathing Pattern: _____

_____

d. Inability to Sustain Spontaneous Ventilation: _____

_____

6. Briefly define the following NANDA nursing diagnoses for alterations in pulse and blood pressure.

a. Altered Tissue Perfusion: _____

_____

b. Risk for Fluid Volume Imbalance: _____

_____

c. Fluid Volume Excess: _____

_____

d. Fluid Volume Deficit: _____

_____

e. Decreased Cardiac Output: _____

_____

7. Describe the use of the following equipment to assess the pulse and blood pressure.

a. Stethoscope: _____

_____

_____

b. Sphygmomanometer: _____

_____

_____

APPLYING YOUR KNOWLEDGE

CRITICAL THINKING QUESTIONS

1. Using a partner, locate the nine sites for pulse assessment. Practice the technique for obtaining radial and apical pulses. Then practice the technique for measuring respirations and assessing blood pressure. Why is it important to be proficient in assessing and reporting vital sign measurements? If you were unsure of one of your vital sign assessments, what would you do?

2. An obese woman in the clinic needs a large blood pressure cuff, and one is not available. The resident tells you, "Just use the cuff you have." What do you do, and why?

3. Using a mannequin in your nursing laboratory, practice taking oral, rectal, and axillary temperatures. Research any new devices for taking temperature, and familiarize yourself with their use. Why do nurses need to be competent in using different methods and devices?

REFLECTIVE PRACTICE USING CRITICAL THINKING SKILLS

Use the following expanded scenario from Chapter 24 in your textbook to answer the questions below.

Scenario: Noah Shoolin is a 2-year-old who is brought to the emergency department by his mother. His mother says he has been running a high fever and has refused to take food or fluids for the past 24 hours. When you attempt to obtain a tympanic temperature, the child begins to scream uncontrollably, crying and pushing the device away from his ear.

1. What might be causing Noah's reaction to the nurse's attempt to assess a tympanic temperature?

_____

_____

_____

2. What would be a successful outcome for Noah?

_____

_____

_____

3. What intellectual, technical, interpersonal, and/or ethical/legal competencies are most likely to bring about the desired outcome?

_____

_____

_____

4. What resources might be helpful for the nurse caring for Noah?

_____

_____

_____

CHAPTER 25

Health Assessment

PRACTICING FOR NCLEX

MULTIPLE CHOICE QUESTIONS

Circle the letter that corresponds to the best answer for each question.

1. Which of the following describes a normal assessment of the eye?
   a. The patient's eyes should not converge when you move your finger toward his/her nose.
   b. The patient's pupils should be black, equal in size, and round and smooth.
   c. The pupils should be pale and cloudy in older adults.
   d. The patient's pupils should dilate when looking at a near object and constrict when looking at a distant object.

2. Which of the following assessment measures is used to assess the location, shape, size, and density of tissues?
   a. Observation
   b. Palpation
   c. Percussion
   d. Auscultation

3. When percussing the stomach, which of the following sounds would most likely be heard?
   a. Tympany
   b. Hyperresonance
   c. Dullness
   d. Flatness

4. A patient who presents with a dusky, bluish skin color is experiencing which of the following conditions?

   a. Flushing
   b. Jaundice
   c. Cyanosis
   d. Pallor

5. Which of the following is a normal finding when assessing internal eye structures?
   a. A uniform yellow reflex
   b. A clear, reddish optic nerve disc
   c. Dark-red arteries and light-red veins
   d. A reddish retina

6. Which of the following are soft, low-pitched sounds heard best over the base of the lungs during inspiration?
   a. Bronchial sounds
   b. Vesicular breath sounds
   c. Bronchovesicular sounds
   d. Adventitious breath sounds

7. A soft, high-pitched, flat sound that is usually percussed over muscle tissue is which of the following?
   a. Flatness
   b. Resonance
   c. Hyperresonance
   d. Dullness

8. Which of the following conditions would be a normal finding when palpating the skin of a patient?
   a. The skin is cool and dry.
   b. When picked up in a fold, the skin fold slowly returns to normal.
   c. The skin is taut and moist to the touch.

d. The texture of the skin varies from smooth and soft to rough and dry.

9. Which of the following eye characteristics is tested by assessing the eight cardinal fields of vision for coordination and alignment?
   a. Visual acuity
   b. Peripheral vision
   c. Extraocular movements
   d. Convergence

10. When assessing the ear canal and tympanic membrane with an otoscope, which of the following findings would be considered normal?
   a. The tympanic membrane should be translucent, shiny, and gray.
   b. The ear canal should be rough and pinkish.
   c. The tympanic membrane should be reddish.
   d. The ear canal should be smooth and white.

11. Mr. Rogers has a large tumor in his left lung. Which assessment technique would be used to determine the size of this tumor?
   a. Auscultation
   b. Palpation
   c. Percussion
   d. Inspection

12. A rubbing, grating sound that is loudest on the lower lateral anterior surface of the thorax and is auscultated during inspiration is known as which of the following?
   a. Wheeze
   b. Friction rub
   c. Rhonchi
   d. Crackles

13. To test the trochlear nerve of a patient, the nurse should do which of the following?
   a. Test pupillary reaction to light and ability to open and close eyelids.
   b. Test vision for acuity and visual fields.
   c. Test ocular movements in all directions.
   d. Test for downward and inward movement of the eye.

14. When a nurse asks a patient to raise her eyebrows, smile and show her teeth, and puff out her cheeks, he is most likely assessing which of the following nerves?
   a. Facial
   b. Vagus

c. Hypoglossal
d. Accessory

15. Which of the following is tested to evaluate the function of specific spinal cord segments?
   a. Motor ability
   b. Balance and gait
   c. Reflexes
   d. Sensory abilities

16. Which of the following assessment techniques would a nurse use to assess the thyroid gland?
   a. Palpation
   b. Inspection
   c. Percussion
   d. Auscultation

17. Which of the following is an accurate description of vesicular breath sounds?
   a. They are high-pitched, harsh sounds, with expiration being longer than inspiration.
   b. They are noisy, strenuous respirations.
   c. They are high-pitched sounds heard on inspiration when there is a narrowing of the upper airway.
   d. They are soft, low-pitched sounds heard best over the base of the lungs during respiration. Inspiration is longer than expiration.

18. A weak, thready pulse found after the nurse palpates peripheral pulses may indicate which of the following conditions?
   a. Hypertension and circulatory overload
   b. Decreased cardiac output
   c. Impaired circulation
   d. Inflammation of a vein

ALTERNATE-FORMAT QUESTIONS

Multiple Response Questions

Circle the letters that correspond to the best answers for each question.

1. Which of the following statements accurately describe a common laboratory or diagnostic procedure? *(Select all that apply.)*
   a. In ultrasonography studies, a computer provides physiologic information and detailed views of fluid-filled soft tissues.
   b. Endoscopic procedures are studies that use a machine with electrodes attached to the body to monitor electric activity.

c. During aspiration procedures, a needle or similar instrument is inserted into a body organ or cavity and fluid or tissue is removed and sent to the laboratory for examination.

d. Studies that involve the administration of radionuclide and subsequent measurement of radiation from an organ to detect functional abnormalities are called nuclear scanning.

e. Blood studies, urine studies, and sputum studies are examples of laboratory procedures.

f. Paracentesis and thoracentesis are examples of endoscopic procedures.

2. Which of the following statements describe the tone that may be percussed at specific body locations? *(Select all that apply.)*

   a. A flat tone may be heard over the thigh.

   b. A dull sound is generally heard over the liver.

   c. Resonance is heard over an emphysematous lung.

   d. Hyperresonance is percussed over the abdominal cavity.

   e. Loud tympany may be heard over a gastric air bubble.

   f. A dull sound would be heard over a puffed-out cheek.

3. Which of the following statements accurately describe the appearance of basic types of skin lesions? *(Select all that apply.)*

   a. A freckle is a palpable, elevated solid mass smaller than 0.5 cm.

   b. Vitiligo is a circumscribed, flat, nonpalpable change in skin color with a lesion larger than 1 cm.

   c. Acne is a pustule filled with pus formed by free fluid in a cavity within skin layers.

   d. A nevus or common mole is fibrous tissue that replaces tissue in the dermis or subcutaneous layer of the skin.

   e. Impetigo is a thin flake of exfoliated dermis.

   f. A fissure is a deep linear crack that extends into the dermis.

4. Which of the following are recommended guidelines for testing peripheral vision? *(Select all that apply.)*

   a. Have the patient stand or sit about 3 feet away.

   b. Have the patient cover one eye with a hand or index card.

c. Ask the patient to look directly at a predetermined spot on the wall behind you.

d. Cover your own eye opposite the patient's closed eye.

e. Hold one arm outstretched to one side equidistant from you and the patient, and move your fingers into the visual fields from various peripheral points.

f. Ask the patient to tell you when the fingers are first seen (you should see the fingers a second before the patient).

5. Which of the following are structures of the tympanic membrane? *(Select all that apply.)*

   a. Junction of incus and stapes

   b. Cochlea

   c. Oval window

   d. Umbo

   e. Stapes and footplate

   f. Short process of malleus

6. Which of the following are recommended guidelines for assessing the thorax and lungs? *(Select all that apply.)*

   a. The patient is asked to stand during the physical assessment.

   b. The thorax is percussed to detect areas of sensitivity, chest expansion during respirations, and vibrations.

   c. Chest expansion is determined by placing your hands over the posterior chest wall, with the fingers at the level of T9 or T10, and asking the patient to take a deep breath while observing the movement of your thumbs.

   d. Palpation is used to detect airflow within the respiratory tract.

   e. During auscultation of breath sounds, the patient is sitting and is asked to breathe slowly and deeply through the mouth while the diaphragm of the stethoscope is placed over the thoracic landmarks.

   f. Percussion may be used to determine lung position and size and to detect the presence of air, liquids, or solids within the lungs.

7. Which of the following are normal age-related thorax and lung variations? *(Select all that apply.)*

   a. Softer auscultated breath sounds are found in newborns and children.

   b. Children have a slower respiratory rate until 8 to 10 years of age.

   c. Newborns and children use abdominal muscles during respirations.

 d. Older adults may have an increased antero-posterior chest diameter.

 e. Older adults may have an increase in the dorsal spinal curve (kyphosis).

 f. Older adults may have increased thoracic expansion.

8. Which of the following are recommended guidelines for performing a peripheral vascular assessment? *(Select all that apply.)*

 a. Assessments are done by inspection and palpation, with the patient sitting or supine.

 b. The techniques used for cardiovascular assessment include inspection, palpation, and auscultation.

 c. The hands are used to palpate the precordium gently for pulsations using the palmar surface with the four fingers spread in a splayed position.

 d. Auscultation used to determine the heart sounds should be performed in a systematic method, beginning at Erb's point and moving to the tricuspid area, the mitral area, the pulmonic area, and finally the aortic area.

 e. During auscultation, the first heart sound is heard as the "lub" of "lub-dub" and is heard best at the apical area.

 f. Bruits, which are normal heart sounds similar to murmurs, are heard over the major blood vessels.

Hot Spot Question

1. Place an X on the figure below to mark the spot where the nurse would auscultate to best hear the S_1 heart sound.

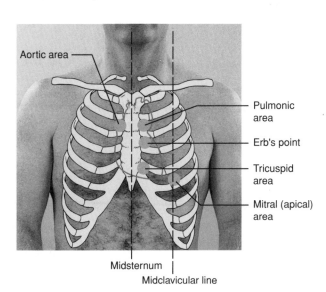

DEVELOPING YOUR KNOWLEDGE BASE

IDENTIFICATION QUESTIONS

1. Locate the organs listed below that are found in the anterior section of the abdominal cavity. Place your answers on the lines provided on the illustration below.

Sigmoid colon
Small intestine
Stomach
Appendix
Bladder
Spleen
Transverse colon
Ascending colon
Cecum
Liver
Descending colon

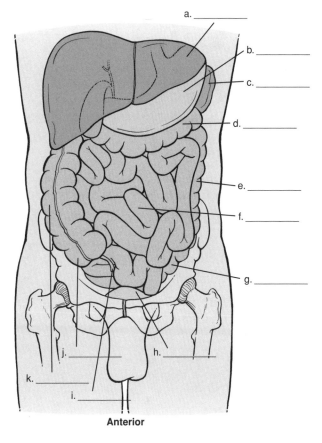

Anterior

2. Locate the following list of internal structures of the ear and place your answers on the lines provided on the illustration below.

Incus
Facial nerve
Cochlea
Semicircular canals

Malleus
Tympanic membrane
Stapes and footplate
Cochlear and vestibular branch
Oval window
Eustachian tube
Round window

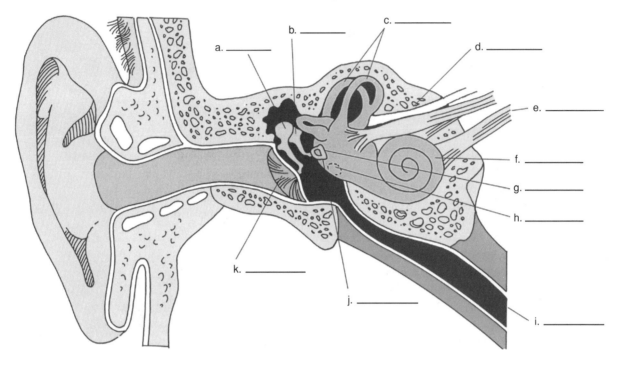

MATCHING EXERCISES

Match the organs listed in Part B with their proper location listed in Part A. Answers may be used more than once.

PART A

a. Right upper quadrant
b. Left upper quadrant
c. Right lower quadrant
d. Left lower quadrant
e. Midline

PART B

1. ___ Liver

2. ___ Stomach

3. ___ Gallbladder

4. ___ Sigmoid colon

5. ___ Cecum

6. ___ Spleen

7. ___ Urinary bladder

8. ___ Left ureter and lower kidney pole

9. ___ Appendix

10. ___ Right kidney and adrenal gland

11. ___ Body of pancreas

12. ___ Left ovary and fallopian tube

Match the terms in Part A with the correct definitions for findings during skin assessment listed in Part B.

PART A

a. Flushing
b. Cyanosis
c. Jaundice
d. Pallor
e. Ecchymosis
f. Petechiae

g. Lesion

h. Turgor

i. Bruits

PART B

13. _____ Yellow color

14. _____ Redness

15. _____ Dusky, blue color

16. _____ Purplish discoloration

17. _____ Diseased or injured tissue

18. _____ Paleness

19. _____ Elasticity of the skin

20. _____ Very small hemorrhagic spots

Match each nerve listed in Part A with its function listed in Part B.

PART A

a. Olfactory (I) nerve

b. Optic (II) nerve

c. Oculomotor (III), trochlear (IV), and abducens (VI) nerves

d. Trigeminal (V) nerve

e. Facial (VII) nerve

f. Acoustic (VIII) nerve

g. Glossopharyngeal (IX) nerve

h. Vagus (X) nerve

i. Accessory (XI) nerve

j. Hypoglossal (XII) nerve

PART B

21. _____ A sensory nerve that is tested by assessing hearing ability

22. _____ A sensory nerve whose function is vision. Vision is tested for acuity and visual fields.

23. _____ A sensorimotor nerve that is assessed by observing the facial muscles for deviation of the jaw to one side and by palpating facial muscles for tone while the patient clenches the jaw

24. _____ A motor nerve that affects the movement and strength of the tongue

25. _____ A sensory nerve whose function is the sense of smell

26. _____ Motor nerves that control the movement of the eyes through the cardinal fields of gaze; pupil size, shape, response to light, and accommodation; and opening of the upper eyelids

27. _____ A sensorimotor nerve that innervates the muscles of the face and functions to provide the taste sensation of the anterior two thirds of the tongue

28. _____ A motor nerve that is assessed by asking the patient to open the mouth and say "aaah" as the upward movement of the soft palate is observed

29. _____ A motor nerve that controls the movement of the head and shoulders

Match the positions listed in Part A with their description and function listed in Part B.

PART A

a. Sitting position

b. Supine position

c. Dorsal recumbent position

d. Sims' position

e. Prone position

f. Lithotomy position

g. Knee–chest position

h. Standing position

PART B

30. _____ The patient kneels, using the knees and chest to bear the weight of the body. The position is used to assess the rectal area.

31. _____ The patient lies on the left or right side with the lower arm behind the body and the upper arm bent at the shoulder and elbow. The knees are both bent, with the uppermost leg at a more acute angle. The position is used to assess the rectum or vagina.

32. _____ The patient is in the dorsal recumbent position with the buttocks at the edge of the examining table and feet supported in stirrups. This position is used to assess the female rectum and genitalia.

33. _____ The patient may sit upright in a chair or on the side of the examining table or bed. This position allows visualization of the upper body and facilitates lung expansion. It is used to take vital signs and assess the head, neck, posterior and anterior thorax and lungs, breasts, heart, and upper extremities.

34. ___ The patient lies on the back with legs separated, knees bent, and soles of the feet flat on the bed. This position is used to assess the head and neck, anterior thorax and lungs, breasts, heart, extremities, and peripheral pulses.

35. ___ The patient lies flat on the back with legs together but extended and slightly bent at the knees. This position is used to assess the head and neck, anterior thorax and lungs, breasts, heart, abdomen, extremities, and peripheral pulses.

36. ___ The patient lies on the abdomen, flat on the bed, with the head turned to one side. This position is used to assess the hip joint and posterior thorax.

SHORT ANSWER

1. Identify five purposes of performing a health assessment.

a. _____

b. _____

c. _____

d. _____

e. _____

2. Briefly describe how the following instruments are used in a health assessment.

a. Ophthalmoscope: _____

_____

b. Otoscope: _____

_____

c. Snellen chart: _____

_____

d. Nasal speculum: _____

_____

e. Vaginal speculum: _____

_____

f. Tuning fork: _____

_____

g. Percussion hammer: _____

_____

3. List four factors that should be considered when deciding on a position for the physical assessment of a patient.

a. _____

b. _____

c. _____

d. _____

4. Describe how you would prepare a patient and the environment for a physical assessment.

a. Patient: _____

_____

b. Environment: _____

_____

5. Complete the table below listing the four assessment techniques; give a brief description of each technique and the types of assessments made.

Technique	Definition	Assessment/Observation
a. Inspection:		
b. Palpation:		
c. Percussion:		
d. Auscultation:		

6. List and describe the four characteristics of sound assessed by auscultation.

   a. _____

   b. _____

   c. _____

   d. _____

7. Briefly describe how you would assess a patient for the following conditions.

   a. Edema: _____

   _____

   b. Dehydration: _____

   _____

8. Describe the procedure for assessing the pupils of a patient for the following.

   a. Reaction to light: _____

   _____

   _____

   b. Accommodation: _____

   _____

   _____

   c. Convergence: _____

   _____

   _____

9. List the steps used to assess bone conduction according to Weber and Rinne.

   a. Weber: _____

   _____

   _____

   b. Rinne: _____

   _____

   _____

10. You are asked to perform a neurologic assessment on a patient. List the equipment you would assemble before performing the assessment. In what position would your patient be placed? _____

   _____

   _____

11. Give an example of a question you may ask to assess a patient's mental status in the following areas.

   a. Orientation: _____

   _____

   b. Immediate memory: _____

   _____

   c. Past memory: _____

   _____

   d. Abstract reasoning: _____

   _____

   e. Language: _____

   _____

12. Complete the following paragraph by filling in the blanks with the correct word.

   During auscultation of the heart, the first heart sound heard is the (a) _____ of "lub-dub." This sound occurs when the (b) _____ and (c) _____ valves close and corresponds with the onset of (d) _____ contraction. This sound is called (e) _____ and is heard best in the (f) _____ area. The second heart sound, (g) _____, occurs at the end of (h) _____ and represents the closure of the (i) _____ and (j) _____ valves. It is the (k) _____ of "lub-dub." These two sounds occur within (l) _____ second(s) or less.

APPLYING YOUR KNOWLEDGE

CRITICAL THINKING QUESTIONS

1. Being prepared is a key factor in conducting a competent health assessment. The nurse must display well-developed cognitive, interpersonal, technical, and ethical skills. Describe what you would do to prepare the patient, the room, and the environment for an examination. How and why would you modify these preparations for the following patients?

   a. A patient who is comatose

   b. A patient who is uncooperative

   c. A patient who does not understand your language

   d. A small child

2. Make a list of all the instruments you would use to perform a health assessment. Arrange the instruments according to the order in which they will be used. Write a definition of each instrument and how it is to be used during the assessment. Rate yourself on your technical ability to use each instrument and technique. Practice using the instruments on a partner until you feel confident. Reflect on:

a. How confident you need to be before you can assess a patient independently

b. When it is safe to "practice" on a patient

REFLECTIVE PRACTICE USING CRITICAL THINKING SKILLS

Use the following expanded scenario from Chapter 25 in your textbook to answer the questions below.

Scenario: Billy Collins, a 9-year-old with a history of allergies, including an allergy to insect stings, is spending a week at summer camp. He suddenly reports to the camp counselor that he was just stung by a bee. The counselor rushes Billy to the nearest emergency health center after helping him self-inject epinephrine. He presents with itching and hives, difficulty breathing, nausea, and palpitations. When his parents arrive, they ask you what more they can do, if anything, to prevent this situation from occurring in the future.

1. What type of health assessments would the nurse caring for Billy conduct?

2. What would be a successful outcome for Billy and his family?

3. What intellectual, technical, interpersonal, and/or ethical/legal competencies are most likely to bring about the desired outcome?

4. What resources might be helpful for this family?

CHAPTER 26

Safety, Security, and Emergency Preparedness

PRACTICING FOR NCLEX

MULTIPLE CHOICE QUESTIONS

Circle the letter that corresponds to the best answer for each question.

1. Which of the following is the major safety problem in healthcare facilities?
   a. Falls
   b. Fires
   c. Violence
   d. Poisoning

2. When deciding whether to use restraints on a patient, the nurse should consider which of the following accurate statements?
   a. According to a recent study, unrestrained older patients were three times more likely to sustain fall-related injuries than restrained older patients.
   b. There are no physiologic hazards associated with the proper use of restraints on older patients.
   c. The Joint Commission stated that restraints can cause physical and psychological harm, loss of dignity, and even death.
   d. Generally, a physician's order is not necessary to apply restraints.

3. When filing a safety event report, the nurse should be aware of which of the following accurate statements?
   a. The safety event report becomes a part of the medical record.
   b. A physician must be present when a safety event report is completed.
   c. Laws governing the completion of a safety event report are uniform throughout the country.
   d. The safety event report is not part of the medical record and should not be mentioned in the documentation.

4. Which of the following statements presents an accurate statistic that should be considered when planning safety for patients?
   a. There is no evidence linking a relationship between childhood sexual abuse and certain physical symptoms in adults, such as gastrointestinal disorders.
   b. Some people are more likely than others to have falls; for instance, some children have multiple mishaps, resulting in fractured bones.
   c. According to the CDC, approximately 81% of all adolescent deaths from motor vehicle accidents involve the use of alcohol and/or other drugs.

d. Because older adults have more experience with their environment, they are less vulnerable to falls.

5. Which of the following statements concerning fires is accurate?

   a. Most people who die in house fires do not die from burns, but from smoke inhalation.

   b. Most home fires are started by the use of candles.

   c. Most fatal home fires occur while people are awake.

   d. Fire is the major safety problem in hospitals and the leading cause of accidental death for the elderly at home.

6. Mrs. Nix, age 86, was admitted to the hospital in a confused and dehydrated state. After she got out of bed and fell, restraints were applied. She began to fight and was rapidly becoming exhausted. She has black-and-blue marks on her wrists from the restraints. Which of the following would be the most appropriate nursing intervention for Mrs. Nix?

   a. Sedate her with sleeping pills and leave the restraints on.

   b. Take the restraints off and stay with her and talk gently to her.

   c. Leave the restraints on and talk with her, explaining that she must calm down.

   d. Talk with Mrs. Nix's family about taking her home because she is out of control.

7. Which of the following would be an alternative to the use of restraints for ensuring patient safety and preventing falls?

   a. Involve family members in the patient's care.

   b. Allow the patient to use the bathroom independently.

   c. Keep the patient sedated with tranquilizers.

   d. Maintain a high bed position so the patient will not attempt to get out unassisted.

ALTERNATE-FORMAT QUESTIONS

Multiple Response Questions

Circle the letters that correspond to the best answers for each question.

1. Which of the following statements accurately describe factors affecting safety in the general population? *(Select all that apply.)*

   a. OSHA has determined that younger construction workers are at particular risk for sustaining a fatal injury owing to their inexperience.

   b. According to Pillitteri, ribavirin, used for respiratory infections in infants and children, may be harmful to a developing fetus.

   c. Carpal tunnel syndrome occurs from exposure to toxins in the environment.

   d. Certain environments have proved to be more hazardous than others and may expose residents to potentially unhealthy substances.

   e. Any limitation in mobility is potentially unsafe.

   f. Stressful situations are more devastating to young adults because they typically have less adaptive and coping capacity.

2. Which of the following statements reflect considerations a nurse should keep in mind when assessing a patient for safety? *(Select all that apply.)*

   a. A person with a history of falls is likely to fall again.

   b. Some people are more prone to have accidents than others.

   c. Fires are responsible for most hospital incidents.

   d. Between 15% and 25% of falls result in fractures or soft tissue injury.

   e. A medication regimen that includes diuretics or analgesics places an individual at risk for falls.

   f. A nurse whose behavior is reasonable and prudent and similar to what would be expected of another nurse in a similar circumstance is still likely to be found liable if a patient falls, especially if an injury results.

3. Which of the following statements accurately describe symptoms produced by a bioterrorism agent? *(Select all that apply.)*

   a. Inhalation anthrax produces fever, fatigue, cough, dyspnea, and pain; the patient's condition may progress to meningitis, septicemia, shock, and death.

   b. Symptoms of the plague ("black death") include a characteristic rash that progresses to crusted scabs in 5 days.

c. Botulism produces skeletal muscle paralysis that progresses symmetrically in a descending manner and muscle weakness that can result abruptly in respiratory failure.

d. Tularemia produces fever and cough; the patient's condition may progress to respiratory failure.

e. Smallpox produces fever, myalgias, conjunctival symptoms, mild hypotension, and petechial hemorrhages; the patient's condition may progress to shock and hemorrhage.

f. Lassa fever, Ebola fever, and yellow fever cause diarrhea, nausea, and respiratory distress.

4. Which of the following are examples of nerve agents? *(Select all that apply.)*

a. Phosgene

b. Tabun

c. Sarin

d. Soman

e. Agent 15

f. Phosphogene oxime

5. Which of the following are acronyms for organizations that are involved in emergency preparedness? *(Select all that apply.)*

a. NDMS

b. FEMA

c. CDC

d. HMO

e. TJC

f. EPO

6. Which of the following would be an age-appropriate method to prevent accidents and promote safety in a preschooler? *(Select all that apply.)*

a. Supervise the child closely to prevent injury.

b. Childproof the house to ensure that poisonous products and small objects are out of reach.

c. Instruct the child to wear proper safety equipment when riding bicycles or scooters.

d. Do not leave the child alone in the bathtub or near water.

e. Provide drug, alcohol, and sexuality education.

f. Practice emergency evacuation measures.

7. Which of the following actions would a nurse perform when properly applying restraints to a patient? *(Select all that apply.)*

a. Check agency policy for the application of restraints and secure a physician's order.

b. Choose the most restrictive type of device that allows the least amount of mobility.

c. Pad bony prominences.

d. For a restraint applied to an extremity, ensure that the restraint is tight enough that a finger cannot be inserted between the restraint and the patient's wrist or ankle.

e. Fasten the restraint to the side rail.

f. Remove the restraint at least every 2 hours or according to agency policy and patient need.

Prioritization Questions

1. Place the following steps for applying restraints to a patient in the order in which they should occur:

a. Explain the reason for use of restraints to the patient and family.

b. Determine the need for restraints and assess patient's physical condition, behavior, and mental status.

c. Fasten restraint to the bed frame, not the bed rail.

d. Apply restraints according to manufacturer's directions.

e. Perform hand hygiene; document reason for restraining patient.

f. Perform hand hygiene.

g. Remove restraint at least every 2 hours; reassure patient at regular intervals and assess for signs of sensory deprivation.

h. Confirm agency policy for application of restraints and secure physician order.

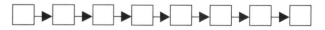

DEVELOPING YOUR KNOWLEDGE BASE

MATCHING EXERCISES

Match the type of poisonous agent in Part A with its common clinical manifestations listed in Part B. List the type of emergency treatment you would use for each agent on the line provided.

PART A

a. Acetaminophen (products containing Tylenol)

b. Caustics (oven cleaner, drain openers, toilet bowl cleaners, rust removers, battery contents, chemicals used for hair permanents)

c. Hydrocarbons (gasoline, kerosene, furniture polish, lamp oil)

d. Iron (vitamin preparations)

e. Lead (paint chips, paint dust)

PART B

1. ____ Nausea, vomiting, diarrhea, abdominal pain, melena, hematemesis, lethargy, coma. Treatment: _____

2. ____ Burning pain in mouth and throat, drooling, edema of lips and mouth, esophageal and gastric burns, vomiting, hemoptysis. Treatment: _____

3. ____ Anorexia, nausea, vomiting, liver toxicity

   Treatment: _____

4. ____ May be asymptomatic; anorexia, abdominal pain, encephalopathy, neurobehavioral deficits. Treatment: _____

5. ____ Gagging, coughing, choking, dyspnea, grunting, nausea, chills, fever, lethargy. Treatment: _____

Match the safety precaution listed in Part B with the appropriate age group listed in Part A. Some answers may be used more than once.

PART A

a. Fetus

b. Infant

c. Toddler and preschooler

d. School-aged child

e. Adolescent

f. Adult

g. Older adult

PART B

6. ____ This age group needs assistance to evaluate activities that are potentially dangerous and to discuss specific interventions that provide for safety at home, at school, and in the neighborhood.

7. ____ Falls, fires, and motor vehicle crashes are significant hazards for this age group, and safety measures should be directed toward preventing these injuries.

8. ____ Education for this group must focus on safe driving skills, the dangers of drug and alcohol use, and creation of a healthy lifestyle as a way to respond to the stress of daily living.

9. ____ A pregnant student requires reinforcement about the risks associated with alcohol consumption, smoking, drug use, and exposure to dangers in the environment.

10. ____ This group needs education about ways to handle the stresses of daily life (e.g., raising a family, handling a demanding career) without relying on drugs and alcohol.

11. ____ Vigilant supervision by parents and guardians is required to anticipate hazards and provide protection for this group, with precautionary devices.

12. ____ Safety care for this group entails never leaving them unattended, using crib rails, and monitoring objects that may be placed in the mouth and swallowed.

CORRECT THE FALSE STATEMENTS

Circle the word "true" or "false" that follows the statement. If you circled "false," change the underlined word or words to make the statement true. Write your answer in the space provided.

1. Nearly <u>one third</u> of older adults fall at home each year.

   True   False _____

2. According to The Joint Commission, caregivers must use at least <u>two</u> patient identifiers (neither to be the patient's room number) whenever administering medications and providing treatments or procedures.

   True   False _____

3. A person with a history of falling is <u>at great risk</u> to fall again.

   True   False _____

4. Most exposures to toxic fumes occur in the
   <u>workplace</u>.

   True   False _____

5. Asphyxiation may occur in any age group, but
   the incidence is greatest among <u>older adults</u>.

   True   False _____

6. Keeping a gun in the home <u>increases</u> the risk
   for domestic homicide.

   True   False _____

7. A <u>rear-facing</u> safety seat is recommended for
   infants who are younger than 1 year old and
   weigh less than 20 pounds.

   True   False _____

8. For the <u>school-aged child</u>, the focus of
   parental responsibility is on childproofing
   the environment.

   True   False _____

9. As the primary reason for applying restraints,
   nurses consistently cite the <u>risk for injury to
   patients and healthcare workers from
   irrational behavior</u>.

   True   False _____

10. Using a restraint on an older person who tends
    to wander is <u>justified to ensure his/her safety</u>.

    True   False _____

11. Nearly half of all drowning victims are
    <u>teenagers</u>.

    True   False _____

12. The number of deaths from accidental
    poisoning has <u>decreased</u> over the years.

    True   False _____

SHORT ANSWER

1. Identify two safety risks for each of the
   following age groups.

   a. Neonates and infants: _____

   b. Toddler and preschooler: _____

   c. School-aged child: _____

   d. Adolescent: _____

   e. Adult: _____

   f. Older adult: _____

2. List two examples of how the following
   factors can affect safety.

   a. Developmental considerations: _____

   b. Lifestyle: _____

   c. Limitation in mobility: _____

   d. Limitation in sensory perception: _____

   e. Limitation in knowledge: _____

   f. Limitation in ability to communicate: ____

   g. Limitation in health status: _____

   h. Limitation in psychosocial state: _____

3. Briefly explain why the following information
   is necessary when assessing the patient for
   safety.

   a. Nursing history: _____

   b. Physical assessment: _____

   c. Accident-prone behavior: _____

   d. The environment: _____

4. Mrs. Vogel, age 72, fell when getting out of bed to use the bathroom in her nursing home. List four characteristics that should be assessed to determine whether this patient is at a greater risk for falls.

   a. _____

   b. _____

   c. _____

   d. _____

5. You are visiting a homebound patient who is staying with her daughter, who also has a toddler at home. You notice that the house is not childproofed and watch in horror as the toddler pulls a bottle of disinfectant out from under the sink while the mother is busy caring for her own mother. How would you prepare and present a plan for this mother to childproof her home?

   _____

   _____

   _____

6. List three questions you could ask a patient to assess for hazards that may cause a child to asphyxiate or choke.

   a. _____

   b. _____

   c. _____

7. Write a sample nursing diagnosis for each of the following situations.

   a. A mother refuses to use a car seat for her child: _____

   _____

   b. An older patient has poor vision and cannot read the label on her medication bottle: _____

   _____

   c. A mother leaves her child unattended in the bathtub while she answers the phone: _____

   _____

   d. A patient tells you she is "clumsy" and has fallen several times in the past few years: _____

   _____

   e. The windows and doors do not operate properly in the home of an older couple, but they cannot afford repairs: _____

   _____

8. List three opportunities a nurse can use to teach students about safety.

   a. _____

   b. _____

   c. _____

9. List five risks associated with the use of restraints.

   a. _____

   b. _____

   c. _____

   d. _____

   e. _____

10. Mrs. Bender is a patient who has been placed in restraints to protect her from falling after other methods have failed. She refused to listen to information about the dangers of falling and repeatedly attempted to go to the bathroom on her own. How would you document the use of restraints on this patient?

   _____

   _____

   _____

   _____

   _____

11. List the information that should be included on a safety event report, when it should be filled out, and who is responsible for recording the event.

   _____

   _____

   _____

   _____

   _____

12. Describe how you would assess a patient for risk for falling by using the Get Up and Go test (Hendrich, 2007). State the time parameters for full mobility, almost complete independence, and impaired mobility.

_____
_____
_____
_____
_____

APPLYING YOUR KNOWLEDGE

CRITICAL THINKING QUESTIONS

1. Visit the homes of friends or relatives who have children of different ages living with them. Ask for permission to inspect their home for safety features that are appropriate to the ages of the children. Check for poison control, fire prevention, fall protection, burn and shock protection, and so on. Share your results with the family, and explain to them what they need to do (if anything) to improve safety in their home. Reflect on the importance that different families attach to safety and its implication for your nursing practice.

2. Many people tend to take safety measures for granted. Draw on your experiences in conversations with nurses to identify safety risks for both nurses and patients in different practice settings. What can you do to minimize these risks?

REFLECTIVE PRACTICE USING CRITICAL THINKING SKILLS

Use the following expanded scenario from Chapter 26 in your textbook to answer the questions below.

Scenario: Bessie Washington, age 77, was recently discharged to her home after suffering a cerebrovascular accident (brain attack). She lives alone in a small one-bedroom apartment and uses a walker to ambulate. A visiting nurse performing a safety assessment notes that she has hardwood floors with throw rugs covering the traffic areas, and old newspapers and magazines are stacked in piles close to heating vents. There are no fire alarms visible in the room. Mrs. Washington tells you, "I have so much stuff crammed into this apartment, I almost fell this morning going from my bedroom to the kitchen."

1. What safety interventions might the nurse implement for this patient?

_____
_____
_____

2. What would be a successful outcome for Mrs. Washington?

_____
_____
_____

3. What intellectual, technical, interpersonal, and/or ethical/legal competencies are most likely to bring about the desired outcome?

_____
_____
_____

4. What resources might be helpful for Mrs. Washington?

_____
_____
_____

CHAPTER 27

Asepsis and Infection Control

PRACTICING FOR NCLEX

MULTIPLE CHOICE QUESTIONS

Circle the letter that corresponds to the best answer for each question.

1. Spherical bacteria belong to which of the following groups?
   a. Bacilli
   b. Cocci
   c. Spirochetes
   d. Vacillates

2. Which of the following is the smallest of all microorganisms and can be seen only through an electron microscope?
   a. Cocci
   b. Spirochetes
   c. Fungi
   d. Virus

3. When an organism is transmitted through personal contact with an inanimate object, such as contaminated blood, the route of transmission is which of the following?
   a. Direct contact
   b. Vectors
   c. Indirect contact
   d. Airborne

4. During which stage of infection is the person most infectious?
   a. Incubation period
   b. Prodromal stage
   c. Full stage of illness
   d. Convalescent period

5. Which of the following is a protective mechanism that eliminates the invading pathogen and allows tissue repair to occur?
   a. Inflammatory response
   b. Immune response
   c. Cellular immune response
   d. Humoral immune response

6. Which of the following is a natural reservoir for tetanus?
   a. Humans
   b. Animals
   c. Soil
   d. Food

7. Mrs. Teal is to have an indwelling urinary catheter inserted. Which of the following would be the precaution taken during this procedure?
   a. Surgical asepsis technique
   b. Medical asepsis technique
   c. Droplet precautions
   d. Strict reverse isolation

ALTERNATE-FORMAT QUESTIONS

Multiple Response Questions

Circle the letter that corresponds to the best answer for each question.

1. Which of the following occur during the prodromal stage of an infection? *(Select all that apply.)*

   a. Specific signs and symptoms of the infection are present.

   b. The signs and symptoms disappear as the person returns to a healthy state.

   c. The person is most infectious during this stage.

   d. Signs and symptoms are present, but they are often vague and nonspecific.

   e. The organisms are growing and multiplying, but symptoms are not present yet.

   f. This stage lasts for 7 to 14 days.

2. Which of the following statements regarding asepsis are accurate? *(Select all that apply.)*

   a. Asepsis includes all activities to prevent infection or break the chain of infection.

   b. Surgical asepsis involves only the procedures and practices that reduce the number and transfer of pathogens.

   c. Surgical asepsis includes practices used to render and keep objects and areas free from microorganisms.

   d. Medical asepsis techniques are appropriate for most procedures in the home.

   e. When practicing medical asepsis, the nurse should place soiled bed linens on the floor.

   f. When practicing surgical asepsis, the nurse should hold sterile objects below waist level to prevent accidental contamination.

3. Which of the following techniques for hand hygiene are recommended by the CDC? *(Select all that apply.)*

   a. Even if a healthcare worker's hands are not visibly soiled with blood or body fluids, handwashing with soap and water is required.

   b. Effective handwashing requires at least a 15-second scrub with plain soap or disinfectant and warm water.

   c. A healthcare worker's nails should not be polished because polish increases the number of microorganisms trapped under the nails.

   d. Artificial nails do not increase the risk for developing a fungal infection in the nail bed.

   e. Wearing gloves eliminates the need for proper hand hygiene.

   f. Gloving does not guarantee complete protection from infectious organisms.

4. Which of the following statements accurately describe the processes of disinfection and sterilization? *(Select all that apply.)*

   a. Disinfection destroys all pathogenic organisms except spores.

   b. The process of sterilization destroys all pathogenic microorganisms, including spores.

   c. The CDC recommends that all supplies, linens, and equipment in a healthcare setting should be treated as if the patient were infectious.

   d. The choice of using a chemical or physical means of sterilization and disinfection is determined by the preference of the healthcare agency.

   e. Articles that are to be sterilized should be rinsed first with hot running water to remove organic material.

   f. Articles that are being sterilized do not need to be washed with soap first.

5. Which of the following actions would a nurse perform when opening a sterile package and preparing a sterile field? *(Select all that apply.)*

   a. Sterile packages should never be opened while held in the hands.

   b. A sterile item should be covered if it is not used immediately.

   c. When opening a sterile wrapped drape, select a work area that is at waist level or higher.

   d. Sterile items should be dropped onto a sterile field from a 12-inch height or added to the field from the side.

   e. When pouring a sterile solution, hold the bottle outside the edge of the sterile field with the label side uppermost and prepare to pour from a height of 4 to 6 inches.

   f. Discard any sterile solution that is not used during a procedure.

6. Which of the following statements accurately describes the proper use of personal protective equipment in a healthcare agency? *(Select all that apply.)*

   a. Only invasive patient procedures require a clean pair of gloves.

   b. Some care activities for an individual patient may necessitate changing gloves more than once.

   c. A waterproof gown may be used more than one time.

   d. Except for respirator, remove PPE at the doorway or in anteroom.

   e. To remove gown: unfasten ties, if at the neck and back, and allow the gown to fall away from shoulders.

   f. When a mask is not being worn, it can be lowered around the neck and brought back over the mouth and nose for reuse.

7. Which of the following are CDC guidelines for maintaining infection-control practices in hospitals? *(Select all that apply.)*

   a. Use airborne precautions for patients who have infections that spread through the air such as tuberculosis, chickenpox, and measles.

   b. Place a patient on airborne precautions in a private room that has monitored negative air pressure, and keep the door open.

   c. Droplet precautions should be used for patients with MRSA, VRE, or VISA.

   d. Wear a mask when working within 3 feet of a patient who is on droplet precautions.

   e. Use contact precautions for patient diagnosed with rubella, mumps, diphtheria, or the adenovirus infection.

   f. Wear gloves whenever you enter the room of a patient on contact precautions.

Prioritization Questions

1. Place the following steps for removing protective equipment in the order in which they should occur when the nurse has completed patient care:

   a. Remove gown.

   b. Remove mask/respirator.

   c. Remove gloves.

   d. Remove goggles/face shield.

   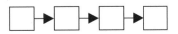

2. Place the following steps of the infection cycle in the order in which an infection would occur:

   a. Portal of exit

   b. Infectious agent

   c. Means of transmission

   d. Reservoir

   e. Portal of entry

   f. Susceptible host

   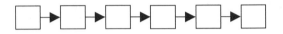

DEVELOPING YOUR KNOWLEDGE BASE

FILL-IN-THE-BLANKS

1. _____ is a disease state that results from the presence of pathogens in or on the body.

2. _____ are the most significant and most commonly observed infection-causing agents in healthcare institutions.

3. Most bacteria require oxygen to live and grow and are, therefore, referred to as _____.

4. Athlete's foot, ringworm, and yeast infections are caused by _____.

5. Microorganisms that commonly inhabit various body sites and are part of the body's natural defense system are referred to as _____.

6. The natural habitats of organisms, such as humans, animals, soil, and food, are examples of _____.

7. The _____ is the point at which organisms enter a new host.

8. The body commonly responds to an antigen by producing a(n) _____.

9. A(n) _____ is an infection, not present on admission, that certain patients in health agencies develop during the course of treatment for other conditions.

MATCHING EXERCISES

Match the terms in Part A with their definitions listed in Part B.

PART A

a. Infection
b. Pathogen
c. Bacteria
d. Gram-positive bacteria
e. Gram-negative bacteria
f. Aerobic bacteria
g. Anaerobic bacteria
h. Host
i. Fungi
j. Normal flora
k. Opportunists
l. Virus
m. Antigen
n. Antibody

PART B

1. _____ Bacteria that are potentially harmful

2. _____ Bacteria that require oxygen to live

3. _____ A disease state that results from the presence of pathogens in or on the body

4. _____ A disease-producing microorganism

5. _____ Microorganisms that commonly inhabit various body sites and are part of the body's natural defense system

6. _____ Plant-like organisms that can cause infection

7. _____ An invading foreign protein such as bacteria, or in some cases the body's own proteins

8. _____ Most significant and commonly observed infection-causing agents in healthcare institutions

9. _____ Bacteria that have chemically more complex cell walls and can be decolorized by alcohol

10. _____ Bacteria that can live without oxygen

11. _____ Bacteria that have thick cell walls that resist colorization and are stained violet

12. _____ The body responds to an antigen by producing this.

Match the diseases in Part B with their mode of transmission listed in Part A. Give an example of how the diseases are transmitted on the line provided. Answers may be used more than once.

PART A

a. Direct contact
b. Indirect contact
c. Vehicle
d. Airborne
e. Vector

PART B

13. _____ AIDS _____
14. _____ Lyme disease _____
15. _____ Tuberculosis _____
16. _____ Wound infection _____
17. _____ Hepatitis _____
18. _____ Abscess _____
19. _____ Boil _____

Match the type of infection in Part A with its definition listed in Part B.

PART A

a. Nosocomial
b. Exogenous
c. Endogenous
d. Iatrogenic

PART B

20. _____ An infection that occurs as a result of treatment or a diagnostic procedure

21. _____ A hospital-acquired infection

22. _____ An infection in which the causative organism is normally harbored within the patient

23. _____ An infection caused by an organism acquired from other persons

CORRECT THE FALSE STATEMENTS

Circle the word "true" or "false" that follows the statement. If you circled "false," change the underlined word or words to make the statement true. Place your answer in the space provided.

1. <u>Gram-negative bacteria</u> have chemically complex walls and can be decolorized by alcohol.

   True   False _____

2. Methicillin-resistant *S. aureus* and vancomycin-resistant *enterococci* are most often transmitted by <u>the hands of healthcare providers</u>.

   True   False _____

3. <u>Wearing gloves</u> is the most effective way to help prevent the spread of organisms.

   True   False _____

4. <u>Resident bacteria</u>, normally picked up by the hands in the course of usual activities of daily living, are relatively few on clean and exposed areas of the skin.

   True   False _____

5. <u>Nonantimicrobial agents</u> are considered adequate for routine mechanical cleansing of the hands and removal of most transient microorganisms.

   True   False _____

6. <u>Sterilization</u> is the process by which all microorganisms, including spores, are destroyed.

   True   False _____

7. In a home environment, contaminated items may be disinfected by placing them in boiling water for <u>10 minutes</u>.

   True   False _____

8. When observing <u>medical asepsis</u>, areas are considered contaminated if they are touched by any object that is not also sterile.

   True   False _____

9. Using <u>body substance isolation precautions</u> eliminates the need for category-specific or disease-specific systems, except for certain airborne diseases that require special precautions.

   True   False _____

SHORT ANSWER

1. List four factors that influence an organism's potential to produce disease.

   a. _____

   b. _____

   c. _____

   d. _____

2. Give an example of a disease that is transmitted by organisms from the following reservoirs.

   a. Other humans: _____

   b. Animals: _____

   c. Soil: _____

3. List three portals of exit in the human body.

   a. _____

   b. _____

   c. _____

4. Give an example of the following means of transmission.

   a. Direct contact: _____

   _____

   b. Indirect contact: _____

   _____

   c. Vectors: _____

   _____

   d. Airborne: _____

   _____

5. Briefly describe the following body defenses against infection.

   a. Inflammatory response: _____

   _____

   _____

   b. Immune response: _____

   _____

   _____

6. List four factors that influence the susceptibility of a host.

   a. _____

   b. _____

c. _____

d. _____

7. Briefly describe the nurse's role in controlling or treating infection in the following stages of the nursing practice.

a. Assessing: _____
_____
_____

b. Diagnosing: _____
_____
_____

c. Planning: _____
_____
_____

d. Implementing: _____
_____
_____

e. Evaluating: _____
_____
_____

8. Give two examples of how you would practice medical asepsis in the following areas.

a. Patient's home: _____
_____

b. Public facilities: _____
_____

c. Community: _____
_____

d. Healthcare facility: _____
_____

9. List three measures healthcare agencies have found to be successful in reducing the incidence of nosocomial infections.

a. _____

b. _____

c. _____

10. Explain why the following factors should be considered when selecting sterilization and disinfection methods.

a. Nature of organisms present: _____
_____

b. Number of organisms present: _____
_____

c. Type of equipment: _____
_____

d. Intended use of equipment: _____
_____

e. Available means for sterilization and disinfection: _____
_____

f. Time: _____
_____

11. Describe the role of the infection-control nurse in the following situations.

a. Hospital: _____
_____

b. Home care setting: _____
_____

12. Zelen is a 35-year-old fireman who sustained third-degree burns on his upper body.

a. Write a nursing diagnosis that relates to his increased risk for skin infection. ____
_____

b. Describe how the nurse can help to control or prevent infection for this patient.
_____
_____

13. In the emergency department, a patient you are treating for lacerations tells you that he was recently diagnosed with TB. Would you use different precautions for this patient than for another emergency department patient? Why?
_____
_____
_____

APPLYING YOUR KNOWLEDGE

CRITICAL THINKING QUESTIONS

1. Try to imagine what it must feel like to be in strict isolation. Then interview a patient whose medical condition necessitated the use of isolation precautions. Find out how it felt to be isolated and, in some cases, feared by healthcare workers. See if anything was done to help alleviate the disorientation and meet the patient's basic needs of love and belonging. What did you learn that would help you to direct your future nursing care for patients in isolation?

2. A nurse is obligated to provide nursing care to all patients regardless of race, creed, religion, and so forth. Should this code also include "regardless of the medical condition of the patient"? Should nurses be able to choose whether or not to take care of a patient who has a contagious disease? Do you believe the precautions being taken with these patients offer adequate protection for the healthcare provider? Should there be consequences for medical personnel who refuse to take care of these patients? Share your responses with your classmates and see if you agree.

REFLECTIVE PRACTICE USING CRITICAL THINKING SKILLS

Use the following expanded scenario from Chapter 27 in your textbook to answer the questions below.

Scenario: Giselle Turheis, age 38, is undergoing chemotherapy treatment for leukemia in the hospital. The staff has placed Ms. Turheis on neutropenic precautions and restricted visitors to her room. The flowers she received from her family were sent home to avoid having standing water in her room. Healthcare workers regularly appear at her bedside in masks and gowns. When the nurse explains the reason for these precautions to Ms. Turheis and her family, Ms. Turheis says, "I know my risk for infection is really high because of my poor immune status, but I feel so out of touch with reality now. And when I get home, how will I respond to my Sunday school students who are used to greeting me with a big hug? I want to be safe, but I know that I need these hugs too!"

1. How might the nurse respond to Ms. Turheis in a manner that respects her human dignity, while at the same time, maintaining a safe environment for her?

   _____

   _____

   _____

2. What would be a successful outcome for Ms. Turheis?

   _____

   _____

   _____

3. What intellectual, technical, interpersonal, and/or ethical/legal competencies are most likely to bring about the desired outcome?

   _____

   _____

   _____

4. What resources might be helpful for Ms. Turheis?

   _____

   _____

   _____

CHAPTER 28

Complementary and Alternative Therapies

PRACTICING FOR NCLEX

MULTIPLE CHOICE QUESTIONS

Circle the letter that corresponds to the best answer for each question.

1. Which of the following is a term generally used to describe "traditional" medical care?
   a. Allopathy
   b. Holism
   c. Integrative care
   d. Homeopathy

2. In which of the following CAT systems is understanding the patient's "dosha" a central theme?
   a. Yoga
   b. Traditional Chinese medicine
   c. Ayurveda
   d. Qi gong

3. A patient who practices a set of exercises consisting of various physical postures designed to promote strength and flexibility is most likely practicing what CAT system?
   a. Qi gong
   b. Yoga
   c. Traditional Chinese medicine
   d. Ayurveda

4. Which of the following systems of medicine is a way of life with emphasis on patient responsibility, education, health maintenance, and disease prevention?
   a. Homeopathy
   b. Chiropractic
   c. Naturopathy
   d. Allopathy

5. Which of the following mind–body techniques promotes parasympathetic activity, helping to reduce sympathetic activity and restore the balance of both systems?
   a. Relaxation
   b. Imagery
   c. Chiropractic
   d. Medication

6. In which of the following spiritual approaches does treatment consist of retrieving lost soul energy, restoring individual's relationship with the spirit world, and then treating symptoms?
   a. Traditional Chinese medicine
   b. Intercessory prayer
   c. Structural therapies
   d. Shamanism

ALTERNATE-FORMAT QUESTIONS

Multiple Response Questions

Circle the letters that correspond to the best answers for each question.

1. Which of the following are tenets of traditional Chinese medicine (TCM)? *(Select all that apply.)*
   a. TCM believes that the interaction of people with their environment is the most significant factor in creating health.

b. The goal of the TCM diagnostic process is to arrive at the pattern of disharmony that is manifesting in the person.

c. TCM believes that qi flows vertically in the body through an intricate structure of meridians.

d. TCM is a system of postures, exercises, breathing techniques, and visualization that regulates qi.

e. TCM is based on the belief of supporting the body while the symptoms are allowed to run their course.

f. In TCM, qi is viewed as either yin or yang energy.

2. Which of the following are scientific premises upon which the practice of Therapeutic Touch is based? *(Select all that apply.)*

a. A human being is a closed energy system.

b. Anatomically, a human being is bilaterally symmetrical.

c. Illness is an imbalance in the individual's energy field.

d. Human beings project an aura that consists of at least seven layers of energy.

e. Human beings have natural abilities to transform and transcend their conditions of living.

f. Neuropeptides are believed to be the messenger molecules that connect the mind and body.

3. Which of the following statements accurately represent the role of CAT in nursing today? *(Select all that apply.)*

a. The nursing profession is expanding its knowledge base to include information that explains selected CAT.

b. Certification is available for nurses wishing to practice holistic nursing.

c. Graduate-level specialization in holistic nursing is available at some universities.

d. It is expected that CAT will eventually replace traditional nursing in many health-care facilities.

e. Practitioners of CAT are strictly regulated by the government.

f. The development of CAT is market and patient driven.

4. Which of the following are locations of chakras? *(Select all that apply.)*

a. Patella

b. Wrist

c. Heart

d. Throat

e. Solar plexus

f. Stomach

5. Which of the following are general characteristics of allopathic medicine? *(Select all that apply.)*

a. Curing is accomplished by internal agents.

b. Illness occurs in either the mind or the body, which are separate entities.

c. Illness is a manifestation of imbalance or disharmony and is a process.

d. Curing occurs quickly and seeks to destroy the invading organism or repair the affected part.

e. Healing is done by the patient.

f. Health is the absence of disease.

6. Which of the following methods would be a CAT approach to an illness? *(Select all that apply.)*

a. Acupuncture

b. Heart medications

c. Rest and fluids

d. Herbs

e. Surgery

f. Decongestants

DEVELOPING YOUR KNOWLEDGE BASE

FILL-IN-THE-BLANKS

1. In traditional Chinese medicine, the characteristics of the _____ are cool, moist, and dark.

2. _____ is the theory and philosophy that focuses on connections and interactions between the parts of the whole.

3. _____ consists of placing very thin, short, sterile needles at particular points believed to be centers of nerve and vascular tissue.

4. _____ involves using all five senses to depict an event or body process unfolding according to a plan.

5. _____ are chemical compounds that contain ingredients believed to promote health.

6. _____ is the technique of using essential oils for medicinal purposes.

MATCHING EXERCISES

Match the CAT in Part A with its description listed in Part B.

PART A

a. Ayurveda

b. Yoga

c. Traditional Chinese medicine

d. Acupuncture

e. Qi gong

f. Homeopathy

g. Naturopathy

PART B

1. ___ Uses thin, short, sterile needles, placed at centers of nerve and vascular tissue

2. ___ Based on the belief of supporting the body while the symptoms are allowed to run their course

3. ___ Consists of a set of exercises that promote health through various physical postures

4. ___ A system of postures, exercises (gentle and dynamic), breathing techniques, and visualization

5. ___ Understanding the patient's basic constitution or "dosha" is the central theme

6. ___ Qi (energy) is the central theme.

SHORT ANSWER

1. Define the following concepts and their basic philosophy of medicine.

a. Allopathy: _____

_____

_____

b. Holism: _____

_____

_____

c. Integrative care: _____

_____

_____

2. Briefly describe the following CATs and related nursing considerations.

a. Ayurveda: _____

_____

Nursing considerations: _____

_____

b. Yoga: _____

_____

Nursing considerations: _____

_____

c. Traditional Chinese medicine: _____

_____

Nursing considerations: _____

_____

d. Qi gong: _____

_____

Nursing considerations: _____

_____

3. Describe three mind–body therapies you might use for a patient experiencing unrelieved pain due to chemotherapy.

a. _____

_____

b. _____

_____

c. _____

_____

4. Describe the four scientific principles used in Therapeutic Touch.

a. _____

b. _____

c. _____

d. _____

5. Describe how the nursing care plan would differ for a patient diagnosed with leukemia when using the following three different spiritual approaches.

a. Shamanism: _____

_____

b. Native American tradition: _____

_____

c. Intercessory prayer: _____

_____

6. Explain why the following therapies might be used to heal patients.

a. Nutritional therapy: _____

_____

b. Aromatherapy: _____

_____

c. Music: _____

_____

d. Humor: _____

_____

7. List and give an example of the four types or domains of CAT described by the NCCAM.

a. _____

_____

b. _____

_____

c. _____

_____

d. _____

_____

APPLYING YOUR KNOWLEDGE

CRITICAL THINKING QUESTIONS

1. Discuss how you might change your nursing plan to include CAT when treating the following patients.

a. A 42-year-old man with end-stage AIDS who is receiving hospice care at home

b. A 7-year-old girl diagnosed with juvenile diabetes who must learn to self-administer insulin

c. A 75-year-old man with Alzheimer's disease who is living in a nursing home

2. Discuss the blended skills you would need to care for a patient when incorporating the following spiritual approaches into the plan of care.

a. Shamanism

b. Native American tradition

c. Intercessory prayer

REFLECTIVE PRACTICE USING CRITICAL THINKING SKILLS

Use the following expanded scenario from Chapter 28 in your textbook to answer the questions below.

Scenario: Sylvia Puentes is a middle-aged woman scheduled to undergo abdominal surgery next week. She comes to the outpatient clinic for preoperative evaluation and laboratory testing. During the nursing interview, she says, "I'm really anxious about the surgery, but I don't want to take any medicines. Is there anything I can do to help me relax?" She also says she would like to learn about new therapies for treating her pain postoperatively.

1. What type of Complementary and Alternative Therapies might the nurse suggest to promote relaxation for Ms. Puentes?

_____

_____

_____

2. What would be a successful outcome for Ms. Puentes?

_____

_____

_____

3. What intellectual, technical, interpersonal, and/or ethical/legal competencies are most likely to bring about the desired outcome?

_____

_____

_____

4. What resources might be helpful for Ms. Puentes?

_____

_____

_____

CHAPTER 29

Medications

PRACTICING FOR NCLEX

MULTIPLE CHOICE QUESTIONS

Circle the letter that corresponds to the best answer for each question.

1. Which of the following is the name assigned to a drug by the manufacturer that first develops it?
   a. Trade name
   b. Official name
   c. Chemical name
   d. Generic name

2. Most drugs are excreted through which of the following organs?
   a. Kidneys
   b. Lungs
   c. Intestines
   d. Skin

3. Which of the following acts designated the United States Pharmacopeia and the National Formulary as official standards of drugs and empowered the federal government to enforce these standards?
   a. Federal Food, Drug, and Cosmetic Act
   b. Food and Drug Administration
   c. Pure Food and Drug Act
   d. Comprehensive Drug Abuse Prevention and Control Act

4. Which of the following statements about patient medications is accurate?
   a. Safe practice dictates that a nurse follows written or verbal orders.

   b. In most settings, student nurses are permitted to accept verbal orders from a physician.
   c. When a patient is admitted to a hospital, all drugs that the physician may have ordered while the patient was at home are continued.
   d. Upon admittance to a hospital, all patient medications from home should be sent home with the family or placed in safekeeping.

5. Which of the following types of medication orders would a physician prescribe for "as needed" pain medication?
   a. Standing order
   b. PRN order
   c. Single order
   d. Stat order

6. A nurse suspects a drug he/she administered to a patient is in error. Who is legally responsible for the error?
   a. Nurse
   b. Physician
   c. Hospital
   d. Pharmacist

7. Which of the following measurement systems uses a grain as the basic unit of weight?
   a. Metric
   b. Apothecary
   c. Household
   d. Decimal

8. If a nurse is preparing medication for a patient and is called away to an emergency, which of the following should he/she do?

   a. Have another nurse guard the preparations.

   b. Put the medications back in the containers.

   c. Have another nurse finish preparing and administering the medications.

   d. Lock the medications in a room and finish them when he/she returns.

9. Before administering a drug to a patient, the nurse should identify the patient by doing which of the following?

   a. Call the patient by name.

   b. Check the patient's ID bracelet.

   c. Check the patient's record.

   d. Check the patient's name with family or significant others.

10. Which means of drug administration would be used in an emergency to achieve rapid absorption and quicker results?

    a. Injection

    b. Oral

    c. Patch

    d. Inhalation

11. Which of the following sites is recommended for adults as a safe site for the majority of intramuscular injections?

    a. Vastus lateralis site

    b. Deltoid muscle site

    c. Ventrogluteal site

    d. Dorsogluteal site

12. Mrs. Harris is a 78-year-old woman admitted to your unit after experiencing symptoms of stroke. When administering the medication prescribed for her, the nurse should be aware that this patient has an increased possibility of drug toxicity due to which of the following age-related factors?

    a. Decreased adipose tissue and increased total body fluid in proportion to total body mass

    b. Increased number of protein-binding sites

    c. Increased kidney function, resulting in excessive filtration and excretion

    d. Decline in liver function and production of enzymes needed for drug metabolism

13. To convert 0.8 grams to milligrams, the nurse should do which of the following?

    a. Move the decimal point 2 places to the right.

    b. Move the decimal point 3 places to the right.

    c. Move the decimal point 2 places to the left.

    d. Move the decimal point 3 places to the left.

14. Mr. Downs is given a dose of gentamicin and has an immediate reaction of hypotension, bronchospasms, and rapid, thready pulse. Which of the following would be the drugs of choice for this situation?

    a. Antibiotic, antihistamines, and Isuprel

    b. Bronchodilators, antihistamines, and vasodilators

    c. Epinephrine, antihistamines, and bronchodilators

    d. Antihistamines, vasodilators, and bronchoconstrictors

15. Mrs. Banks has an order for Chloromycetin, 500 mg every 6 hours. The drug comes in 250-mg capsules. Which of the following would be the correct dosage?

    a. 1 tab

    b. 2 tabs

    c. 3 tabs

    d. 4 tabs

16. An oral medication has been ordered for Mr. Moran, who has a nasogastric tube in place. Which of the following nursing activities would increase the safety of medication administration?

    a. Check the tube placement before administration.

    b. Have Mr. Moran swallow the pills around the tube.

    c. Flush the tube with 30 to 40 mL saline before medication administration.

    d. Bring the liquids to room temperature before administration.

17. When giving an intramuscular injection using the Z-track technique, the nurse should use which of the following techniques?

    a. Use a needle at least 1 inch long.

    b. Apply pressure to the injection site.

c. Inject the medication quickly, and steadily withdraw the needle.

d. Do not massage the site because it may cause irritation.

ALTERNATE-FORMAT QUESTIONS

Multiple Response Questions

Circle the letters that correspond to the best answers for each question.

1. Which of the following statements accurately describe the influence of specific factors on the absorption of a drug? *(Select all that apply.)*

   a. Injected medications are usually absorbed more rapidly than oral medications.

   b. Liquid preparations have to be dissolved in the gastrointestinal fluids.

   c. The unionized form of drugs is absorbed more readily.

   d. Acidic drugs are well absorbed in the stomach.

   e. Food in the stomach always delays the absorption of medications.

   f. A trough level is the point when a drug is at its highest concentration.

2. Which of the following statements accurately describe an adverse drug effect? *(Select all that apply.)*

   a. A drug allergy is always manifested immediately after the patient receives the medication.

   b. An anaphylactic reaction is a life-threatening immediate reaction to a drug that results in respiratory distress, sudden severe bronchospasm, and cardiovascular collapse.

   c. Drug tolerance occurs when the body cannot metabolize one dose of a drug before another dose is administered.

   d. A cumulative effect occurs when the body becomes accustomed to a particular drug over a period of time.

   e. An idiosyncratic effect is any abnormal or peculiar response to a drug that may manifest itself by over response, under response, or a response different from the expected outcome.

   f. An antagonistic effect occurs when the combined effect of two or more drugs acting simultaneously produces an effect that is less than that of each drug alone.

3. Which of the following is a type of order that a physician might write? *(Select all that apply.)*

   a. A standing order to be carried out as specified until canceled by another order

   b. A prn order for pain medication

   c. A single order to be carried out only once at a specified time

   d. A stat order to be carried out at a predetermined later date

   e. A double order to increase the dosage of the medication being administered

   f. A floating order to administer medication as needed

4. Which of the following factors should a nurse consider when administering medications to an older adult? *(Select all that apply.)*

   a. An increased number of protein-binding sites

   b. An increased difficulty with the penetration of fat-soluble drugs

   c. Altered peripheral venous tone

   d. A decline in liver function

   e. A decline in enzyme production needed for drug metabolism

   f. An increased gastric emptying time

5. Which of the following actions would a nurse be expected to perform when instilling eyedrops correctly? *(Select all that apply.)*

   a. Wash hands and put on gloves.

   b. Clean the eyelids and eyelashes of any drainage with cotton balls soaked in clean water.

   c. Tilt the patient's head back slightly if sitting or place the head on a pillow if lying down.

   d. Have the patient look up and focus on something on the ceiling.

   e. Place the thumb near the margin of the lower eyelid and exert pressure upward over the bony prominence of the cheek.

   f. Squeeze the container and allow the prescribed number of drops to fall into the cornea.

6. Which of the following actions would a nurse be expected to perform when instilling eardrops correctly? *(Select all that apply.)*

   a. Make sure the solution to be instilled is at room temperature.

   b. Clean the external ear with cotton balls moistened with normal saline solution.

c. Place the patient on the affected side in bed.

d. Draw up the amount of solution needed in the dropper and return any excess medication to the stock bottle.

e. Straighten the auditory canal by pulling the cartilaginous portion of the pinna up and back in an adult and down and back in an infant or child under 3 years.

f. Hold the dropper in the ear with its tip above the auditory canal.

7. Which of the following actions would a nurse be expected to perform when administering a subcutaneous injection correctly? *(Select all that apply.)*

a. If using the outer aspect of the upper arm, place the patient's arm over the chest with the outer area exposed.

b. Remove the needle cap with the dominant hand, pulling it straight off.

c. Grasp and bunch the area surrounding the injection site or spread the skin at the site.

d. Inject the needle quickly at an angle of 45 to 90 degrees.

e. If blood appears when aspirating, withdraw the needle and reinject it at another site.

f. After removing the needle, massage the area gently with the alcohol swab unless it is a subcutaneous heparin or insulin injection site.

8. Which of the following are components of a medication order? *(Select all that apply.)*

a. The full name of the patient

b. The date and sometimes the time when the order is written

c. Preferably the brand name of the drug to be administered

d. The dosage of the drug, stated in either the apothecary or metric system

e. The route by which the drug is to be administered, only if there is more than one route possible

f. The signature of the nurse carrying out the order

Fill-in-the-Blank Questions

A physician has ordered medications in certain amounts. You have them on hand but in different quantities. Make the necessary conversions and write what you will give to each patient on the line provided.

1. Order: gentamicin 60 mg. On hand: gentamicin 80 mg/2 cc. Give patient: _____

2. Order: Mestinon 30 mg. On hand: Mestinon 60 mg/tab. Give patient: _____

3. Order: amitriptyline 75 mg. On hand: amitriptyline 25 mg/tab. Give patient: _____

4. Order: phenylbutazone 250 mg. On hand: phenylbutazone 500 mg/tab. Give patient: _____

5. Order: Pro-Banthine 15 mg. On hand: Pro-Banthine 5 mg/tab. Give patient: _____

6. Order: penicillin V 250 mg. On hand: penicillin V 500 mg/tab. Give patient: _____

7. Order: Lanoxin 0.125 mg. On hand: Lanoxin 0.250 mg/tab. Give patient: _____

8. Order: metaproterenol sulfate 20 mg. On hand: metaproterenol sulfate 10 mg/tab. Give patient: _____

9. Order: ACTH 40 mg. On hand: ACTH 10 mg/cc. Give patient: _____

DEVELOPING YOUR KNOWLEDGE BASE

MATCHING EXERCISES

Match the types of drug preparations in Part A with their descriptions listed in Part B.

PART A

a. Capsule

b. Elixir

c. Liniment

d. Lotion

e. Ointment

f. Tablet

g. Pill

h. Powder

i. Solution

j. Suppository

k. Suspension

l. Syrup

m. Enteric coated

PART B

1. _____ Small, solid dose of medication; compressed or molded; may be any size or shape, or enteric coated

2. _____ Powder or gel form of an active drug enclosed in a gelatinous container

3. _____ Medication mixed with alcohol, oil, or soap, which is rubbed on the skin

4. _____ Finely divided, undissolved particles in a liquid medium; should be shaken before use

5. _____ Medication in a clear liquid containing water, alcohol, sweeteners, and flavoring

6. _____ An easily melted medication preparation in a firm base, such as gelatin, that is inserted into the body

7. _____ Drug particles in a solution for topical use

8. _____ Mixture of a powdered drug with a cohesive material; may be round or oval

9. _____ A drug dissolved in another substance

10. _____ Single drug or mixture of finely ground drugs

11. _____ Medication combined with water and sugar solution

12. _____ Tablet or pill that prevents stomach irritation

Match the types of injections listed in Part A with their injection site listed in Part B.

PART A

a. Subcutaneous injection

b. Intramuscular injection

c. Intradermal injection

d. Intravenous injection

e. Intra-arterial injection

f. Intracardial injection

g. Intraperitoneal injection

h. Intraspinal injection

i. Intraosseous injection

PART B

13. _____ Corium

14. _____ Bone

15. _____ Muscle tissue

16. _____ Artery

17. _____ Heart tissue

18. _____ Vein

19. _____ Peritoneal cavity

20. _____ Subcutaneous tissue

SHORT ANSWER

1. List three categories for drug classification.

   a. _____

   b. _____

   c. _____

2. Explain the following processes by which drugs alter cell physiology.

   a. Drug–receptor interactions: _____

   _____

   b. Drug–enzyme interactions: _____

   _____

3. Give an example of how the following factors affect drug action.

   a. Developmental stage of patient: _____

   _____

   b. Weight: _____

   _____

c. Sex: _____

_____

d. Genetic and cultural factors: _____

_____

e. Psychological factors: _____

_____

f. Pathology: _____

_____

g. Environment: _____

_____

h. Time of administration: _____

_____

4. Give three examples of situations in which you would question a medical order.

a. _____

b. _____

c. _____

5. Briefly describe the following three types of medication supply systems.

a. Stock supply system: _____

_____

b. Individual supply system: _____

_____

c. Unit-dose system: _____

_____

6. List the three checks and five rights of administering medication.

a. Three checks: _____

_____

_____

b. Five rights: _____

_____

_____

_____

7. Your patient tells you she refuses to take the medication prescribed for her because it tastes "disgusting." List three techniques you could use to mask the taste.

a. _____

b. _____

c. _____

8. Explain how the following factors would affect the type of equipment a nurse would choose for an injection.

a. Route of administration: _____

_____

b. Viscosity of the solution: _____

_____

c. Quantity to be administered: _____

_____

d. Body size: _____

_____

e. Type of medication: _____

_____

9. List four steps that should be followed when a medication error occurs.

a. _____

b. _____

c. _____

d. _____

10. Describe the use of the following types of prepackaged medications.

a. Ampules: _____

_____

b. Vials: _____

_____

c. Prefilled cartridges: _____

_____

11. Transcribe the following medication orders on the patient medication record below and sign for the medications you would administer in a 24-hour period. Be prepared to discuss administration guidelines.

Tenormin, 50 mg, PO od

HydroDIURIL, 50 mg, PO od

NPH Insulin U100, 45 units SQ daily in AM

Regular Insulin U100, 10 units SQ stat

Cipro, 500 mg, PO q12h

Timoptic 0.25% gtt OD bid

Dalmane, 30 mg, PO hs, prn

Nitro-paste ½ inch, q8h to chest wall

Tylenol with codeine #2, PO q4h, prn

Colace, 100 mg, PO od

Medical Administration Record

Ord date	PRN MEDS.		
		Date	
		Time	
		Init / Site	
		Date	
		Time	
		Init / Site	

SINGLE ORDERS—PREOPERATIVES

Ord date	Medication—Dosage—Route of Admin	Date/Time	Site/Initials

INJECTION SITES MUST BE CHARTED

Ord date	ROUTINE MEDICATIONS Medication—Dosage—Route of Admin	Hr	Date/Time						

12. You are preparing Jim Toole for discharge. He will be taking the following medications at home: Xanax, Zantac, and Cipro. Use the chart below to identify the information you will need to teach him about these medications. Use a pharmacology text for medication information.

Method	Xanax	Zantac	Cipro
Dosage			
Route of administration			
Frequency/schedule			
Desired effects			
Possible adverse effects			
Signs and symptoms of toxic drug effects			
Special instructions			
Recommended course of action with problems			

APPLYING YOUR KNOWLEDGE

CRITICAL THINKING QUESTIONS

1. Think about your responsibilities when administering medication and then describe how you would respond in the following situations:

   a. A physician who is in a hurry prescribes a medication for your patient. After he leaves, you read the order and don't understand why your patient would need the medication prescribed. Because you are legally responsible for medications administered, what would you do?

   b. You bring a medication to a patient, who tells you, "That's not my pill." What would you do?

2. Medication errors are not uncommon and may be lethal. Interview several nurses about their experiences with errors and what contributes to them. Think about how nurses individually and collectively can act to reduce errors. Develop a plan with your classmates to help minimize these errors.

REFLECTIVE PRACTICE USING CRITICAL THINKING SKILLS

Use the following expanded scenario from Chapter 29 in your textbook to answer the questions below.

Scenario: François Baptiste is an elderly man with a wound infection requiring intravenous antibiotic therapy. He is scheduled to receive his next dose at 10 a.m. The medication delivered by the pharmacy is labeled with the correct drug and dose, but with another patient's name. The nurse checks the patient identification band, and notes that it does not match the medication label.

1. How might the nurse use blended nursing skills to respond to this medication error.

   _____

   _____

   _____

2. What would be a successful outcome for this patient?

   _____

   _____

   _____

3. What intellectual, technical, interpersonal, and/or ethical/legal competencies are most likely to bring about the desired outcome?

   _____

   _____

   _____

CHAPTER 30

Perioperative Nursing

PRACTICING FOR NCLEX

MULTIPLE CHOICE QUESTIONS

Circle the letter that corresponds to the best choice for each question.

1. Which of the following types of anesthesia is administered by injecting a local anesthetic around a nerve trunk supplying the area of surgery?

   a. Nerve block

   b. Subdural block

   c. Surface anesthesia

   d. Local infiltration with lidocaine

2. When obtaining a consent form from a patient scheduled to undergo surgery, the nurse should consider which of the following facts?

   a. A consent form is legal, even if the patient is confused or sedated.

   b. The form that is signed is not a legal document and would not hold up in court.

   c. In emergency situations, the doctor may obtain consent over the telephone.

   d. The responsibility for securing informed consent from the patient lies with the nurse.

3. A 9-month-old baby is scheduled for heart surgery. When preparing this patient for surgery, the nurse should consider which of the following surgical risks associated with infants?

   a. Prolonged wound healing

   b. Potential for hypothermia or hyperthermia

   c. Congestive heart failure

   d. Gastrointestinal upset

4. Mr. Lemke, age 42, is scheduled for elective hernia surgery. While taking a medical history for Mr. Lemke, you find out he is taking antibiotics for an infection. To which of the following surgical risks would Mr. Lemke be predisposed because of his use of antibiotics?

   a. Hemorrhage

   b. Electrolyte imbalances

   c. Cardiovascular collapse

   d. Respiratory paralysis

5. When preparing a patient who has diabetes mellitus for surgery, the nurse should be aware of which of the following potential surgical risks associated with this disease?

   a. Fluid and electrolyte imbalance

   b. Slow wound healing

   c. Respiratory depression from anesthesia

   d. Altered metabolism and excretion of drugs

6. Mr. Pete is an obese 62-year-old man scheduled for heart surgery. Which of the following surgical risks related to obesity should be considered when performing an assessment for this patient?

   a. Delayed wound healing and wound infection

   b. Alterations in fluid and electrolyte balance

   c. Respiratory distress

   d. Hemorrhage

7. When teaching a postoperative patient about pain control, the nurse should consider which of the following statements?

   a. When giving pain medication p.r.n., the patient should ask for the medication when the pain becomes severe.

   b. The nurse is responsible for ordering and administering pain medications.

   c. Medications for pain usually are given by injection for the first few days or as long as the patient is NPO.

   d. Alternate pain control methods, such as TENS and PCA, should not be used after surgery.

8. To prevent postoperative complications, which of the following measures should be taken after surgery?

   a. The patient should be instructed to avoid coughing if possible to minimize damage to the incision.

   b. The patient should take shallow breaths to prevent collapse of the alveoli.

   c. The patient should be instructed to do leg exercises to increase venous return.

   d. The patient should not be turned in bed until the incision is no longer painful.

9. Which of the following is the most common postanesthesia recovery emergency?

   a. Respiratory obstruction

   b. Cardiac distress

   c. Wound infection

   d. Dehydration

10. Mr. Fischer has returned to your unit after cardiac surgery. Which of the following interventions would be appropriate to prevent cardiovascular complications for him?

    a. Position him in bed with pillows placed under his knees to hasten venous return.

    b. Keep him from ambulating until the day after surgery.

    c. Implement leg exercises and turn him in bed every 2 hours.

    d. Keep him cool and uncovered to prevent elevated temperature.

11. Which of the following interventions should be carried out by the nurse when a postoperative patient is in shock?

    a. Remove extra coverings on the patient to keep temperature down.

    b. Place the patient in a flat position with legs elevated 45 degrees.

    c. Do not administer any further medication.

    d. Place the patient in the Trendelenburg or "shock" position.

12. Which of the following is a recommended physical preparation for a patient undergoing surgery?

    a. Shave the area of the incision with a razor.

    b. Empty the patient's bowel of feces.

    c. Do not allow the patient to eat or drink anything for 8 to 12 hours before surgery.

    d. Be sure the patient is well nourished and hydrated.

13. Which of the following preoperative medications would be prescribed to decrease pulmonary and oral secretions and prevent laryngospasm?

    a. Narcotic analgesics

    b. Anticholinergics

    c. Neuroleptanalgesic agents

    d. Histamine-receptor antihistaminics

14. Which of the following positions would be used in minimally invasive surgery of the lower abdomen or pelvis?

    a. Trendelenburg position

    b. Sims' position

    c. Lithotomy position

    d. Prone position

15. Which of the following would be an appropriate reaction to a patient experiencing pulmonary embolus?

    a. Try to overhydrate the patient with fluids.

    b. Instruct the patient to perform Valsalva's maneuver.

    c. Place the patient in semi-Fowler's position.

    d. Assist the patient to ambulate every 2 to 3 hours.

16. Your postsurgical patient is experiencing decreased lung sounds, dyspnea, cyanosis, crackles, restlessness, and apprehension. Which of the following conditions would you diagnose?

    a. Atelectasis

    b. Pneumonia

    c. Pulmonary embolus

    d. Thrombophlebitis

ALTERNATE-FORMAT QUESTIONS

Multiple Response Questions

Circle the letters that correspond to the best answers for each question.

1. Which of the following actions would be performed in the postoperative phase of the perioperative period? *(Select all that apply.)*
   a. The nurse prepares the patient for home care.
   b. The physician informs the patient that surgical intervention is necessary.
   c. The patient is transferred to the recovery room.
   d. The patient is admitted to the recovery area.
   e. The patient begins to emerge from anesthesia.
   f. The patient participates in a rehabilitation program after surgery.

2. Which of the following examples of surgery would be classified as surgical procedures based on purpose? *(Select all that apply.)*
   a. Control of hemorrhage
   b. Breast biopsy
   c. Cleft palate repair
   d. Colostomy
   e. Tracheostomy
   f. Breast reconstruction

3. Regional anesthesia may be accomplished through which of the following methods? *(Select all that apply.)*
   a. Inhalation
   b. Spinal block
   c. Intravenous
   d. Oral route
   e. Nerve block
   f. Epidural block

4. Which of the following pieces of information must be provided to a patient to obtain informed consent? *(Select all that apply.)*
   a. A description of the procedure or treatment, along with potential alternative therapies
   b. The name and qualifications of the nurse providing perioperative care

   c. The underlying disease process and its natural course
   d. Explanation of the risks involved and how often they occur
   e. Explanation that a signed consent form is binding and cannot be withdrawn
   f. Customary insurance coverage for the procedure

5. Which of the following statements accurately describe the surgical risks related to the developmental stage of the patient? *(Select all that apply.)*
   a. Infants are at a greater risk from surgery than are middle-aged adults.
   b. Infants experience a slower metabolism of drugs that require renal biotransformation.
   c. Muscle relaxants and narcotics have a shorter duration of action in infants.
   d. Older adults have decreased renal blood flow and a reduced bladder capacity, necessitating careful monitoring of fluid and electrolyte status and input and output.
   e. Older adults have an increased gastric pH and require monitoring of nutritional status during the perioperative period.
   f. Older adults have an increased hepatic blood flow, liver mass, and enzyme function that prolongs the duration of medication effects.

6. Which of the following statements accurately describe how preexisting disease states affect surgical risk? *(Select all that apply.)*
   a. Cardiovascular diseases increase the risk for dehydration after surgery.
   b. Patients with respiratory disease may experience alterations in acid–base balance after surgery.
   c. Kidney and liver diseases influence the patient's response to anesthesia.
   d. Endocrine diseases increase the risk for hyperglycemia after surgery.
   e. Endocrine diseases increase the risk for slow surgical wound healing.
   f. Pulmonary disorders increase the risk for hemorrhage and hypovolemic shock after surgery.

7. Which of the following statements accurately describe the effects the patient's medications may have on surgical risk? *(Select all that apply.)*

   a. Diuretics may precipitate hemorrhage.

   b. Anticoagulants may cause electrolyte imbalances.

   c. Diuretics may cause respiratory depression from anesthesia.

   d. Tranquilizers may increase the hypotensive effect of anesthetic agents.

   e. Adrenal steroids may cause respiratory paralysis.

   f. Abrupt withdrawal from adrenal steroids may cause cardiovascular collapse in long-term users.

8. Which of the following are significant abnormal findings related to presurgical screening tests? *(Select all that apply.)*

   a. An elevated white blood cell count, indicating an infection

   b. Decreased hematocrit and hemoglobin level, indicating bleeding or anemia

   c. Increased hyperkalemia or hypokalemia, indicating possible renal failure

   d. Elevated blood urea nitrogen or creatinine levels, indicating an increased risk for cardiac problems

   e. Abnormal urine constituents, indicating infection or fluid imbalances

   f. Increased hemoglobin level, indicating infection

9. Which of the following nursing interventions would be appropriate for a patient recovering from a surgical procedure? *(Select all that apply.)*

   a. Teach the patient to suppress urges to cough in order to protect the incision.

   b. Encourage the patient to take frequent shallow breaths to improve lung expansion and volume.

   c. Place the patient in a semi-Fowler's position to perform deep-breathing exercises every 1 to 2 hours for the first 24 to 48 hours after surgery and as necessary thereafter.

   d. Encourage the patient to lie still in bed with the incision facing upward to prevent putting pressure on the stitches.

   e. Teach the patient the appropriate leg exercises to increase venous blood return from the legs.

   f. Encourage the patient to use incentive spirometry 10 times each waking hour for the first 5 days after surgery.

Prioritization Questions

1. Place the following guidelines for teaching a patient deep breathing in the order in which they would be performed:

   a. Ask the patient to inhale through the nose gently and completely.

   b. Place the patient in semi-Fowler's position with the neck and shoulders supported.

   c. Ask the patient to exhale gently and completely.

   d. Repeat this exercise three times every 1 to 2 hours.

   e. Ask the patient to place the hands over the rib cage so he/she can feel the chest rise as the lungs expand.

   f. Ask the patient to exhale as completely as possible through the mouth with lips pursed (as if whistling).

   g. Ask the patient to hold his or her breath for 3 to 5 seconds and mentally count "one, one thousand, two, one thousand, etc."

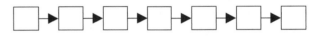

2. Place the following guidelines for teaching a patient effective coughing in the order in which they would be performed:

   a. Ask the patient to "hack out" for three short breaths.

   b. Repeat the exercise every 2 hours while awake.

   c. Place the patient in a semi-Fowler's position, leaning forward and provide a pillow or bath blanket to splint the incision.

   d. Ask the patient to cough deeply once or twice and take another deep breath.

   e. Ask the patient to take a quick breath with mouth open.

   f. Ask the patient to inhale and exhale deeply and slowly through the nose three times.

   g. Ask the patient to take a deep breath and hold it for 3 seconds.

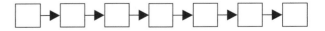

DEVELOPING YOUR KNOWLEDGE BASE

FILL-IN-THE-BLANKS

1. _____ is the name for the wide variety of nursing interventions carried out before, during, and after surgery.

2. Surgical procedures are usually classified according to _____, _____, and _____.

3. Surgery that is planned and based on the patient's choice is classified as _____.

4. Surgery is classified as minor or major based on _____.

5. _____ anesthesia does not cause narcosis but results in analgesia and reflex loss.

6. The three stages of general anesthesia are _____, _____, and _____.

7. A patient who is scheduled for a colonoscopy would most likely receive what type of sedation? _____.

8. _____ is a patient's voluntary agreement to undergo a particular procedure or treatment after receiving the appropriate information from the physician.

9. Two common forms of advance directives are _____ and _____.

MATCHING EXERCISES

Match the type of nurse listed in Part A with the role he/she performs listed in Part B. Answers may be used more than once.

PART A

a. Scrub nurse
b. Circulating nurse
c. RNFA
d. APN
e. PA

PART B

1. ___ Member of the sterile team who maintains surgical asepsis while draping and handling instruments and supplies

2. ___ Actively assists the surgeon by providing exposure, hemostasis, and wound closure

3. ___ Coordinates care activities and collaborates with physicians and nurses in all phases of perioperative and postanesthesia care

4. ___ Assesses the patient on admission to the operating room and collaborates in safely positioning the patient on the operating bed

5. ___ Integrates case management, critical paths, and research into care of the surgical patient

6. ___ Assists with monitoring the patient during surgery, provides additional supplies, and maintains environmental safety

SHORT ANSWER

1. Briefly describe the time period for the following stages of the perioperative period.

   a. Preoperative phase: _____

   b. Intraoperative phase: _____

   c. Postoperative phase: _____

2. Give a brief description of the following types of surgery.

   a. Based on urgency: _____

   b. Based on degree of risk: _____

   c. Based on purpose: _____

3. Describe the following three phases of anesthesia.

   a. Induction: _____

   b. Maintenance: _____

   c. Emergence: _____

4. Your patient is undergoing surgery to remove a lump from her breast. List four areas of information that should be given to the patient when securing informed consent.

   a. _____

   b. _____

   c. _____

   d. _____

5. Indicate how each of the following diseases places the patient at greater risk for postoperative complications.

   a. Cardiovascular disease: _____

   _____

   _____

   b. Pulmonary disorders: _____

   _____

   _____

   c. Kidney and liver function disorders: _____

   _____

   _____

   d. Metabolic disorders: _____

   _____

   _____

6. Explain how you would help your patient overcome the following fears experienced in the preoperative phase.

   a. Fear of the unknown: _____

   _____

   b. Fear of pain and death: _____

   _____

   c. Fear of changes in body image and self-concept: _____

   _____

7. Describe the nurse's role in providing screening tests for the preoperative patient.

   _____

   _____

   _____

8. Describe how you would prepare a preoperative patient for the following conditions.

   a. Surgical events and sensations: _____

   _____

   b. Pain management: _____

   _____

9. Describe how you would prepare a patient on the day of surgery in the following areas.

   a. Hygiene and skin preparation: _____

   _____

   _____

   b. Elimination: _____

   _____

   _____

   c. Nutrition and fluids: _____

   _____

   _____

   d. Rest and sleep: _____

   _____

   _____

10. Give three examples of expected outcomes for a patient during the intraoperative phase.

   a. _____

   b. _____

   c. _____

11. List the five phases that signify the return of CNS function.

   a. _____

   b. _____

   c. _____

   d. _____

   e. _____

12. Prepare a teaching plan for a postoperative patient who is moving into a home healthcare setting. Include the family in your planning.

   _____

   _____

   _____

   _____

13. Give an example of how the following factors may present a greater surgical risk for some patients.

a. Developmental considerations: _____

_____

b. Medical history: _____

_____

c. Medications: _____

_____

d. Previous surgery: _____

_____

e. Perceptions and knowledge of surgery: ___

_____

f. Lifestyle: _____

_____

g. Nutrition: _____

_____

h. Use of alcohol, illicit drugs, nicotine: ____

_____

i. Activities of daily living: _____

_____

j. Occupation: _____

_____

k. Coping patterns: _____

_____

l. Support systems: _____

_____

m. Sociocultural needs: _____

_____

14. Explain what a nurse in the PACU would assess when checking a patient in the postoperative phase using the following guidelines.

a. Vital signs: _____

_____

_____

b. Color and temperature of skin: _____

_____

c. Level of consciousness: _____

_____

d. Intravenous fluids: _____

_____

e. Surgical site: _____

_____

f. Other tubes: _____

_____

g. Pain management: _____

_____

h. Position and safety: _____

_____

i. Comfort: _____

_____

15. Give an example of two nursing interventions you would institute for a postoperative patient to help alleviate the following problems that interfere with comfort.

a. Nausea and vomiting: _____

_____

b. Thirst: _____

_____

c. Hiccups: _____

_____

d. Surgical pain: _____

_____

APPLYING YOUR KNOWLEDGE

CRITICAL THINKING QUESTIONS

1. Prepare a preoperative assessment for the patients described below. Develop a nursing care plan for each patient based on the data collected. Be sure to include preoperative care, intraoperative care, and postoperative care in your planning.

a. A 52-year-old man who smokes a pack of cigarettes a day is scheduled to undergo heart bypass surgery. The patient is overweight and says he rarely finds time to exercise.

b. A 35-year-old woman is scheduled to undergo surgery to remove a colon tumor. She underwent radiation therapy 6 weeks before the surgery date. She has a family history of colon cancer.
Reflect on how individual differences in patients influence their need for nursing and nursing's perioperative priorities.

2. Make a list of common postoperative complications. Describe how you would monitor the patient for these complications and what nursing measures you would take to prevent them. Be sure to include cardiovascular complications, shock, hemorrhage, thrombophlebitis, respiratory complications, pneumonia, atelectasis, and wound complications. Think of personal and system variables that might influence your effectiveness.

REFLECTIVE PRACTICE USING CRITICAL THINKING SKILLS

Use the following expanded scenario from Chapter 30 in your textbook to answer the questions below.

Scenario: Molly Greenbaum is a 38-year-old woman diagnosed with recurring vaginal cysts. Her physician recommends a vaginal hysterectomy to be performed on an outpatient basis. She arrives at the hospital at 6:30 a.m. and is scheduled for surgery later in the day. The patient, with tears in her eyes and wringing her hands, says, "I really didn't sleep very much last night. I kept thinking about the surgery." She tells you she has been unable to sleep or eat properly since receiving the news,

2 weeks ago, that she needed a hysterectomy. She asks the nurse, "What if I don't feel like a woman anymore? What will this do to my sex life? Is this operation really necessary?"

1. How might the nurse use blended nursing skills to implement the perioperative plan of care in a manner that respects Ms. Greenbaum's human dignity and addresses her fears and concerns about the surgical experience?

_____

_____

_____

2. What would be a successful outcome for this patient?

_____

_____

_____

3. What intellectual, technical, interpersonal, and/or ethical/legal competencies are most likely to bring about the desired outcome?

_____

_____

_____

4. What resources might be helpful for Ms. Greenbaum?

_____

_____

_____

Hygiene

PRACTICING FOR NCLEX

MULTIPLE CHOICE QUESTIONS

Circle the letter that corresponds to the best answer for each question.

1. Which of the following would be the appropriate treatment for acne?
   a. The infected areas should be gently squeezed to release the infection.
   b. A person with acne should wash his/her skin less frequently to avoid removing beneficial oils.
   c. Foods that are found to aggravate the condition should be eliminated.
   d. Cosmetics and emollients should be used to cover the condition.

2. When caring for a patient with dentures, which of the following should the nurse tell the patient?
   a. Keeping dentures out for long periods of time permits the gum line to change, affecting denture fit.
   b. Dentures should be wrapped in tissue or a disposable wipe when out of the mouth and stored in a disposable cup.
   c. Dentures should never be stored in water because the plastic material may warp.
   d. A brush and nonabrasive powder should be used to clean the dentures and hot water should be used to rinse them.

3. Which of the following is an appropriate guideline for providing perineal care for a patient?
   a. Always proceed from the most contaminated area to the least contaminated area.
   b. Do not retract the foreskin in an uncircumcised male.
   c. Dry the cleaned areas and apply an emollient as indicated.
   d. Powder the area to prevent the growth of bacteria.

4. Which of the following is an appropriate measure when providing foot care for a patient?
   a. Soak the feet in a solution of mild soap and tepid water.
   b. Rinse the feet, dry thoroughly, and apply moisturizer on the tops and bottoms.
   c. For diabetic patients, trim the nails with nail clippers.
   d. Cut off any corns or calluses.

5. When bathing your patient, you notice she has a rash on her arms. Which of the following would be an appropriate nursing intervention?
   a. Avoid washing the area because cleansing agents will only make the rash worse.
   b. Use a tepid bath to relieve inflammation and itching.
   c. Do not use over-the-counter products on unknown rashes.
   d. Use a moisturizing lotion on a wet rash to prevent itching.

6. When caring for the skin of patients of different age groups, which of the following should the nurse consider?

   a. An infant's skin and mucous membranes are protected from infection by a natural immunity.

   b. Secretions from skin glands are at their maximum from age 3 on.

   c. The skin becomes thicker and more leathery with aging and is prone to wrinkles and dryness.

   d. An adolescent's skin ordinarily has enlarged sebaceous glands and increased glandular secretions.

ALTERNATE-FORMAT QUESTIONS

Multiple Response Questions

Circle the letters that correspond to the best answers for each question.

1. Which of the following actions are appropriate steps when making an unoccupied bed? *(Select all that apply.)*

   a. First, adjust the bed to the high position and drop the side rails.

   b. Fold reusable linens on the bed in fourths and hang them over a clean chair.

   c. Snugly roll the soiled linens into the bottom sheet and place on the floor next to the bed.

   d. Place the bottom sheet with its center fold in the center of the bed and place the draw-sheet with its center fold in the center of the bed.

   e. Tuck the bottom sheets securely under the head of the mattress, forming a corner according to agency policy.

   f. Place the pillow at the head of the bed with the closed end facing toward the window.

2. Which of the following statements accurately describe appropriate environmental care for a hospitalized patient? *(Select all that apply.)*

   a. Patients should not store their personal items in the bedside stand because nurses need to open and close the stand to obtain bath basin, lotion, and other items.

   b. Patient beds should be positioned at the appropriate height with the wheels unlocked.

   c. Principles of surgical asepsis should be followed at the bedside.

   d. Soiled dressings or anything with a strong odor should not be placed in the waste receptacle in the patient's room.

   e. In general, room temperature should be between 20° and 23°C (68° and 74°F).

   f. Nurses should avoid carrying out conversations immediately outside the patient's room.

3. Which of the following statements accurately describe findings that may be made when performing a physical assessment of the oral cavity? *(Select all that apply.)*

   a. Caries may exist in the teeth, resulting from the failure to remove plaque.

   b. Gingivitis may be present involving the alveolar tissues.

   c. Hard deposits called tartar may be found on the teeth if plaque is allowed to build up.

   d. Stomatitis may be noted as an inflammation of the tongue.

   e. Cheilosis may present as reddened fissures at the angles of the mouth.

   f. Oral malignancies may be present in the form of a dry oral mucosa.

4. Which of the following are recommended guidelines when performing oral care? *(Select all that apply.)*

   a. Use a hard toothbrush to remove plaque from the teeth.

   b. Ideally, brush teeth immediately after eating or drinking.

   c. Never clean the tongue with a toothbrush.

   d. If desired, use an automatic toothbrush to remove debris and plaque from teeth.

   e. Never use water-spray units to assist with oral hygiene.

   f. If desired, use salt and sodium bicarbonate as cleaning agents for short-term use.

5. Which of the following are appropriate nursing measures when caring for a patient's eyes and ears? *(Select all that apply.)*

   a. Clean the eye from the inner canthus to the outer canthus using a wet, warm washcloth; cotton ball; or compress.

   b. Use artificial tear solution or normal saline twice a day when the blink reflex is decreased or absent.

   c. Use a protective shield if necessary to keep the lids closed when the blink reflex is absent.

   d. Use boric acid to remove excess secretions from the eyes.

   e. Clean the patient's external ear with a washcloth-covered finger.

   f. Use cotton-tipped swabs to clean the inner ear and to remove cerumen.

Prioritization Question

1. Place the following steps for assisting a patient with the removal and cleansing of dentures in the order in which they should be performed:

   a. Rinse thoroughly with water and return dentures to patient.

   b. Apply gentle pressure with a 4″ × 4″ gauze to grasp upper denture plate and remove. Place it immediately in the denture cup.

   c. Apply petroleum jelly to lips if needed.

   d. Perform hand hygiene. Don disposable gloves.

   e. Offer mouthwash so patient can rinse his or her mouth before replacing dentures.

   f. Lift the lower denture using slight rocking motion, remove, and place in the denture cup.

   g. If patient prefers, add denture cleanser to the cup with water and follow directions on preparation or brush all areas with toothbrush and paste. Place paper towels or washcloth in sink while brushing.

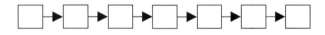

DEVELOPING YOUR KNOWLEDGE BASE

FILL-IN-THE-BLANKS

1. _____ is an inflammation of the tissue that surrounds the teeth.

2. Absence or loss of hair on the head is called baldness or _____.

3. Infestation with lice is called _____.

4. The care provided to a patient shortly before he/she retires to bed (assistance with toileting, washing face and hands, and oral care) is known as _____ care.

5. A self-contained bathing system consisting of a plastic bag containing 8 to 10 premoistened washcloths is called a _____.

MATCHING EXERCISES

Match the oral diseases/conditions in Part A with their definitions listed in Part B.

PART A

a. Stomatitis

b. Gingivitis

c. Periodontitis

d. Halitosis

e. Plaque

f. Tartar

g. Glossitis

h. Cheilosis

 i. Dry oral mucosa

j. Oral malignancies

k. Caries

 l. *Candida albicans*

PART B

1. ____ A strong mouth odor

2. ____ A marked inflammation of the gums involving the alveolar tissues

3. ____ Ulceration of the lips, most often caused by vitamin B complex deficiencies

4. ____ Lumps or ulcers

5. ____ Inflammation of the oral mucosa with numerous causes (bacteria, virus, mechanical trauma, irritants, nutritional deficiencies, and systemic infection)

6. ____ May be related to dehydration or may be caused by mouth breathing, an alteration in salivary functioning, or certain medications

7. ____ Hard deposits at the gum lines that attack the fibers that fasten teeth to the gums and eventually attack bone tissue

8. ____ An inflammation of the tissue that surrounds the teeth

9. ____ An invisible, destructive bacterial film that builds up on everyone's teeth and eventually leads to the destruction of tooth enamel

10. ____ An inflammation of the tongue

11. ____ The formation of cavities

CORRECT THE FALSE STATEMENTS

Circle the word "true" or "false" that follows the statement. If you circled "false," change the underlined word or words to make the statement true. Place your answer in the space provided.

1. The <u>sebaceous glands</u> secrete cerumen, which consists of a heavy oil and brown pigment, into the external ear canals.

   True   False _____

2. Fluid loss through fever, vomiting, or diarrhea reduces the fluid volume of the body and is called <u>dehydration</u>.

   True   False _____

3. Jaundice, a condition caused by excessive bile pigments in the skin, results in a <u>grayish</u> skin color.

   True   False _____

4. A <u>bag bath</u> consists of a plastic bag containing 10 washcloths that have been moistened with a nonrinsable cleaner and water mixture and that are warmed for a short time before use.

   True   False _____

5. Before leaving the patient's bedside, the nurse should ensure that the bed is in its <u>highest</u> position.

   True   False _____

6. The odor of perspiration occurs when <u>bacteria</u> act on the skin's normal secretions.

   True   False _____

7. <u>Dry</u> skin is especially bothersome during adolescence.

   True   False _____

8. Pressure ulcers are areas of cellular necrosis caused by <u>increased blood circulation</u> to the involved area.

   True   False _____

9. Hard contact lenses should be removed before sleeping and <u>should not be worn more than 12 to 16 hours</u>.

   True   False _____

10. Another name for baldness is <u>alopecia</u>.

    True   False _____

11. <u>Pediculus humanus capitis</u> infests the body.

    True   False _____

12. A physician who treats foot disorders is known as a <u>pediatrician</u>.

    True   False _____

13. Depending on the patient's self-care abilities, the nurse offers assistance with toileting, oral care, bathing, back massage, special skin care measures, cosmetics, dressing, and positioning for comfort during the <u>afternoon care</u> schedule.

    True   False _____

SHORT ANSWER

1. Briefly describe how the following factors may influence personal hygiene behaviors.

   a. Culture: _____

   _____

   b. Socioeconomic class: _____

   _____

   c. Spiritual practices: _____

   _____

   d. Developmental level: _____

   _____

   e. Health state: _____

   _____

   f. Personal preference: _____

   _____

2. List four specific activities necessary to meet daily needs that may be addressed as self-care deficits.

   a. _____

   b. _____

   c. _____

   d. _____

3. A mother brings her 6-month-old baby to a well-baby clinic for immunizations. Upon examining the infant, you notice dirt accumulated in the skin folds and a scaly scalp. Write a sample diagnosis for the infant's hygiene deficit. Develop a nursing care plan for the infant and mother that includes teaching hygiene. _____

_____

_____

_____

4. Describe the activities the nurse would perform in the following scheduled care time periods.

   a. Early morning care: _____

   _____

   _____

   b. Morning care: _____

   _____

   _____

   c. Afternoon care: _____

   _____

   _____

   d. Hour of sleep care: _____

   _____

   _____

   e. As-needed care: _____

   _____

   _____

5. List five benefits of bathing.

   a. _____

   b. _____

   c. _____

   d. _____

   e. _____

6. Describe how you would prepare a bed bath for a patient who is able to wash himself.

   _____

   _____

   _____

7. List four advantages of a towel bath.

   a. _____

   b. _____

   c. _____

   d. _____

8. List three benefits of a back rub.

   a. _____

   b. _____

   c. _____

9. Describe how the following conditions should be controlled in order to provide a comfortable environment for the patient.

   a. Ventilation: _____

   _____

   _____

   b. Odors: _____

   _____

   _____

   c. Room temperature: _____

   _____

   _____

   d. Lighting and noise: _____

   _____

   _____

10. You are visiting a patient at home who is recovering from heart surgery. When you prepare a bed bath for the patient, you notice her skin is dry and flaky. List four interventions you could use for this patient to prevent injury and irritation.

   a. _____

   b. _____

   c. _____

   d. _____

11. Describe the conditions you would look for when assessing the following areas.

   a. Lips: _____

   _____

b. Buccal mucosa: _____

_____

c. Gums: _____

_____

d. Tongue: _____

_____

e. Hard and soft palates: _____

_____

f. Eye: _____

_____

g. Ear: _____

_____

h. Nose: _____

_____

12. Describe how you would clean the following areas for a patient.

a. Eye: _____

_____

b. Ear: _____

_____

c. Nose: _____

_____

13. Briefly describe the care necessary for the following corrective devices.

a. Contact lenses: _____

_____

_____

b. Artificial eye: _____

_____

_____

c. Hearing aids: _____

_____

_____

d. Dentures: _____

_____

_____

14. List four variables known to cause nail and foot problems.

a. _____

b. _____

c. _____

d. _____

APPLYING YOUR KNOWLEDGE

CRITICAL THINKING QUESTIONS

1. Think about nurses' responsibility to assist patients with daily hygiene. Then reflect on how you would respond in the following situations. See if your classmates would respond as you do.

a. A same-age, opposite-sex patient requires total assistance with hygiene.

b. A patient confined to bed but able to assist with hygiene refuses to do so.

c. An elderly incontinent patient refuses your offer to assist her with perineal care.

2. Interview patients of different backgrounds or cultures to find out how they perform their daily hygiene routine. Note how their routine is similar to or different from your personal routine. What would you do to assist these people if they were placed in your care?

REFLECTIVE PRACTICE USING CRITICAL THINKING SKILLS

Use the following expanded scenario from Chapter 31 in your textbook to answer the questions below.

Scenario: Sonya Delamordo is an older Hispanic woman who has had a stroke, resulting in right-sided paralysis. She is being discharged from the hospital and will now live with her daughter, who will be her primary caretaker. Her daughter, who is eager to help her mother, asks numerous questions about how to keep her mother clean. She tells the nurse she is worried about being able to take care of her mother's fine hair, as well as her dentures and hearing aids.

1. What patient teaching should be implemented to help meet the hygienic needs of Ms. Delamordo?

   _____

   _____

   _____

2. What would be a successful outcome for this patient?

   _____

   _____

   _____

3. What intellectual, technical, interpersonal, and/or ethical/legal competencies are most likely to bring about the desired outcome?

   _____

   _____

   _____

4. What resources might be helpful for Ms. Delamordo and her daughter?

   _____

   _____

   _____

PATIENT CARE STUDY

Read the following patient care study and use your nursing process skills to answer the questions below.

Scenario: Dominic Gianmarco, a 78-year-old retired man with a history of Parkinson's disease, lives alone in a small home. He was recently hospitalized for problems with cardiac rhythm, and a pacemaker was installed. The home healthcare nurse visits 1 week after he was discharged to monitor his recovery and compliance with his medication regimen. The nurse observes that Mr. Gianmarco is disheveled and there are multiple stains on his clothing. Several food items are in various stages of preparation on the kitchen counter, and some appear to have spoiled. Mr. Gianmarco has several days' growth of beard and a body odor is apparent. He is pleasant and oriented to place and person but cannot identify the time or day of the week: "I lose track of what day it is. Time is not important when you are my age. The most important thing to me right now is to be able to take care of myself and stay in this house near my friends." There is a walker visible in a corner of the living room, but Mr. Gianmarco ambulates slowly around the house with a minimum of difficulty and does not use the walker. He comments that he keeps busy "reading, watching old movies, and going to senior citizen activities with friends who stop by for me." His daughter, who lives several hours away, visits him every weekend and prepares his medications for the week in a plastic container that is easy for him to open. The nurse observes that all the medications appeared to have been taken to date: "I don't mess around with my medicines. One helps my ticker and the others keep me from shaking so much."

1. Identify pertinent patient data by placing a single underline beneath the objective data in the case study and a double underline beneath the subjective data.

2. Complete the Nursing Process Worksheet on page 193 to develop a three-part diagnostic statement and related plan of care for this patient.

3. Write down the patient and personal nursing strengths you hope to draw upon as you assist this patient to better health.

   Patient strengths: _____

   _____

   _____

   Personal strengths: _____

   _____

   _____

4. Pretend that you are performing a nursing assessment of this patient after the plan of care is implemented. Document your findings.

   _____

   _____

   _____

NURSING PROCESS WORKSHEET

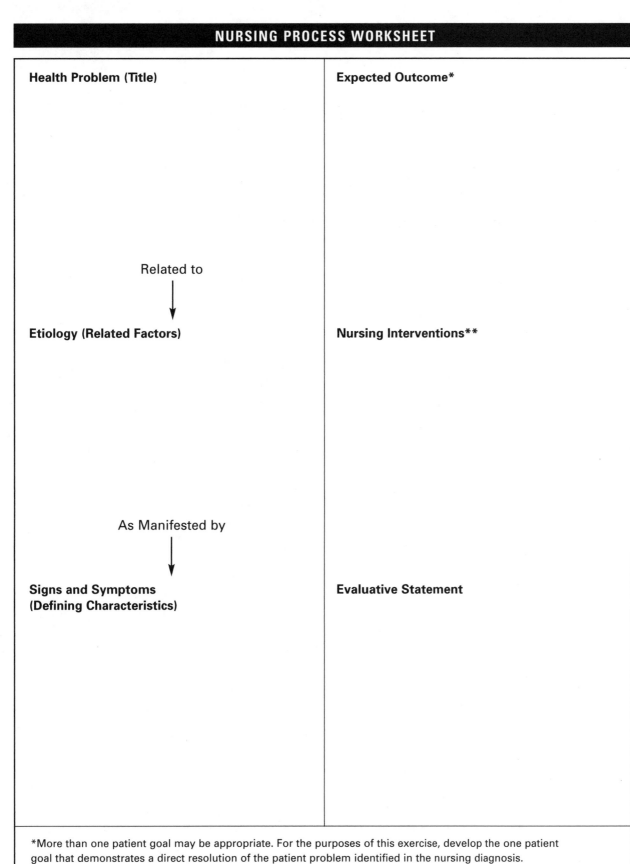

Health Problem (Title)

Related to
↓

Etiology (Related Factors)

As Manifested by
↓

**Signs and Symptoms
(Defining Characteristics)**

Expected Outcome*

Nursing Interventions**

Evaluative Statement

*More than one patient goal may be appropriate. For the purposes of this exercise, develop the one patient
goal that demonstrates a direct resolution of the patient problem identified in the nursing diagnosis.
**Be sure you are able to list the scientific rationale for each nursing intervention you ordered.

CHAPTER 32

Skin Integrity and Wound Care

PRACTICING FOR NCLEX

MULTIPLE CHOICE QUESTIONS

Circle the letter that corresponds to the best answer for each question.

1. A patient who is being treated for self-inflicted wounds admits to the nurse that she is anorexic. Which of the following criteria would alert the healthcare worker to her nutritional risk?

   a. Albumin level of 3.5 mg/dL
   b. Total lymphocyte count of 1,500/mm^3
   c. Body weight decrease of 5%
   d. Arm muscle circumference 90% of standard

2. A patient with a pressure ulcer on his back should be treated by which of the following methods?

   a. A foam wedge should be used to keep body weight off his back.
   b. A ring cushion should be used to protect reddened areas from additional pressure.
   c. The amount of time the head of the bed is elevated should be increased.
   d. Positioning devices and techniques should be used to maintain posture and distribute weight evenly for the patient in a chair.

3. When cleaning a wound, the nurse should adhere to which of the following protocols?

   a. The wound should be cleaned with each dressing change.
   b. Friction should be used with cleaning materials to loosen dead cells.
   c. Povidone–iodine or hydrogen peroxide should be used to fight infection in the wound.
   d. Irrigating devices should not be used on wounds because they damage the cells needed for healing.

4. Which of the following recommendations for wound dressing is accurate?

   a. Use wet-to-dry dressings continuously.
   b. Keep the intact, healthy skin surrounding the ulcer moist because it is susceptible to breakdown.
   c. Select a dressing that absorbs exudate, if it is present, but still maintains a moist environment.
   d. Pack wound cavities tightly with dressing material.

5. You are giving a back rub to an older patient at home and notice a stage II pressure ulcer. Which of the following treatments would you suggest for this patient?

   a. Treat the ulcer using pressure-relieving devices.
   b. Use a wet-to-dry dressing on the wound.
   c. Cover the wound with a nonadherent dressing and change every 8 to 12 hours.
   d. Maintain a moist healing environment with a saline or occlusive dressing to promote natural healing.

6. Which of the following drains provide sinus tract and would be used after incision and drainage of an abscess, in abdominal surgery?

    a. T-tube

    b. Jackson-Pratt

    c. Penrose

    d. Hemovac

7. A patient's pressure ulcer is superficial and presents clinically as an abrasion, blister, or shallow crater. It would be categorized as which of the following stages?

    a. Stage I

    b. Stage II

    c. Stage III

    d. Stage IV

8. Which of the following is an effect of applying heat to a body part?

    a. Constriction of peripheral blood vessels

    b. Reduced blood flow to tissues

    c. Increased venous congestion

    d. Increased supply of oxygen and nutrients to the area

9. Which of the following patients would be at greatest risk for developing a pressure ulcer?

    a. A newborn

    b. A patient with cardiovascular disease

    c. An older patient with arthritis

    d. A critical care patient

10. Which of the following patients would most likely develop a pressure ulcer from shearing forces?

    a. A patient sitting in a chair who slides down

    b. A patient who lifts himself up on his elbows

    c. A patient who lies on wrinkled sheets

    d. A patient who must remain on his back for long periods of time

11. A large wound with considerable tissue loss allowed to heal naturally by formation of granulation tissue would be classified as which of the following categories of wound healing?

    a. Primary intention

    b. Secondary intention

    c. Tertiary intention

    d. None of the above

12. Which of the following vitamins is needed for collagen synthesis, capillary formation, and resistance to infection?

    a. Vitamin A

    b. Vitamin B

    c. Vitamin C

    d. Vitamin K

ALTERNATE-FORMAT QUESTIONS

Multiple Response Questions

Circle the letters that correspond to the best answers for each question.

1. Which of the following statements accurately describe the effect of various factors on wound healing? *(Select all that apply.)*

    a. Children heal more rapidly than older adults.

    b. Adequate blood flow is essential for wound healing.

    c. People who are thin may heal more slowly due to the small amounts of subcutaneous and tissue fat in their bodies.

    d. Vitamins B and D are essential for re-epithelialization and collagen synthesis.

    e. People who are taking corticosteroid drugs are at high risk for delayed healing.

    f. Radiation increases bone marrow function, resulting in increased leukocytes and a decreased risk for infection.

2. Which of the following statements accurately describe the complications that may occur during wound healing? *(Select all that apply.)*

    a. Symptoms of wound infection are usually apparent within 1 to 2 weeks after the injury or surgery.

    b. Dehiscence is present when there is a partial or total disruption of wound layers.

    c. During evisceration, the viscera protrude through the incisional area.

    d. Patients who are thin are at greater risk for these complications owing to a thinner layer of tissue cells.

    e. An increase in the flow of serosanguineous fluid from the wound between postoperative days 4 and 5 is a sign of an impending evisceration.

    f. Postoperative fistula formation is most often the result of delayed healing, commonly manifested by drainage from an opening in the skin or surgical site.

3. Which of the following generally occur during normal wound healing? *(Select all that apply.)*

   a. The edges of a healing surgical wound appear clean and well approximated, with a crust along the edges.

   b. It takes approximately 2 weeks for the edges of the wound to appear normal and heal together.

   c. Increased swelling and drainage may occur during the first 5 days of the wound.

   d. The wound should not feel hot upon palpation.

   e. The inflammatory response results in the formation of exudate in the wound.

   f. Incisional pain during wound healing is usually most severe for the first 3 to 5 days and then progressively diminishes.

4. Which of the following statements describe the proper use of the various types of dressings? *(Select all that apply.)*

   a. A Surgipad is often used to cover an incision line directly.

   b. Transparent dressings are applied over ABDs to help keep the wound dry.

   c. Op-Site is often used over intravenous sites, subclavian catheter insertion sites, and noninfected healing wounds.

   d. Using appropriate aseptic techniques when changing dressings is crucial.

   e. Gauze dressings are commonly used to cover wounds.

   f. Telfa is applied to the wound to keep drainage from passing through and being absorbed by the outer layer.

5. Which of the following interventions might a nurse be expected to perform when providing competent care for a patient with a draining wound? *(Select all that apply.)*

   a. Administer a prescribed analgesic 30 to 45 minutes before changing the dressing, if necessary.

   b. Change the dressing midway between meals.

   c. Apply a protective ointment or paste, if appropriate, to cleaned skin surrounding the draining wound.

   d. Apply another layer of protective ointment or paste on top of the previous layer when changing dressings.

   e. Apply an absorbent dressing material as the first layer of the dressing.

   f. Apply a nonabsorbent material over the first layer of absorbent material.

6. Which of the following are characteristics of Y (yellow) wounds? *(Select all that apply.)*

   a. They reflect the color of normal granulation tissue.

   b. They are characterized by oozing from the tissue covering the wound.

   c. They should be cleansed by irrigating the wound and using wet-to-moist dressings and absorptive dressings.

   d. The nurse should consult with the physician about using a topical antimicrobial medication to decrease the growth of bacteria.

   e. They are covered with thick eschar.

   f. They are usually treated by using sharp, mechanical, or chemical débridement.

7. Which of the following statements accurately describe a factor in the development of a pressure ulcer? *(Select all that apply.)*

   a. Pressure ulcers usually occur over bony prominences where body weight is distributed over a small area without much subcutaneous tissue.

   b. Most pressure ulcers occur over the trochanter and calcaneus.

   c. Generally, a pressure ulcer will not appear within the first 2 days in a person who has not moved for an extended period of time.

   d. The major predisposing factor for a pressure ulcer is internal pressure applied over an area, which results in occluded blood capillaries and poor circulation to the tissues.

   e. The skin can tolerate considerable pressure without cell death, but for short periods only.

   f. The duration of pressure, compared to the amount of pressure, plays a larger role in pressure ulcer formation.

8. Which of the following statements accurately describe the formation of pressure ulcers? *(Select all that apply.)*

   a. Reactive hyperemia is considered a stage I pressure ulcer.

   b. A stage II pressure ulcer is superficial and may present as a blister or abrasion.

c. Damage to the subcutaneous tissue indicates a stage III lesion.

d. A stage III pressure ulcer presents with full-thickness skin loss.

e. If eschar is present, it may be difficult to stage a pressure ulcer.

f. The first indication that a pressure ulcer may be developing is reddening of the skin over the area under pressure.

9. Which of the following would be appropriate actions for the nurse to take when cleaning and dressing a pressure ulcer? *(Select all that apply.)*

a. Clean the wound with each dressing change using aggressive motions to remove necrotic tissue.

b. Use povidone–iodine or hydrogen peroxide to irrigate and clean the ulcer.

c. Use whirlpool treatments, if ordered, until the ulcer is considered clean.

d. Keep the ulcer tissue moist and the surrounding skin dry.

e. Select a dressing that absorbs exudate, if present, but still maintains a moist environment for healing.

f. Pack wound cavities densely with dressing material to promote tissue healing.

10. Which of the following are effects of the application of heat in wound care? *(Select all that apply.)*

a. The application of heat dilates peripheral blood vessels.

b. The application of heat decreases tissue metabolism.

c. The application of heat increases blood viscosity and capillary permeability.

d. The application of heat reduces muscle tension and helps relieve pain.

e. Extensive, prolonged heat increases cardiac output and pulse rate.

f. Extensive, prolonged heat increases blood pressure.

11. Which of the actions would a nurse be expected to perform when using cold therapy during wound care? *(Select all that apply.)*

a. Apply an ice bag for 1 hour and then remove it for about an hour before reapplying it.

b. Place a hypothermia blanket on the bed and cover it with a sheet so the patient's skin does not come in direct contact with the cold blanket.

c. Monitor the patient's rectal temperature every 15 minutes and all vital signs every 30 minutes when using a hypothermia blanket.

d. Change cold compresses frequently, continuing the application for 1 hour, and repeating the application every 2 to 3 hours as ordered.

e. Avoid wringing out cold compresses to prevent diminishing the effect of the cold.

f. In a home setting, use a bag of frozen vegetables (such as peas), if desired, as a substitute for a cold compress.

Prioritization Question

1. Place the following steps to collecting a wound culture in the order in which they should be performed.

a. Using aseptic technique, don sterile gloves and clean wound. Remove sterile gloves.

b. Explain the procedure to patient; gather equipment; perform hand hygiene.

c. Apply clean dressing to wound.

d. Perform hand hygiene. Remove all equipment and make patient comfortable.

e. Remove gloves from inside out, and discard them in plastic waste bag. Perform hand hygiene.

f. Twist cap to loosen swab in Culturette tube, or open separate swab and remove cap from culture tube, keeping inside uncontaminated. Don clean glove or new sterile glove, if necessary.

g. Label specimen container appropriately, attach laboratory requisition to tube with a rubber band or place tube in plastic bag with requisition attached; send to lab within 20 minutes.

h. Carefully insert swab into wound and roll gently. Use another swab if collecting specimen from another site.

i. Place swab in Culturette tube, being careful not to touch outside of container. Twist cap to secure; if using Culturette tube, crush ampule of medium at bottom of tube.

j. Don clean disposable gloves. Remove dressing and assess wound and drainage.

k. Record collection of specimen, appearance of wound, and description of drainage in chart.

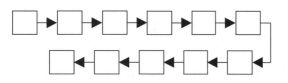

DEVELOPING YOUR KNOWLEDGE BASE

FILL-IN-THE-BLANKS

1. Wounds that result from surgery, intravenous therapy, and lumbar punctures are commonly known as _____.

2. Swelling and pain that occur from an incision are caused by an accumulation of _____.

3. In the inflammatory cellular phase of a wound, _____ or _____ cells arrive first to ingest bacteria and cellular debris.

4. New tissue found in a wound that is highly vascular, bleeds easily, and is formed in the proliferative phase is known as _____ tissue.

5. An abnormal passage from an internal organ to the skin or from one internal organ to another is known as a(n) _____.

6. Which antiseptic cleaning agent is usually used to clean a wound? _____

7. Anchoring a bandage by wrapping it around the body part with complete overlapping of the previous bandage turn is the _____ method of bandage wrapping.

8. A(n) _____ is a wound with a localized area of tissue necrosis.

MATCHING EXERCISES

Match the term in Part A with the correct definition in Part B.

PART A

a. Dehiscence

b. Ischemia

c. Eschar

d. Wound

e. Exudate

f. Granulation tissue

g. Epithelialization

h. Scar

i. Hemorrhage

j. Evisceration

k. Serous wound drainage

l. Sanguineous wound drainage

m. Purulent wound drainage

n. Red wounds

o. Yellow wounds

p. Black wounds

q. Dressing

PART B

1. ____ The partial or total disruption of wound layers

2. ____ New tissue, pink-red in color, composed of fibroblasts and small blood vessels that fill an open wound when it starts to heal

3. ____ Used as a protective cover over a wound

4. ____ The protrusion of viscera through the incisional area

5. ____ Composed of fluid and cells that escape from the blood vessels and are deposited in or on tissue surfaces

6. ____ Wounds in the proliferative stage of healing that are the color of granulation tissue

7. ____ Wound drainage that is composed of the clear, serous portion of the blood and drainage from serous membranes

8. ____ Wounds that are covered with thick eschar, which is usually black but may be brown, gray, or tan

9. ____ May occur from a slipped suture, a dislodged clot from stress at the suture line, infection, or the erosion of a blood vessel by a foreign body (such as a drain)

10. ____ Wound drainage that is made up of white blood cells, liquefied dead tissue debris, and both dead and live bacteria

11. ____ Wounds that are characterized by oozing from the tissue covering the wound, often accompanied by purulent drainage

12. ____ Necrotic tissue

13. ____ A disruption in the normal integrity of the skin

14. ____ Avascular collagen tissue that does not sweat, grow hair, or tan in sunlight

15. ____ Wound drainage that consists of large numbers of red blood cells and looks like blood

Match the wound care dressings and wraps in Part A with their definition/indication listed in Part B. Some answers may be used more than once.

PART A

a. Telfa

b. Gauze dressings

c. Sof-Wick

d. ABDs, Surgipads

e. Transparent dressings

f. Bandages

g. Binders

h. Roller bandages

PART B

16. ____ Strips of cloth, gauze, or elasticized material used to wrap a body part

17. ____ A special gauze that covers the incision line and allows drainage to pass through and be absorbed by the center absorbent layer

18. ____ Wraps designed for a specific body part

19. ____ Used to prevent outer dressings from adhering to the wound and causing further injury when removed

20. ____ Commonly used to cover wounds; they come in various sizes and are commercially packaged as single units or in packs.

21. ____ Placed over the smaller gauze to absorb drainage and protect the wound from contamination or injury

22. ____ Precut halfway to fit around drains or tubes

23. ____ Applied directly over a small wound or tube, these dressings are occlusive, decreasing the possibility of contamination while allowing visualization of the wound.

24. ____ They may be made of cloth (flannel or muslin) or an elasticized material that fastens together with Velcro.

25. ____ The type of dressing often used over intravenous sites, subclavian catheter insertion sites, and healing wounds

SHORT ANSWER

1. List six major functions of the skin.

   a. _____

   b. _____

   c. _____

   d. _____

   e. _____

   f. _____

2. Describe how the following mechanisms contribute to pressure ulcer development.

   a. External pressure: _____

   b. Friction and shearing forces: _____

   _____

3. Give an example of how the following factors affect the likelihood that a patient will develop a pressure ulcer.

   a. Nutrition: _____

   _____

   b. Hydration: _____

   _____

   c. Moisture on the skin: _____

   _____

   d. Mental status: _____

   _____

   e. Age: _____

   _____

   f. Immobility: _____

   _____

4. When visiting a patient recovering from a stroke in her home, you notice a pressure ulcer developing on her coccyx. Develop a nursing care plan for this patient that involves the family in the treatment of the ulcer.

_____

_____

_____

_____

5. Briefly describe the phases of wound healing.

   a. Hemostasis: _____

   _____

   _____

   b. Inflammatory phase: _____

   _____

   _____

   c. Proliferative phase: _____

   _____

   _____

   d. Maturation phase: _____

   _____

   _____

6. List three goals for patients who are at risk for impaired skin integrity.

   a. _____

   b. _____

   c. _____

7. Give two examples of interview questions that could be asked to assess a patient's skin integrity in the following areas.

   a. Overall appearance of the skin: _____

   _____

   _____

   b. Recent changes in skin condition: _____

   _____

   _____

   c. Activity/mobility: _____

   _____

   _____

   d. Nutrition: _____

   _____

   _____

   e. Pain: _____

   _____

   _____

   f. Elimination: _____

   _____

   _____

8. Describe how you would assess the following aspects of wound healing.

   a. Appearance: _____

   _____

   b. Wound drainage: _____

   _____

   c. Pain: _____

   _____

   d. Sutures and staples: _____

   _____

9. List the purposes for wound dressings. _____

   _____

   _____

10. Describe the RYB color classification and care of open wounds.

   a. R = red = protect: _____

   _____

   _____

   b. Y = yellow = cleanse: _____

   _____

   _____

   c. B = black = débride: _____

   _____

   _____

11. Briefly describe the use of the following methods of applying heat and any advantages or disadvantages.

   a. Hot water bags or bottles: _____

   _____

   b. Electric heating pad: _____

   _____

   c. Aquathermia pad: _____

   _____

   d. Heat lamps: _____

   _____

   e. Heat cradles: _____

   _____

   f. Hot packs: _____

   _____

   g. Warm moist compresses: _____

   _____

   h. Sitz baths: _____

   _____

   i. Warm soaks: _____

   _____

APPLYING YOUR KNOWLEDGE

CRITICAL THINKING QUESTIONS

1. Develop a nursing plan to assist the following patients who are at high risk for pressure ulcers.

   a. A comatose 35-year-old man

   b. A frail elderly man who is confined to bed

   c. A 20-year-old woman who is in a lower body cast

   d. A premature baby on life support

   What knowledge and skills do you need to prevent pressure ulcers in these patients?

2. Follow the wound care for three patients with different types of wounds (e.g., gunshot wound, a wound from surgery, a pressure ulcer). Help the nurse assess the wound each day and apply the dressings. Interview the patients to see how the wound has affected their mobility, sensory perception, activity,

nutrition, and exposure to friction and shear. Keep a log of the daily changes in the wound.

REFLECTIVE PRACTICE USING CRITICAL THINKING SKILLS

Use the following expanded scenario from Chapter 32 in your textbook to answer the questions below.

Scenario: Sam Bentz is a 56-year-old man admitted to the hospital for aggressive treatment of a bone infection that has not responded to usual methods. His wife has been taking care of him at home for the past 3 weeks. She states that the medicines the doctor prescribed made her husband feel sick to his stomach and occasionally made him throw up. She says her husband spent most of his day in bed and had no energy to get up to wash or eat. Mr. Bentz is 5 feet 4 inches tall and weighs more than 300 pounds. During the nursing assessment, he says, "Last time I was here, my skin got really irritated and I developed several skin wounds."

1. What nursing intervention would be appropriate to prevent skin irritation and the development of pressure ulcers for Mr. Bentz?

   _____

   _____

   _____

2. What would be a successful outcome for this patient?

   _____

   _____

   _____

3. What intellectual, technical, interpersonal, and/or ethical/legal competencies are most likely to bring about the desired outcome?

   _____

   _____

   _____

4. What resources might be helpful for Mr. Bentz and his wife?

   _____

   _____

   _____

PATIENT CARE STUDY

Read the following patient care study and use your nursing process skills to answer the questions below.

Scenario: Mrs. Chijioke, an 88-year-old woman who has lived alone for years, was brought to the hospital after neighbors found her lying at the bottom of her cellar steps. She had broken her hip and underwent hip repair surgery 3 days ago. The nurse assigned to care for Mrs. Chijioke noticed during the patient's bath that the skin of her coccyx, heels, and elbows was reddened. The skin returned to a normal color when pressure was relieved in these areas. There was no edema, nor was there induration or blistering. Although Mrs. Chijioke can be lifted out of bed into a chair, she spends most of the day in bed, lying on her back with an abductor pillow between her legs. At 5 feet tall and 89 pounds, Mrs. Chijioke looks lost in the big hospital bed. Her eyes are bright, and she usually attempts a warm smile, but she has little physical strength and lies seemingly motionless for hours. Her skin is wrinkled and paper thin, and her arms are bruised from unsuccessful attempts at intravenous therapy. She was dehydrated on admission because she had spent almost 48 hours crumpled at the bottom of her steps before being found by her neighbors, and she was clearly in need of nutritional, fluid, and electrolyte support.

A long-time diabetic, Mrs. Chijioke is now spiking a fever (39.0°C, or 102.2°F), which concerns her nurse.

1. Identify pertinent patient data by placing a single underline beneath the objective data in the patient care study and a double underline beneath the subjective data.

2. Complete the Nursing Process Worksheet on page 203 to develop a three-part diagnostic statement and related plan of care for this patient.

3. Write down the patient and personal nursing strengths you hope to draw upon as you assist this patient to better health.

   Patient strengths: _____

   _____

   _____

   Personal strengths: _____

   _____

   _____

4. Pretend that you are performing a nursing assessment of this patient after the plan of care is implemented. Document your findings.

   _____

   _____

   _____

NURSING PROCESS WORKSHEET

Health Problem (Title)

Expected Outcome*

Related to

↓

Etiology (Related Factors)

Nursing Interventions**

As Manifested by

↓

**Signs and Symptoms
(Defining Characteristics)**

Evaluative Statement

*More than one patient goal may be appropriate. For the purposes of this exercise, develop the one patient goal that demonstrates a direct resolution of the patient problem identified in the nursing diagnosis.
**Be sure you are able to list the scientific rationale for each nursing intervention you ordered.

CHAPTER 33

Activity

PRACTICING FOR NCLEX

MULTIPLE CHOICE QUESTIONS

Circle the letter that corresponds to the best answer for each question.

1. Joints are classified according to which of the following criteria?
   a. Bone type they connect
   b. Amount of movement they permit
   c. Size of the joint
   d. Amount of space between the bones

2. Which of the following terms describes the lateral movement of a body part toward the midline of the body?
   a. Adduction
   b. Abduction
   c. Circumduction
   d. Extension

3. An object has greater stability under which of the following conditions?
   a. A wide base of support and high center of gravity
   b. A narrow base of support and high center of gravity
   c. A wide base of support and low center of gravity
   d. A narrow base of support and low center of gravity

4. Which of the following postural reflexes informs the brain of the location of a limb or body part as a result of joint movements stimulating special nerve endings in muscles, tendons, and fascia?
   a. Labyrinthine sense
   b. Extensor reflexes
   c. Optic reflexes
   d. Proprioceptor sense

5. The CNS part that integrates semivoluntary movements, such as walking, swimming, and laughing, is which of the following?
   a. Basal ganglia
   b. Cerebral motor cortex
   c. Cerebellum
   d. Pyramidal pathways

6. A patient who is bedridden may experience which of the following conditions?
   a. Increase in the movement of secretions in the respiratory tract
   b. Increase in circulating fibrinolysin
   c. Predisposition to renal calculi
   d. Increased metabolic rate

7. Which of the following parts of the CNS assists the motor cortex and basal ganglia by making body movements smooth and coordinated?
   a. Cerebral motor cortex
   b. Cerebellum
   c. Basal ganglia
   d. Pyramidal pathways

8. On assessing an ambulatory patient, you observe that both arms swing freely in alternation with leg swings. You are assessing which of the following?

   a. Alignment
   b. Joint function
   c. Gait
   d. Muscle tone

9. Mr. Drennan will be ambulating for the first time since his cardiac surgery. Which of the following should the nurse consider when assisting Mr. Drennan?

   a. Patients who are fearful of walking should be told to look at their feet when walking to ensure correct positioning.
   b. Patients who can lift their legs only 1 to 2 inches off the bed do not have sufficient muscle power to permit walking.
   c. Nurses should never assist patients with ambulation without a physical therapist present.
   d. If an ambulating patient whom a nurse is assisting begins to fall, the nurse should slide the patient down his/her own body to the floor, carefully protecting the patient's head.

10. The ribs are an example of which of the following types of bones?

    a. Long bones
    b. Short bones
    c. Flat bones
    d. Irregular bones

11. Which of the following traumas to the musculoskeletal system is a break in the continuity of the structure of a bone or cartilage?

    a. Fracture
    b. Sprain
    c. Strain
    d. Dislocation

12. Swimming, jogging, and bicycling are examples of which of the following types of exercises?

    a. Isotonic exercises
    b. Isometric exercises
    c. Isokinetic exercises
    d. Stretching exercises

13. Mr. Bellas is a 40-year-old man in a sedentary job who is beginning an exercise program. Which of the following effects will exercise have on his cardiovascular system?

    a. Decreased efficiency of the heart
    b. Decreased heart rate and blood pressure
    c. Decreased blood flow to all body parts
    d. Decreased circulating fibrinolysin

14. The joint between the trapezium and metacarpal of the thumb is an example of which of the following types of joints?

    a. Gliding joint
    b. Condyloid joint
    c. Pivot joint
    d. Saddle joint

15. A body that is in correct alignment when standing maintains which of the following positions?

    a. The chest is held upward and backward.
    b. The abdominal muscles are held downward and the buttocks upward.
    c. The knees are slightly bent.
    d. The base of support is on the soles of the feet.

ALTERNATE-FORMAT QUESTIONS

Multiple Response Questions

Circle the letters that correspond to the best answers for each question.

1. Which of the following are examples of isometric exercise? *(Select all that apply.)*

   a. Jogging
   b. Range-of-motion exercises
   c. Contracting the quadriceps
   d. Kegel exercises
   e. Bicycling
   f. Contracting and releasing the gluteal muscles

2. Which of the following statements accurately describe typical body movements? *(Select all that apply.)*

   a. Dorsiflexion is the backward bending of the hand or foot.
   b. Internal rotation is a body part turning on its axis away from the midline of the body.

   c. Rotation is the turning of a body part on the axis provided by its joint.

   d. Flexion is the state of being in a straight line

   e. Inversion is the movement of the sole of the foot inward.

   f. Plantar flexion refers to the flexion of the hand.

3. Which of the following are effects of exercise on body systems? *(Select all that apply.)*

   a. Increases resting heart rate and blood pressure

   b. Increases intestinal tone

   c. Increases efficiency of metabolic system

   d. Increases blood flow to kidneys

   e. Decreases appetite

   f. Decreases rate of carbon dioxide excretion

4. Which of the following are effects of immobility on body systems? *(Select all that apply.)*

   a. Increased cardiac workload

   b. Increased depth of respiration

   c. Increased rate of respiration

   d. Decreased urinary stasis

   e. Increased risk for renal calculi

   f. Increased risk for electrolyte imbalance

5. Which of the following are normal findings when assessing a patient's mobility status? *(Select all that apply.)*

   a. Increased joint mobility

   b. Independent maintenance of correct alignment

   c. Scissors gait

   d. Head, shoulders, and hips aligned in bed

   e. Full range of motion

   f. Fasciculations

6. Which of the following are recommended nursing interventions for problems related to mobility? *(Select all that apply.)*

   a. For increased cardiac workload, instruct the patient to lie in the prone position.

   b. For ineffective breathing patterns, encourage shallow breathing and coughing.

   c. For orthostatic hypotension, have the patient sleep sitting up or in an elevated position.

   d. For impaired physical mobility, perform ROM exercises every 2 hours.

   e. For constipation, increase fluid intake and roughage.

   f. For impaired skin integrity, reposition the patient in correct alignment at least every 1 to 2 hours.

7. Which of the following are accurate guidelines when teaching crutch walking to patients? *(Select all that apply.)*

   a. Keep elbows close to sides.

   b. Prevent crutches from getting closer than 3 inches to the feet.

   c. Use the four-point gait for patients who may bear weight on both feet.

   d. Use the swing-to gait for patients who may bear weight on one foot.

   e. Use the two-point gait for patients who may not bear weight on either foot.

   f. When climbing stairs, advance the unaffected leg past the crutches, then place weight on the crutches, then advance the affected leg and then the crutches.

8. Which of the following are accurate steps when assisting with passive ROM exercises? *(Select all that apply.)*

   a. Raise the bed to the highest position.

   b. Adjust the bed to the flat position or as low as the patient can tolerate.

   c. Begin ROM exercises at the patient's head and move down one side of the body at a time.

   d. Perform each exercise 10 to 15 times.

   e. Move each joint in a smooth, rhythmic manner.

   f. Use a flat palm to support joints during ROM exercises.

DEVELOPING YOUR KNOWLEDGE BASE

IDENTIFICATION

1. Identify the bed positions illustrated below by placing the names of the positions on the lines provided.

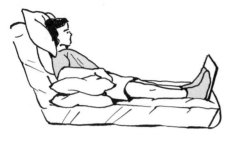

a. _____

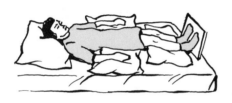

b. _____

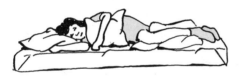

c. _____

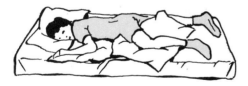

d. _____

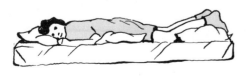

e. _____

MATCHING EXERCISES

Match the type of joint listed in Part A with the examples listed in Part B.

PART A

a. Ball-and-socket joint
b. Condyloid joint
c. Gliding joint
d. Hinge joint
e. Pivot joint
f. Saddle joint

PART B

1. ___ The joints between the axis and atlas and the proximal ends of the radius and ulna

2. ___ Carpal bones of the wrist; tarsal bones of the feet

3. ___ The joint between the trapezium and metacarpal of the thumb

4. ___ Wrist joint

5. ___ Shoulder and hip joints

Match the term used to describe body positions and movements in Part A with its definition listed in Part B.

PART A

a. Abduction
b. Adduction
c. Circumduction
d. Flexion
e. Extension
f. Hyperextension
g. Dorsiflexion
h. Plantar flexion
i. Rotation
j. Internal rotation
k. External rotation
l. Pronation
m. Supination
n. Inversion
o. Eversion

PART B

6. ___ The assumption of a prone position

7. ___ Lateral movement of a body part away from the midline of the body

8. ___ Backward bending of the hand or foot

9. ___ Movement of the sole or foot outward

10. ___ The state of being bent

11. ___ A body part turning on its axis away from the midline of the body

12. ___ Lateral movement of a body part toward the midline of the body

13. ___ Movement of the sole of the foot inward

14. ___ Movement of the distal part of the limb to trace a complete circle while the proximal end of the bone remains fixed

15. ___ The assumption of a supine position

16. ___ A body part turning on its axis toward the midline of the body

17. ___ Flexion of the foot

18. ___ The state of being in a straight line

19. ___ The turning point of a body part on the axis provided by its joint

Match the condition related to muscle mass listed in Part A with its definition listed in Part B.

PART A

a. Atrophy
b. Hypertrophy
c. Muscle tone
d. Flaccidity
e. Spasticity
f. Paresis
g. Hemiparesis
h. Paraplegia
i. Quadriplegia

PART B

20. ___ Increased muscle mass resulting from exercise or training

21. ___ Increased tone that interferes with movement

22. ___ Impaired muscle strength or weakness

23. ___ Muscle mass that is decreased through disuse or neurologic impairment

24. ___ Paralysis of the arms and legs

25. ___ The slight residual tension that remains in a resting normal muscle with an intact nerve supply

26. ___ Decreased tone that results from disuse or neurologic impairment

27. ___ Weakness of half of the body

CORRECT THE FALSE STATEMENTS

Circle the word "true" or "false" that follows the statement. If you circled "false," change the underlined word or words to make the statement true. Place your answer in the space provided.

1. The bones of the jaw and spinal column would be classified as <u>short bones</u>.

   True   False _____

2. In a <u>gliding joint</u>, articular surfaces are flat; flexion–extension and abduction–adduction are permitted.

   True   False _____

3. <u>Ligaments</u> are tough, fibrous bands that bind joints together and connect bones and cartilage.

   True   False _____

4. It is a <u>nerve impulse</u> that stimulates muscles to contract.

   True   False _____

5. <u>Body dynamics</u> are the efficient use of the body as a machine and as a means of locomotion.

   True   False _____

6. <u>Tonus</u> is the term used to describe the state of slight contraction or the usual state of skeletal muscles.

   True   False _____

7. The <u>narrower</u> a base of support and the lower the center of gravity, the greater the stability of the object.

   True   False _____

8. The <u>labyrinthine</u> sense informs the brain of the location of a limb or body part as a result of joint movements stimulating special nerve endings in muscles, tendons, and fascia.

True   False _____

9. The <u>cerebral motor cortex</u> integrates semivoluntary movements such as walking, swimming, and laughing.

True   False _____

10. Rehabilitative exercises for knee or elbow injuries are examples of <u>isokinetic</u> exercises.

True   False _____

11. <u>Atelectasis</u> is an incomplete expansion or collapse of lung tissue.

True   False _____

12. <u>Footdrop</u> is a complication of immobility in which the foot cannot maintain itself in the perpendicular position, heel–toe gait is impossible, and the patient experiences extreme difficulty in walking.

True   False _____

13. Should a patient faint or begin to fall while walking, the nurse should stand with his/her feet apart to create a wide base of support and rock the pelvis out on the side <u>opposite</u> the patient.

True   False _____

14. When a patient stands between the back legs of a walker, the walker should extend from the floor to the patient's hip joint; the patient's elbows should be flexed about <u>30 degrees</u>.

True   False _____

15. A nurse should <u>lift</u> an object to be moved to reduce the energy needed to overcome the pull of gravity.

True   False _____

SHORT ANSWER

1. Briefly explain the effects of exercise and immobility on the body systems listed in the table below. Write your answers in the spaces provided in the table below.

Body System	Effects of Exercise	Effects of Immobility
Cardiovascular		
Respiratory		
Gastrointestinal		
Urinary		
Musculoskeletal		
Metabolic		
Integumentary		
Psychological Well-Being		

2. List three functions performed by the muscles through contraction.

   a. _____

   b. _____

   c. _____

3. Describe the following points of attachment of muscle to bone.

   a. Point of origin: _____

   _____

   b. Point of insertion: _____

   _____

4. Describe the four steps the nervous system completes to stimulate muscles to contract.

   a. _____
   _____

   b. _____
   _____

   c. _____
   _____

   d. _____
   _____

5. Briefly describe the following concepts of body mechanics.

   a. Body alignment or posture: _____
   _____

   b. Balance: _____
   _____

   c. Coordinated body movement: _____
   _____

6. List four guidelines for the use of body mechanics when a person is at work.

   a. _____
   _____

   b. _____
   _____

   c. _____
   _____

d. _____
_____

7. Briefly describe how the following types of exercise provide health benefits to patients, and give an example of each.

   a. Aerobic exercises: _____
   _____

   b. Stretching exercises: _____
   _____

   c. Strength and endurance exercises: _____
   _____

   d. Activities of daily living: _____
   _____

8. List four psychological benefits of regular exercise.

   a. _____

   b. _____

   c. _____

   d. _____

9. Briefly describe how the following devices are used to promote correct alignment or alleviate discomfort on body parts.

   a. Pillows: _____
   _____

   b. Mattresses: _____
   _____

   c. Adjustable bed: _____
   _____

   d. Bed side rails: _____
   _____

   e. Trapeze bar: _____
   _____

   f. Cradle: _____
   _____

   g. Sandbags: _____
   _____

   h. Trochanter rolls: _____
   _____

   i. Hand/wrist splints or rolls: _____
   _____

10. Describe how you would teach a patient the following exercises.

   a. Quadriceps drills: _____
   _____
   _____

   b. Pushups: _____
   _____
   _____

   c. Dangling: _____
   _____
   _____

11. Mrs. Mulherin is a 60-year-old woman admitted to a healthcare facility for degenerative joint disease. Explain how you would assess, diagnose, and plan an exercise program for this patient.

   a. Physical assessment: _____
   _____
   _____
   _____
   _____

   b. Diagnosis: _____
   _____
   _____
   _____
   _____

   c. Exercise program: _____
   _____
   _____
   _____
   _____

12. Give two examples of normal and abnormal findings when assessing the mobility status of a patient in the following areas.

   a. General ease of movement:
   Normal: _____
   _____
   Abnormal: _____
   _____

   b. Gait and posture:
   Normal: _____
   _____
   Abnormal: _____
   _____

   c. Alignment:
   Normal: _____
   _____
   Abnormal: _____
   _____

   d. Joint structure and function:
   Normal: _____
   _____
   Abnormal: _____
   _____

   e. Muscle mass, tone, and strength:
   Normal: _____
   _____
   Abnormal: _____
   _____

   f. Endurance:
   Normal: _____
   _____
   Abnormal: _____
   _____

APPLYING YOUR KNOWLEDGE

CRITICAL THINKING QUESTIONS

1. Visit a center for rehabilitative medicine and observe how the physical therapists assist patients to become mobile. Interview several patients to find out how the lack of mobility has affected their lives. See if you can help with some of the exercise routines, and try some of the exercises yourself. Develop a nursing care plan to incorporate what you learned about mobility and exercise into your own patient care routine.

2. Using a partner, practice putting each other into the following positions: Fowler's, supine, prone, lateral side-lying, and Sims'. What did this teach you about the experience of being positioned that will be helpful in your practice? Assess each position for health risks that may arise from the following factors: comfort level, body alignment, and pressure points. Write down the advantages and disadvantages of each position.

3. Try maneuvering on a busy street on crutches or in a wheelchair. How does impaired mobility affect your ability to perform everyday chores? How did the public react to your impaired mobility? What effects might a permanent disability have on patients, and how can you promote their coping?

REFLECTIVE PRACTICE USING CRITICAL THINKING SKILLS

Use the following expanded scenario from Chapter 33 in your textbook to answer the questions below.

Scenario: Kelsi Lester is a 10-year-old girl admitted to the pediatric unit as a result of a skiing accident. Unconscious for 2 days, she may or may not regain consciousness. She is on complete bed rest and requires frequent positioning to maintain correct body alignment and range of motion. Her parents are nearby and express concerns about the redness developing around her shoulder blades. They ask, "Is there anything we can do to make our daughter more comfortable?"

1. What patient teaching might the nurse incorporate into the plan of care to help Kelsi's parents minimize the complications of immobility for their daughter?

_____

_____

_____

2. What would be a successful outcome for this patient?

_____

_____

_____

3. What intellectual, technical, interpersonal, and/or ethical/legal competencies are most likely to bring about the desired outcome?

_____

_____

_____

4. What resources might be helpful for the Lester family?

_____

_____

_____

PATIENT CARE STUDY

Read the following patient care study and use your nursing process skills to answer the questions below.

Scenario: Robert Witherspoon, a 42-year-old university professor, presents for a checkup shortly after his father's death. His father died of complications of coronary artery disease. Mr. Witherspoon is 5 feet 9 inches tall, weighs 235 pounds, has a decided "paunch," and reports that until now he has made no time for exercise because he preferred to use his free time reading or listening to classical music. He enjoys French cuisine, including rich desserts, and has a cholesterol level of 310 mg/dL (normal is 150 to 250 mg/dL). He admits being frightened by his father's death and is appropriately concerned about his elevated cholesterol level. "I guess I've never given much thought to my health before, but my Dad's death changed all that," he tells you. "I know that coronary artery disease runs in families, and I can tell you that I'm not ready to pack it all in yet. Tell me what I have to do to fight this thing." He admits that he used to tease a colleague—who lowered his own cholesterol from 290 to 200 mg/dL by diet and exercise alone—by accusing him of being a fitness freak. "Now, I'm recognizing the wisdom of his health behaviors and wondering if diet and exercise won't do the trick for me. Can you help me design an exercise program that will work?"

1. Identify pertinent patient data by placing a single underline beneath the objective data in the patient care study and a double underline beneath the subjective data.

2. Complete the Nursing Process Worksheet on page 214 to develop a three-part diagnostic statement and related plan of care for this patient.

3. Write down the patient and personal nursing strengths you hope to draw on as you assist this patient to better health.

Patient strengths: _____

_____

_____

Personal strengths: _____

_____

_____

4. Pretend that you are performing a nursing assessment of this patient after the plan of care has been implemented. Document your findings.

_____

_____

_____

NURSING PROCESS WORKSHEET

Health Problem (Title)

Expected Outcome*

Related to

↓

Etiology (Related Factors)

Nursing Interventions**

As Manifested by

↓

**Signs and Symptoms
(Defining Characteristics)**

Evaluative Statement

*More than one patient goal may be appropriate. For the purposes of this exercise, develop the one patient
goal that demonstrates a direct resolution of the patient problem identified in the nursing diagnosis.
**Be sure you are able to list the scientific rationale for each nursing intervention you ordered.

Rest and Sleep

PRACTICING FOR NCLEX

MULTIPLE CHOICE QUESTIONS

Circle the letter that corresponds to the best answer for each question.

1. You notice that a patient admitted to your unit sleeps for an abnormally long time. This patient may have suffered damage to which of the following areas of the brain?
   a. Cerebral cortex
   b. Hypothalamus
   c. Medulla
   d. Midbrain

2. Wakefulness occurs when which of the following is activated with stimuli from the cerebral cortex and peripheral sensory organs?
   a. Reticular activating system
   b. Bulbar synchronizing region
   c. Circadian rhythm
   d. Medulla

3. Which of the following is a characteristic of REM sleep?
   a. Small muscles are immobile, as in paralysis.
   b. Pulse is slow and regular.
   c. Body temperature decreases.
   d. Eyes dart back and forth quickly.

4. When an individual's sleep–wake patterns follow the inner biologic clock, which of the following conditions exists?
   a. Circadian rhythm
   b. Circadian synchronization

   c. Bulbar synchronization
   d. Sleep cycle

5. Which of the following instruments receives and records electrical currents from the brain?
   a. Electroencephalograph
   b. Electrooculogram
   c. Electromyograph
   d. Electrocardiogram

6. The arousal threshold is usually greatest in which of the following stages of NREM sleep?
   a. Stage I
   b. Stage II
   c. Stage III
   d. Stage IV

7. In normal adults, the REM state consumes what percentage of nightly sleep?
   a. 5% to 10%
   b. 10% to 20%
   c. 20% to 25%
   d. 25% to 35%

8. On which of the following patients should a sleep history be obtained?
   a. Only patients who have been suffering from a sleep disorder
   b. Patients who suffer from a sleep disorder or have been unconscious
   c. Patients who suffer from a sleep disorder or who are spending time in the CCU
   d. All patients admitted to a healthcare agency

9. A patient who has been diagnosed with hypothyroidism is admitted to a nursing home. On performing a sleep history on this patient, you find out that the patient is suffering from fatigue, lethargy, depression, and difficulty executing the tasks of everyday living. This patient is probably experiencing which of the following types of sleep deprivation?

   a. REM deprivation

   b. NREM deprivation

   c. Total sleep deprivation

   d. Insomnia

10. Most authorities agree that an individual's sleep–wake cycle is fully developed by what age?

   a. 9 months to 1 year

   b. 1 year to 18 months

   c. 2 to 3 years

   d. 4 to 6 years

11. Which of the following interventions would be recommended for a patient with insomnia?

   a. Nap frequently during the day to make up for the lost sleep at night.

   b. Eliminate caffeine and alcohol in the evening because both are associated with disturbances in the normal sleep cycle.

   c. Exercise vigorously before bedtime to promote drowsiness.

   d. Avoid food high in carbohydrates before bedtime.

12. Mrs. Leister, a new patient in the medical–surgical unit, complains of difficulty sleeping. She is scheduled for an exploratory laparotomy in the morning. Your diagnosis is Sleep Pattern Disturbance: Insomnia related to fear of impending surgery. Which one of the following steps is the most appropriate in planning care for this diagnosis?

   a. Help her maintain her normal bedtime routine and time for sleep.

   b. Provide an opportunity for her to talk about her concerns.

   c. Use tactile relaxation techniques, such as a back massage.

   d. Bring her a warm glass of milk at bedtime.

ALTERNATE-FORMAT QUESTIONS

Multiple Response Questions

Circle the letters that correspond to the best answers for each question.

1. Which of the following statements accurately describe the physiology of sleep? *(Select all that apply.)*

   a. The reticular activating system (RAS) extends upward through the medulla, the pons, and the midbrain and into the hypothalamus.

   b. The bulbar synchronizing region facilitates reflex and voluntary movements as well as cortical activities related to a state of alertness.

   c. During sleep, the RAS experiences few stimuli from the cerebral cortex and the periphery of the body.

   d. The medulla has control centers for several involuntary activities of the body, one of which concerns sleeping and waking.

   e. GABA appears to be necessary for inhibition.

   f. Injury to the hypothalamus may cause a person to remain awake for long periods of time.

2. Which of the following are characteristics of REM sleep? *(Select all that apply.)*

   a. The person is in a transitional stage between wakefulness and sleep.

   b. The person can be aroused with relative ease.

   c. The person reaches the greatest depth of sleep, called delta sleep.

   d. Respirations are irregular and sometimes interspersed with apnea.

   e. Metabolism and body temperature increase.

   f. It constitutes about 20% to 25% of sleep.

3. Which of the following statements accurately describe developmental patterns of sleep? *(Select all that apply.)*

   a. Newborns sleep an average of 16 hours per day.

   b. NREM sleep constitutes much of the sleep cycle of a young infant.

   c. The need for sleep in toddlers increases with age due to the more active state they are in.

d. 12 hours is the average amount of sleep needed by preschoolers.

e. Sleep needs generally decrease when physical growth peaks.

f. An average of 5 to 7 hours of sleep is generally adequate for older adults.

4. Which of the following statements accurately describe factors that affect sleep patterns? *(Select all that apply.)*

a. Excessive exercise promotes fatigue and improves the quality of sleep.

b. Sleep disorders are the major problem associated with shift work.

c. Sleep is not affected by watching television or participating in stimulating outside activities.

d. A small protein and carbohydrate snack is recommended to promote sleep.

e. Large quantities of alcoholic beverages have been found to limit REM and delta sleep.

f. Nicotine has a relaxing effect, and smokers usually have an easier time falling asleep.

5. Which of the following describe the influences of illness on sleep patterns? *(Select all that apply.)*

a. Gastric secretions decrease during REM sleep.

b. The pain associated with disease of the coronary arteries and myocardial infarction is more likely during NREM sleep.

c. Epilepsy seizures are more likely to occur during NREM sleep.

d. Liver failure and encephalitis tend to cause a reversal in day–night sleeping habits.

e. Hypothyroidism tends to increase the amount of NREM sleep.

f. The administration of a larger mid-afternoon dose of asthma medication may prevent attacks that occur at night during sleep.

6. Which of the following are recommended interventions for patients experiencing insomnia who are undergoing stimulus control? *(Select all that apply.)*

a. Recommend that the patient use the bedroom for sex and sleep only.

b. Instruct the patient to leave the bedroom if he/she cannot get to sleep within 15 to 20 minutes; he/she should return to the bedroom when sleepy.

c. Instruct the patient to get up the same time every day, no matter what time he/she fell asleep.

d. Allow the patient to nap during the day if he/she could not sleep during the night.

e. Instruct the patient to exercise moderately 1 hour before going to bed.

f. Encourage the patient to consume one or two alcoholic drinks to help him/her relax before bedtime.

7. Which of the following are types of sleep therapies to treat insomnia? *(Select all that apply.)*

a. Sleep modification

b. Sleep hygiene

c. Cognitive behavioral therapy

d. Multifaceted therapy

e. Stimulus control

f. Multicomponent therapy

8. Which of the following statements accurately describe common sleep disorders? *(Select all that apply.)*

a. Sleep apnea refers to periods of absent breathing between snoring intervals.

b. Patients with restless arm syndrome cannot lie still and experience unpleasant crawling or tingling sensations in the arms.

c. Sleep deprivation results from increased NREM sleep and generally progresses to total sleep deprivation if untreated.

d. Bruxism or sleepwalking is a common type of somnambulism.

e. Enuresis involves bedwetting during sleep and is a form of somnambulism.

f. Sleep-related eating disorder is a type of parasomnia in which the patient eats food but does not remember eating in the morning.

Prioritization Question

1. Place the following stages of a sleep cycle in the order in which they would normally occur.

a. NREM stage III

b. NREM stage I

c. NREM stage II

d. Wakefulness

e. REM

f. NREM stage IV

g. 2nd NREM stage II

h. 2nd NREM stage III

i. 3rd NREM stage II

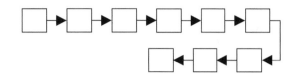

DEVELOPING YOUR KNOWLEDGE BASE

FILL-IN-THE-BLANKS

1. Which two systems in the brainstem are believed to work together to control the cyclic nature of sleep? _____

2. Stages III and IV, representing about 10% of total sleep time, are deep-sleep states termed _____ or slow-wave sleep.

3. _____ are patterns of waking behavior that appear during sleep.

4. _____ is characterized by difficulty falling asleep, intermittent sleep, or early awakening from sleep.

5. _____ is a condition characterized by excessive sleep, particularly during the day.

6. _____ is a condition characterized by an uncontrollable desire to sleep.

MATCHING EXERCISES

Match the sleep disorder listed in Part A with its appropriate definition listed in Part B.

PART A

a. Insomnia

b. Hypersomnia

c. Narcolepsy

d. Sleep apnea

e. Parasomnia

f. Somnambulism

g. Enuresis

h. Bruxism

i. Sleep deprivation

j. Nocturnal myoclonus

PART B

1. ___ Bedwetting during sleep

2. ___ Difficulty in falling asleep, intermittent sleep, or early awakening from sleep

3. ___ A condition characterized by an uncontrollable desire to sleep

4. ___ Grinding teeth during sleep

5. ___ A condition characterized by excessive sleep, particularly during the day

6. ___ Periods of no breathing between snoring intervals

7. ___ Sleepwalking

8. ___ Decrease in the amount, consistency, and quality of sleep

9. ___ Marked muscle contraction that results in the jerking of one or both legs during sleep

Match the stage of NREM sleep listed in Part A with the characteristics of that stage listed in Part B. Some answers may be used more than once, and some questions may have more than one answer.

PART A

a. Stage I

b. Stage II

c. Stage III

d. Stage IV

PART B

10. ___ The depth of sleep increases, and arousal becomes increasingly difficult.

11. ___ It is a transitional stage between wakefulness and sleep.

12. ___ Involuntary muscle jerking may occur and waken the person.

13. ___ The person reaches the greatest depth of sleep, called delta sleep.

14. ___ The person falls into a deep sleep from which he/she cannot be aroused with ease.

15. ___ Constitutes about 10% of sleep

16. ___ Constitutes 50% to 55% of sleep

17. ___ Metabolism slows and the body temperature is low.

18. ___ Constitutes about 5% of sleep

CORRECT THE FALSE STATEMENTS

Circle the word "true" or "false" that follows the statement. If you circled "false," change the underlined word or words to make the statement true. Place your answer in the space provided.

1. During sleep, stimuli from the cortex are <u>minimal</u>.

   True   False _____

2. Sleep stages III and IV are deep-sleep states termed <u>delta sleep, or slow-wave sleep</u>.

   True   False _____

3. If a person is awakened from sleep at any time, he/she will return to sleep again by starting <u>at the point in the cycle where he/she was when disturbed</u>.

   True   False _____

4. Most people go through <u>8 to 10</u> cycles of sleep each night.

   True   False _____

5. On average, infants sleep <u>10 to 14</u> hours each day.

   True   False _____

6. During times of stress, REM sleep <u>decreases</u> in amount, which tends to add to anxiety and stress.

   True   False _____

7. A small <u>protein</u> snack before bedtime is recommended for patients with insomnia.

   True   False _____

8. Exercise that occurs within a 2-hour interval before normal bedtime <u>stimulates</u> sleep.

   True   False _____

9. The administration of a <u>larger mid-afternoon dose</u> of asthma medication may prevent attacks that commonly occur at night during sleep.

   True   False _____

10. <u>Parasomnias</u> are patterns of waking behavior that appear during sleep.

    True   False _____

11. <u>Narcolepsy</u> refers to periods of no breathing between snoring intervals.

    True   False _____

SHORT ANSWER

1. List three benefits of sleep.

   a. _____

   b. _____

   c. _____

2. List the average amount of sleep required for the following age groups.

   a. Infants: _____

   b. Growing children: _____

   c. Adults: _____

   d. Older adults: _____

3. Briefly describe how the following factors influence sleep.

   a. Physical activity: _____

   _____

   b. Psychological stress: _____

   _____

   c. Motivation: _____

   _____

   d. Culture: _____

   _____

   e. Diet: _____

   _____

   f. Alcohol and caffeine: _____

   _____

   g. Smoking: _____

   _____

   h. Environmental factors: _____

   _____

   i. Lifestyle: _____

   _____

   j. Exercise: _____

   _____

   k. Illness: _____

   _____

   l. Medications: _____

   _____

4. List the information that should be determined in a sleep history when a sleep disturbance is noted.

_____

_____

_____

_____

5. Describe four physical findings that either confirm that a patient is getting sufficient rest to provide energy for the day's activities or validate the existence of a sleep disturbance that is decreasing the quantity or quality of sleep.

a. _____

b. _____

c. _____

d. _____

6. Describe how you would prepare a restful environment for a home healthcare patient who is experiencing a sleep disorder.

_____

_____

_____

7. Write a sample nursing diagnosis for the following sleep problems.

a. Mr. Smith is admitted to the hospital for surgery. He normally has no problem falling asleep, but the noise of the hospital and the need for periodic treatments keep him awake at night.

_____

_____

b. Mr. Loper, a 74-year-old patient in a long-term care facility, is bored during the day and takes a nap in the afternoon and early evening. He cannot sleep at night.

_____

_____

c. Dr. Harris, a resident working varying shifts in the emergency room, complains that he is sleepy all the time but cannot sleep when he lies down after work.

_____

_____

d. Mrs. Maher, age 28, consumes four alcoholic drinks when watching television at night before bedtime. After eliminating the alcohol from her diet, she complains of waking after a short period and not being able to fall back to sleep.

_____

_____

e. Mrs. Eichorn, age 45, has two teenage sons who are often out late at night. She cannot get to sleep until they are both home safely, and even then she continues to worry about them.

_____

_____

8. Describe how each of the following is affected by REM sleep.

a. Eyes: _____

b. Muscles: _____

c. Respirations: _____

d. Pulse: _____

e. Blood pressure: _____

f. Gastric secretions: _____

g. Metabolism: _____

h. Sleep cycle: _____

9. List three measures a nurse can take to help alleviate a patient's sleep problem.

a. _____

b. _____

c. _____

10. Give an example of a question you would ask a patient to assess for the following sleep factors.

a. Usual sleeping and waking times: _____

_____

b. Number of hours of undisturbed sleep: ___

_____

c. Quality of sleep: _____

_____

d. Number and duration of naps: _____

e. Energy level: _____

_____

f. Means of relaxing before bedtime: _____

_____

g. Bedtime rituals: _____

_____

h. Sleep environment: _____

_____

i. Pharmacologic aids: _____

_____

j. Nature of a sleep disturbance: _____

_____

k. Onset of a disturbance: _____

_____

l. Causes of a disturbance: _____

_____

m. Severity of a disturbance: _____

_____

n. Symptoms of a disturbance: _____

_____

o. Interventions attempted and results: _____

_____

APPLYING YOUR KNOWLEDGE

CRITICAL THINKING QUESTIONS

1. Visit a busy hospital unit at night. Assess the factors on the ward that would contribute to a patient's sleep deficit. What could be done to change the hospital environment to promote healthy sleeping patterns in the occupants?

2. Develop a sleep teaching tool that explains the typical sleep patterns and requirements for patients of all ages (infants to older adults). Include common factors that disrupt sleep patterns, total amount of sleep required, and possible interventions to minimize sleep pattern disturbances. Interview individuals who have tried your interventions and evaluate the likelihood that your teaching tool will resolve sleep problems.

3. Interview several friends or relatives to find out what they do to prepare for a restful night's sleep. Do they have any bedtime routines that are different from yours? What are some methods they use when they cannot fall asleep? Discuss the effect of lack of sleep on their work performance the following day.

REFLECTIVE PRACTICE USING CRITICAL THINKING SKILLS

Use the following expanded scenario from Chapter 34 in your textbook to answer the questions below.

Scenario: Charlie Bittner is an 86-year-old man who has recently been admitted to a long-term care facility. He tells his daughter that "even though I go to bed around 9 p.m., I don't fall asleep until after midnight and then I'm up twice to go to the bathroom and have a lot of trouble falling back to sleep." His daughter has mentioned to the nurse that her father spends a lot of time napping during the day.

1. What nursing interventions might the nurse employ to help alleviate Mr. Bittner's sleep disturbances?

_____

_____

_____

2. What would be a successful outcome for this patient?

_____

_____

_____

3. What intellectual, technical, interpersonal, and/or ethical/legal competencies are most likely to bring about the desired outcome?

_____

_____

_____

4. What resources might be helpful for Mr. Bittner?

_____

_____

_____

PATIENT CARE STUDY

Read the following patient care study and use your nursing process skills to answer the questions below.

Scenario: Gina Cioffi, a 23-year-old graduate nurse, has been in her new position as a critical care staff nurse in a large tertiary-care medical center for 3 months. "I was so excited about working three 12-hour shifts a week when I started this job, thinking I'd have lots of time for other things I want to do, but I'm not so sure anymore," she says. "I've been doing extra shifts when we're short-staffed because the money is so good, and right now it seems I'm always tired and all I think about all day long is how soon I can get back to bed. Worst of all, when I do finally get into bed, I often can't fall asleep, especially if things have been busy at work and someone 'went bad.' Does everyone else feel like me?" Looking at Gina, you notice dark circles under her eyes and are suddenly struck by the change in her appearance from when she first started working. At that time, she "bounced into work" looking fresh each morning, and her features were always animated. Now, her skin is pale, her hair and clothes look rumpled, and the "brightness" that was so characteristic of her earlier is strikingly absent. With some gentle questioning, you discover that she frequently goes out with new friends she has made at the hospital when her shift is over, and sometimes goes for 48 hours without sleep. "I know I've gotten myself into a rut.

How do I get out of it? I used to think my sleep habits were bad at school, but this is a hundred times worse because there never seems to be time to crash. I just have to keep on going."

1. Identify pertinent patient data by placing a single underline beneath the objective data in the case study and a double underline beneath the subjective data.

2. Complete the Nursing Process Worksheet on page 223 to develop a three-part diagnostic statement and related plan of care for this patient.

3. Write down the patient and personal nursing strengths you hope to draw on as you assist this patient to better health.

Patient strengths: _____

_____

_____

Personal strengths: _____

_____

_____

4. Pretend that you are performing a nursing assessment of this patient after the plan of care is implemented. Document your findings.

_____

_____

_____

NURSING PROCESS WORKSHEET

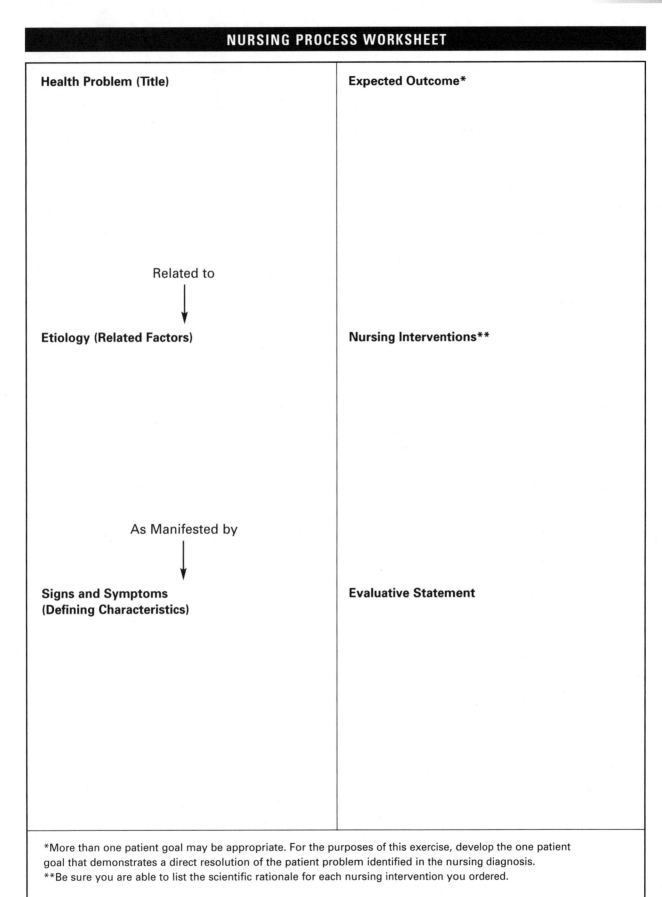

Health Problem (Title)

Expected Outcome*

Related to

↓

Etiology (Related Factors)

Nursing Interventions**

As Manifested by

↓

**Signs and Symptoms
(Defining Characteristics)**

Evaluative Statement

*More than one patient goal may be appropriate. For the purposes of this exercise, develop the one patient goal that demonstrates a direct resolution of the patient problem identified in the nursing diagnosis.
**Be sure you are able to list the scientific rationale for each nursing intervention you ordered.

Comfort

PRACTICING FOR NCLEX

MULTIPLE CHOICE QUESTIONS

Circle the letter that corresponds to the best answer for each question.

1. Pain that is poorly localized and originates in body organs is known as which of the following?
   a. Cutaneous pain
   b. Somatic pain
   c. Visceral pain
   d. Perceived pain

2. You are visiting a patient at home who is recovering from a bowel resection. She complains of constant pain and discomfort and displays signs of depression. When assessing this patient for pain, you should be aware of which of the following facts about pain?
   a. As her primary healthcare giver, you are the authority on the existence and nature of your patient's pain sensation.
   b. The pain your patient is experiencing is probably an emotional or psychological problem due to depression.
   c. A placebo should be administered to the patient to see whether the pain is manufactured or psychogenic before starting drug therapy.
   d. The patient is the only authority on the existence and nature of her pain, and pain management therapy should be reviewed and revised if necessary.

3. Which of the following is a powerful vasodilator that increases capillary permeability and constricts smooth muscles, playing a role in the chemistry of pain at the injury site?
   a. Bradykinin
   b. Prostaglandins
   c. Substance P
   d. Serotonin

4. Pain receptors consisting of free nerve endings that are involved in fast-conducting, acute, well-localized pain include which of the following?
   a. C fibers
   b. Gamma fibers
   c. B fibers
   d. A-delta fibers

5. The highest level of integration of sensory impulses of pain occurs in which of the following regions?
   a. Cortex
   b. Medulla
   c. CNS
   d. Spinal cord

6. A patient who recently underwent amputation of a leg complains of pain in the amputated part. The nurse should explain to the patient which of the following?
   a. The pain cannot exist because the leg has been amputated.
   b. The pain is a phenomenon known as "ghost pain."

c. The pain is a real experience for the patient.

d. The patient is experiencing central pain syndrome.

7. The fact that a person can tolerate a higher temperature as water is gradually heated than if the hand had been plunged into hot water without any preparation can be explained by which of the following theories?

a. Threshold of pain theory

b. Adaptation theory

c. Gate control theory

d. Regulation by neuromodulators

8. Which of the following means of pain control can be generally explained on the basis of the gate control theory?

a. Biofeedback

b. Distraction

c. Hypnosis

d. Acupuncture

9. Aspirin, acetaminophen, and ibuprofen are examples of which of the following types of pharmaceutical agents that relieve pain?

a. NSAIDs

b. Opioids

c. Nonopioid analgesics

d. Adjuvant drugs

10. A patient complains of severe pain following a mastectomy. A good choice of analgesic for this patient would be which of the following?

a. Acetaminophen

b. Aspirin

c. Morphine

d. Methadone

11. A p.r.n. drug regimen is an effective means of administering pain medication in which of the following cases?

a. A patient experiencing acute pain

b. A patient in the early postoperative period

c. A patient experiencing chronic pain

d. A patient in the postoperative stage with occasional pain

12. Your patient is experiencing acute pain following the amputation of a limb. Which of the following nursing interventions should you keep in mind when treating this patient?

a. Treat the pain only as it occurs to prevent drug addiction.

b. Encourage the use of nondrug complementary therapies as adjuncts to the medical regimen.

c. Increase and decrease the serum level of the analgesic as needed.

d. Do not provide analgesia if there is any doubt about the likelihood of pain occurring.

13. Which of the following groups of opioids are produced at neural synapses at various points in the CNS pathway and are powerful pain-blocking chemicals?

a. Dymorphins

b. Endorphins

c. Enkephalins

d. Bradykinins

14. When assessing a patient for pain, the nurse should consider which of the following facts about pain?

a. Patients frequently complain about pain that is not there to get attention.

b. People with pain should be taught to have a high tolerance for pain.

c. All real pain has an identifiable, physical cause.

d. Having an emotional reaction to pain does not mean the pain is a result of an emotional problem.

15. Three days after surgery, Mrs. Dodds continues to have moderate to severe incisional pain. According to the gate control theory, the nurse should do which of the following?

a. Administer pain medications in smaller doses but more frequently.

b. Decrease external stimuli in the room during painful episodes.

c. Reposition Mrs. Dodds and gently massage her back.

d. Advise Mrs. Dodds that she should try to sleep following administration of pain medication.

16. When treating a young boy who is in pain but cannot vocalize this pain, which of the following measures should the nurse employ?

a. Ignore the boy's pain if he is not complaining about it.

  b. Ask the boy to draw a cartoon about the color or shape of his pain.

  c. Medicate the boy with analgesics to reduce the anxiety of experiencing pain.

  d. Distract the boy so he does not notice his pain.

17. After sedating a patient, you assess that he is frequently drowsy and drifts off during conversations. What number on the sedation scale would best describe your patient's sedation level?

  a. 1

  b. 2

  c. 3

  d. 4

ALTERNATE-FORMAT QUESTIONS

Multiple Response Questions

Circle the letters that correspond to the best answers for each question.

1. Which of the following are characteristics of acute pain? *(Select all that apply.)*

  a. It is generally rapid in onset.

  b. It generally lasts for 6 months or longer.

  c. It varies in intensity from mild to severe.

  d. It is protective in nature.

  e. People with acute pain generally experience periods of remission.

  f. An example is the pain associated with cancer.

2. Which of the following statements accurately describe the nature of the pain experience? *(Select all that apply.)*

  a. Patients are able to describe chronic pain because it is generally localized.

  b. Approximately 75% of all patients with cancer have adequate pain control.

  c. Individuals with chronic pain may be viewed, in general, by healthcare personnel as hysterical personalities, malingerers, or hypochondriacs.

  d. Acute pain is often perceived as meaningless and may lead to withdrawal and depression.

  e. Pain that is resistant to therapy is referred to as intractable.

  f. Pain in people whose tissue injury is nonprogressive or healed is termed chronic nonmalignant pain.

3. Which of the following statements accurately describe the stages of the pain process? *(Select all that apply.)*

  a. The activation of pain receptors is referred to as transmission.

  b. A damaged cell releases histamine, which excites nerve endings.

  c. Bradykinin is a hormone-like substance that sends additional pain stimuli to the central nervous system.

  d. No specific pain organs or cells exist in the body.

  e. Pain sensations from the viscera course along the autonomic system.

  f. Stimulation of sensory receptors and the intactness of their nerve supply are necessary conditions for pain.

4. Which of the following are accurate descriptors of the gate control theory? *(Select all that apply.)*

  a. Nerve fibers of small diameter conduct excitatory pain stimuli away from the brain.

  b. Nerve fibers of a large diameter inhibit the transmission of pain impulses from the spinal cord to the brain.

  c. There is a gating mechanism that is believed to be located in substantia gelatinosa cells in the dorsal horn of the spinal cord.

  d. The exciting and inhibiting signals at the gate in the spinal cord determine the impulses that eventually reach the brain.

  e. A large amount of sensory information can be processed by the nervous system at any given moment.

  f. When too much information is sent through the nervous system, cells in the spinal column take over, as if opening a gate.

5. Which of the following statements regarding the perception of pain are accurate? *(Select all that apply.)*

  a. The perception of pain involves the sensory process that occurs when a stimulus for pain is present.

  b. The perception of pain does not include the person's interpretation of the pain.

  c. The pain threshold is the highest intensity of a stimulus that causes the subject to recognize pain.

d. The pain threshold varies from person to person, but many studies conclude that males have lower thresholds than females.

e. The sensation of pain is regulated or modified by neuromodulators.

f. Endorphins are powerful pain-blocking chemicals that have prolonged analgesic effects, produce euphoria, and may be released when certain measures are used to relieve pain.

6. Which of the following are physiologic responses to pain? *(Select all that apply.)*

a. Exaggerated weeping and restlessness

b. Protecting the painful area

c. Increased blood pressure

d. Muscle tension and rigidity

e. Nausea and vomiting

f. Grimacing and moaning

DEVELOPING YOUR KNOWLEDGE BASE

FILL-IN-THE-BLANKS

1. A patient who experiences acute pain following a noxious stimulus is experiencing _____ pain.

2. A patient who has pain related to a surgical incision is experiencing _____ pain.

3. A patient who complains of pain that is poorly localized following abdominal surgery is most likely experiencing _____ pain.

4. A person who experiences a "head rush" from eating ice cream too fast is experiencing _____.

5. A patient who has sharp pains in his left arm following a myocardial infarction is experiencing _____ pain.

MATCHING EXERCISES

Match the type of pain listed in Part A with its definition listed in Part B.

PART A

a. Nociceptive pain

b. Cutaneous pain

c. Somatic pain

d. Visceral pain

e. Neuropathic pain

f. Allodynia

g. Psychogenic pain

h. Referred pain

i. Acute pain

j. Chronic pain

k. Intractable pain

PART B

1. ____ Pain that results from an injury to, or abnormal functioning of, peripheral nerves or the central nervous system

2. ____ Pain that is resistant to therapy and persists despite a variety of interventions

3. ____ Pain that occurs following a normally weak or nonpainful stimulus, such as a light touch or a cold drink

4. ____ Pain that may be limited, intermittent, or persistent but that lasts for 6 months or longer and interferes with normal functioning

5. ____ Pain that is usually acute and transmitted following normal processing of noxious stimuli

6. ____ Pain that is diffuse or scattered and originates in tendons, ligaments, bones, blood vessels, and nerves

7. ____ Pain for which no physical cause can be found

8. ____ Superficial pain that usually involves the skin or subcutaneous tissue

9. ____ Pain that is poorly localized and originates in body organs, the thorax, cranium, and abdomen

10. ____ Pain that is perceived in an area distant from its point of origin

Match the examples in Part B with the type of pain listed in Part A. Answers may be used more than once.

PART A

a. Cutaneous pain

b. Deep somatic pain

c. Visceral pain

d. Referred pain

PART B

11. ____ Pain associated with cancer of the uterus

12. ____ Pain associated with a myocardial infarction

13. ____ Pain associated with a knee injury

14. ____ Pain associated with burns

15. ____ Pain associated with a brain tumor

16. ____ Pain associated with a gash in the skin

17. ____ Pain associated with a broken leg

18. ____ Pain associated with ulcers

Match the term for nonpharmacologic pain relief listed in Part A with its definition listed in Part B.

PART A

a. Imagery

b. Relaxation techniques

c. TENS

d. Cutaneous stimulation

e. Placebo

f. Hypnosis

g. Acupuncture

h. Biofeedback

i. Acupressure

j. Therapeutic touch

k. Distraction

PART B

19. ____ Involves using one's hands to consciously direct an energy exchange from the practitioner to the patient

20. ____ Involves four elements: assuming a comfortable position with the body in good alignment, being in quiet surroundings, repeating certain words, and adopting a passive attitude when distracting thoughts enter the individual's consciousness

21. ____ Involves stimulating the skin's surface to relieve pain; can be explained by the gate control theory

22. ____ Requires the patient to focus attention on something other than the pain

23. ____ An example of mind–body interaction used to decrease pain that involves one or all of the senses and focusing on a mental picture

24. ____ Involves the application of pressure or massage or both to usual acupuncture sites

25. ____ A noninvasive alternative technique that involves electrical stimulation of large-diameter fibers to inhibit the transmission of painful impulses carried over small-diameter fibers

26. ____ A technique that influences a subconscious condition by means of suggestion

27. ____ A technique that uses a machine with a signal to help the patient learn by trial and error to control the supposedly involuntary body mechanisms that may cause pain

28. ____ A technique that uses needles of various lengths to prick specific parts of the body to produce insensitivity to pain

SHORT ANSWER

1. Read each of the situations below and use the table on page 229 to describe behavioral, physiologic, and affective responses to pain that you might observe in these patients:

   Situation A: Mrs. Novinger tells you that she frequently gets migraine headaches and feels one coming on.

   Situation B: Ryan Goode, age 3, reached out to pet a stray cat, who hissed and scratched his forearm.

   Situation C: Mrs. Carol Chung underwent a cesarean birth 2 days ago and is using her call light to request something for her incisional pain.

   Situation D: Joseph Miles, age 79, has a long history of degenerative joint disease and tells you this is a "bad morning" for his joints: "I think the weather must be affecting my arthritis."

   Write a three-part diagnosis statement for each of these patients using the assessment data in the table on page 229.

   Situation A: _____

   Situation B: _____

   Situation C: _____

   Situation D: _____

Situation	Behavioral	Physiologic	Affective
A			
B			
C			
D			

2. Briefly describe the events that occur when the threshold of pain has been reached and there is injured tissue.

_____

_____

_____

3. Explain why referred pain can be transmitted to a cutaneous (skin) site different from its origin.

_____

_____

4. Explain the mechanics of the gate control theory and how it is believed to control pain.

_____

_____

_____

_____

5. Describe the following types of pain and give an example of each from your own experience with patients.

  a. Acute pain: _____

  _____

  b. Chronic pain: _____

  _____

  c. Intractable pain: _____

  _____

6. Give an example of how the following factors may influence a patient's pain experience.

  a. Culture: _____

  _____

  b. Ethnicity: _____

  _____

  c. Family, gender, or age: _____

  _____

  d. Religious beliefs: _____

  _____

  e. Environment and support people: ____

  _____

  f. Anxiety and other stressors: _____

  _____

  g. Past pain experience: _____

  _____

7. List two experiences you have had with pain management for patients. Note your response to their pain and the effectiveness of your pain management techniques. Which pain control measures were most effective, and what could you have done differently to provide better pain control?

  a. _____

  _____

  _____

b. _____
_____
_____

8. Describe how you would respond to a patient who tells you the following about his/her pain experience.

a. "I know you'll know when I'm in pain and will do something to relieve it." _____
_____

b. "If I ask for something for pain, I'm afraid I may become addicted." _____
_____

c. "It's natural to have pain when you get older. It's just something I've learned to live with." _____
_____

9. Give an example of an interview question you could use to assess a patient for the following characteristics of pain.

a. Duration of pain: _____
_____

b. Quantity and intensity of pain: _____
_____

c. Quality of pain: _____
_____

d. Physiologic indicators of pain: _____
_____

10. State your opinion of the use of placebos to satisfy a person's demand for a drug. Is lying to the patient ever justifiable? How could this action affect the nurse–patient relationship? What, if anything, would you say to a physician who prescribed a placebo for your patient?
_____
_____
_____
_____

11. How would you modify your means of assessing for pain in the following patients?

a. A patient with a cognitive impairment: ___
_____

b. A 5-year-old patient: _____
_____

c. An older patient: _____
_____

APPLYING YOUR KNOWLEDGE

CRITICAL THINKING QUESTIONS

1. Think back to the last time you experienced acute pain (e.g., a toothache, headache, backache). If you were at work, were you able to concentrate on anything but the pain? How did the people around you respond to your pain? What measures did you take to relieve the pain, and how successful were they? Interview several patients who are experiencing acute pain. How are they coping psychologically and physically with the pain? What comfort measures work best for them? How has medication helped to control their pain? How can you use this knowledge to improve your care?

2. Find a tool to assess pain. Be sure it includes physical assessment, pain scales, location and duration of the pain, coping measures, pain management, and the effect of pain on daily living. Use this tool to assess the pain of individuals with similar problems (e.g., migraine, cramps, arthritis) and look for factors to explain their different experiences.

3. You notice a young woman who is experiencing intense pain. When you ask the nurses about this patient, they tell you she is in end-stage cancer and has received all the pain medication she has been prescribed. They could not administer more medication without a doctor's order. How would you react to this patient? What would you do to provide alternative comfort measures? Would you be an advocate for this patient and attempt to have more medication prescribed? How might who you are and your competence in pain management affect this woman's last days?

REFLECTIVE PRACTICE USING CRITICAL THINKING SKILLS

Use the following expanded scenario from Chapter 35 in your textbook to answer the questions below.

Scenario: Carla Potter is a 26-year-old white woman. She experiences "bad cramps" and periodic fatigue, anxiety, irritability, and mood swings approximately 1 week before the start of her menses. She told the nurse practitioner that her job as a computer programmer is stressful and these monthly symptoms are affecting her job performance and relationships. She asks the nurse if there is anything available to control these symptoms.

1. What nursing interventions might the nurse use to help minimize the effects of premenstrual syndrome on Ms. Potter?

   _____
   _____
   _____

2. What would be a successful outcome for this patient?

   _____
   _____
   _____

3. What intellectual, technical, interpersonal, and/or ethical/legal competencies are most likely to bring about the desired outcome?

   _____
   _____
   _____

4. What resources might be helpful for Ms. Potter?

   _____
   _____
   _____

PATIENT CARE STUDY

Read the following case study and use your nursing process skills to answer the questions below.

Scenario: Tabitha Wilson is a 24-month-old infant with AIDS who is hospitalized with infectious diarrhea. She is well known to the pediatric staff, and there is real concern that she might not pull through this admission. She has suffered many of the complications of AIDS and is no stranger to pain. At present, the skin on her buttocks is raw and excoriated, and tears stream down her face whenever she is moved. Her blood pressure also shoots up when she is touched. The severity of her illness has left her extremely weak and listless, and her foster mother reports that she no longer recognizes her child. When alone in her crib, she seldom moves, and she moans softly. Several nurses have expressed great frustration caring for Tabitha because they find it hard to perform even simple nursing measures like turning, diapering, and weighing her when they see how much pain these procedures cause.

1. Identify pertinent patient data by placing a single underline beneath the objective data in the case study and a double underline beneath the subjective data.

2. Complete the Nursing Process Worksheet on page 232 to develop a three-part diagnostic statement and related plan of care for this patient.

3. Write down the patient and personal nursing strengths you hope to draw on as you assist this patient to better health.

   Patient strengths: _____
   _____
   _____

   Personal strengths: _____
   _____
   _____

4. Pretend that you are performing a nursing assessment of this patient after the plan of care is implemented. Document your findings.

   _____
   _____
   _____

NURSING PROCESS WORKSHEET

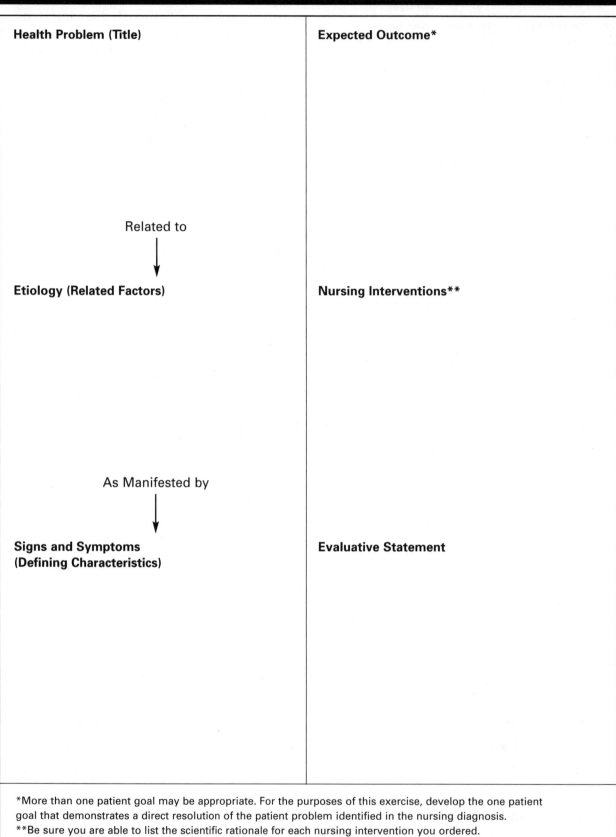

Health Problem (Title)

Expected Outcome*

Related to

↓

Etiology (Related Factors)

Nursing Interventions**

As Manifested by

↓

**Signs and Symptoms
(Defining Characteristics)**

Evaluative Statement

*More than one patient goal may be appropriate. For the purposes of this exercise, develop the one patient goal that demonstrates a direct resolution of the patient problem identified in the nursing diagnosis.
**Be sure you are able to list the scientific rationale for each nursing intervention you ordered.

CHAPTER 36

Nutrition

PRACTICING FOR NCLEX

MULTIPLE CHOICE QUESTIONS

Circle the letter that corresponds to the best answer for each question.

1. When assessing the nutritional requirements of an adult, which of the following facts about nutrition should be considered?
   a. Most nutrients work better alone than they do together.
   b. Nutrient needs remain the same throughout the life cycle.
   c. All nutrients are synthesized in the body.
   d. Nonessential nutrients do not have to be supplied though exogenous sources.

2. Which of the following nutrients supplies energy to the body?
   a. Proteins
   b. Vitamins
   c. Minerals
   d. Water

3. Of the following factors, which increases BMR?
   a. Aging
   b. Fever
   c. Fasting
   d. Sleep

4. Mrs. Blase is an obese patient who visits a weight control clinic. When considering a weight-reduction plan for this patient, the nurse should consider which of the following guidelines?

   a. To lose 1 pound/week, the daily intake should be decreased by 200 calories.
   b. One pound of body fat equals approximately 5,000 calories.
   c. Psychological reasons for overeating should be explored, such as eating as a release for boredom.
   d. Obesity is very treatable, and 50% of obese people who lose weight maintain the weight loss for 7 years.

5. Which of the following is the most abundant and least expensive source of calories in the world?
   a. Carbohydrates
   b. Fats
   c. Proteins
   d. Milk

6. Which of the following sugars must be broken down by enzymes in the intestinal tract before they can be absorbed?
   a. Glucose
   b. Fructose
   c. Galactose
   d. Lactose

7. Which of the following is the primary function of carbohydrates?
   a. To supply energy
   b. To form antibodies
   c. To maintain body tissues
   d. To provide the blood-clotting factor

8. Which of the following foods provides a complete protein?
   a. Vegetables
   b. Meats
   c. Grains
   d. Legumes

9. Which of the following vitamins is water soluble?
   a. Vitamin A
   b. Vitamin B
   c. Vitamin E
   d. Vitamin C

10. Men have a higher need than women for which of the following nutrients due to their larger muscle mass?
    a. Carbohydrates
    b. Minerals
    c. Proteins
    d. Vitamins

11. Which of the following procedures is appropriate when aspirating fluid from small-bore feeding tubes?
    a. Use a small syringe and insert 10 mL of air.
    b. If fluid is obtained when aspirating, measure its volume and pH and flush the tube with water.
    c. Continue to instill air until fluid is aspirated.
    d. Place the patient in the Trendelenburg position to facilitate the fluid aspiration process.

12. Checking the placement of a gastrostomy or jejunostomy tube requires regular comparisons of which of the following?
    a. Tube length
    b. Gastric fluid
    c. pH
    d. Air pressure

13. If a patient can attempt eating regular meals during the day and is prepared to ambulate and resume activities, supplemental feedings should be provided by which of the following methods?
    a. Continuous feeding
    b. Intermittent feeding
    c. Cyclic feeding
    d. Ambulatory feeding

14. When performing nursing actions associated with successful tube feedings, the nurse should do which of the following?
    a. Check tube placement by adding food dye to the tube feed as a means of detecting aspirated fluid.
    b. Check the residual before each feeding or every 4 to 8 hours during a continuous feeding.
    c. Assess for bowel sounds at least four times per shift to ensure the presence of peristalsis and a functional intestinal tract.
    d. Prevent contamination during enteral feedings by using an open system.

15. A nutritional therapy for patients who have nonfunctional gastrointestinal tracts or who are comatose would most likely be accomplished by which of the following?
    a. Enteral feeding pump
    b. PEG
    c. Nasointestinal tube
    d. TPN

16. Which of the following is the best indicator that a patient needs TPN?
    a. Serum albumin level of 2.5 g/dL or less
    b. Residual of more than 100 mL
    c. Absence of bowel sounds
    d. Presence of dumping syndrome

ALTERNATE-FORMAT QUESTIONS

Multiple Response Questions

Circle the letters that correspond to the best answers for each question.

1. Which of the following nutrients supply energy to the body? *(Select all that apply.)*
   a. Vitamins
   b. Minerals
   c. Carbohydrates
   d. Protein
   e. Water
   f. Lipids

2. Which of the following factors increase BMR? *(Select all that apply.)*
   a. Growth
   b. Aging
   c. Prolonged fasting

d. Infections

e. Emotional tension

f. Sleep

3. Which of the following statements accurately describe the action of carbohydrates in the body? *(Select all that apply.)*

   a. Carbohydrates are more difficult to digest than protein or fat.

   b. Ninety percent of carbohydrate is digested.

   c. The percentage of carbohydrates decreases as fiber intake increases.

   d. All carbohydrates are converted to glucose for transport through the blood or for use as energy.

   e. The period between when carbohydrates are consumed and when they are used for energy varies from 10 to 24 hours.

   f. All carbohydrates, except for indigestible fiber, provide 12 cal/g regardless of the source.

4. Which of the following statements regarding the function of protein in the body are accurate? *(Select all that apply.)*

   a. Within the body, more than a thousand different proteins are made by combining amounts and proportions of the 22 amino acids.

   b. Proteins are required for the formation of all body structures.

   c. Dietary protein may be labeled complete or incomplete based on its fiber content.

   d. Dietary protein is broken down into amino acid particles by pancreatic enzymes in the small intestine.

   e. Amino acid particles are absorbed through the intestinal mucosa to be transported to the gallbladder.

   f. The body's protein tissues are in a constant state of flux.

5. Which of the following statements accurately reflect the effects of fat in the diet? *(Select all that apply.)*

   a. Fats in the diet are soluble in water and, therefore, soluble in blood.

   b. Ninety-five percent of the lipids in the diet are in the form of triglycerides.

   c. Food fats contain mixtures of saturated and unsaturated fatty aids depending on the amount of nitrogen in fat molecules.

   d. Most animal fats are considered unsaturated, and most vegetable fats are considered saturated.

   e. Saturated fats tend to raise serum cholesterol levels.

   f. Fat digestion occurs largely in the small intestine.

6. Which of the following are functions of regulatory nutrients? *(Select all that apply.)*

   a. Vitamins, minerals, and water are regulatory nutrients because they are needed by the body for the metabolism of energy nutrients.

   b. Vitamins are inorganic compounds needed by the body in moderate amounts.

   c. Vitamins are essential in the diet because most are either not synthesized in the body or not made in sufficient quantities.

   d. Minerals are inorganic elements found in all body fluids and tissues in the form of salts or combined with organic compounds.

   e. Calcium, phosphorus, and magnesium are microminerals because they are needed by the body in amounts of less than 100 mg/day.

   f. Water accounts for 35% to 50% of the adult's total weight.

7. Which of the following are daily recommended food servings for specific food groups according to the MyPyramid Food Guide? *(Select all that apply.)*

   a. 1 cup of fats or sweets

   b. 1 cup of fruit

   c. 12 oz. grains

   d. 2½ cups vegetables

   e. 3 cups milk

   f. 5½ oz. meats or beans

8. Which of the following statements accurately describe factors that influence nutrient requirements? *(Select all that apply.)*

   a. During adulthood, there is an increase in the basal metabolic rate with each decade.

   b. Because of the changes related to aging, the caloric needs of the older adult increase.

   c. During pregnancy and lactation, nutrient requirements increase.

   d. Nutritional needs per unit of body weight are greater in infancy than at any other time in life.

e. Men and women differ in their nutrient requirements.

f. Trauma, surgery, and burns decrease nutrient requirements.

9. Which of the following are accurate guidelines for preventing complications with enteral feedings? (*Select all that apply.*)

a. Elevate the head of the bed at least 30 degrees during the feeding and for at least 1 hour afterward.

b. Give large, infrequent feedings.

c. Flush the tube before and after feeding.

d. Clean and moisten the nares every 4 to 8 hours.

e. Change the delivery set every other day according to agency policy.

f. Check the residual before intermittent feedings and every 8 hours during continuous feedings.

Fill-in-the-Blank Questions

1. What would be the BMI for a 220-pound man who is 6 feet 3 inches tall? _____

2. According to U.S. guidelines, what would be the daily caloric requirement for a sedentary male whose IBW is 165? _____

3. Approximately what range (in grams) of carbohydrates is needed daily to prevent ketosis? _____

4. Most healthcare experts recommend that protein intake should contribute what percentage of total caloric intake? _____

5. What percentage of an adult's total body weight is water? _____

6. Using the rule of thumb, determine the IBW for a 5-foot, 3-inch woman. _____

7. Using the rule of thumb, determine the IBW for a 5-foot, 8-inch man. _____

DEVELOPING YOUR KNOWLEDGE BASE

MATCHING EXERCISES

Match the nutrient in Part A with the type of function it performs listed in Part B. Answers will be used more than once.

PART A

a. Carbohydrates
b. Protein
c. Fat

PART B

1. ___ Spares protein so it can be used for other functions

2. ___ Insulates the body

3. ___ Stimulates tissue growth and repair

4. ___ Prevents ketosis from inefficient fat metabolism

5. ___ Helps regulate fluid balance through oncotic pressure

6. ___ Cushions internal organs

7. ___ Delays glucose absorption

8. ___ Is necessary for absorption of fat-soluble vitamins

9. ___ Detoxifies harmful substances

10. ___ Forms antibodies

Match the vitamins and minerals listed in Part A with the signs/symptoms of their deficiency listed in Part B.

PART A

a. Vitamin C
b. Vitamin B complex
c. Riboflavin
d. Niacin
e. Vitamin B_6
f. Folate
g. Vitamin B_{12}
h. Vitamin A
i. Vitamin D
j. Vitamin K
k. Calcium
l. Sodium
m. Potassium
n. Iron
o. Fluoride

PART B

11. ___ Pellagra, dermatitis

12. ___ Scurvy, hemorrhage, delayed wound healing

13. ___ Hemorrhagic disease of newborn, delayed blood clotting

14. ___ Hypokalemia, muscle cramps and weakness, irregular heartbeat

15. ___ Microcytic anemia, pallor, decreased work capacity, fatigue, weakness

16. ___ Beriberi, mental confusion, fatigue

17. ___ Anemia, CNS problems

18. ___ Pernicious anemia

19. ___ Night blindness, rough skin

20. ___ Hyponatremia, muscle cramps, cold and clammy skin

21. ___ Tooth decay, risk for osteoporosis

22. ___ Retarded bone growth, bone malformation

23. ___ Tetany, osteoporosis

24. ___ Ariboflavinosis, symptoms related to inflammation and poor wound healing

Match the function in Part B with the mineral listed in Part A. List one food source for each mineral on the line provided at the end of the sentence.

PART A

a. Calcium
b. Phosphorus
c. Magnesium
d. Sulfur
e. Sodium
f. Selenium
g. Chlorine
h. Iron
i. Iodine
j. Zinc
k. Copper
l. Manganese
m. Fluoride
n. Chromium
o. Molybdenum

PART B

25. ___ Promotes certain enzyme reactions and detoxification reactions _____

26. ___ Bone and tooth formation, blood clotting, nerve transmission, muscle contraction _____

27. ___ Component of HCl in stomach; fluid balance; acid–base balance _____

28. ___ Component of thyroid hormones _____

29. ___ Major ion of extracellular fluid; fluid balance; acid–base balance _____

30. ___ Aids in iron metabolism and activity of enzymes _____

31. ___ Tooth formation and integrity; bone formation and integrity _____

32. ___ Antioxidant _____

33. ___ Oxidizes sulfur and products of sulfur metabolism _____

34. ___ Bone and tooth formation; acid–base balance; energy metabolism _____

35. ___ Oxygen transported by way of hemoglobin; constituent of enzyme systems _____

36. ___ Tissue growth; sexual maturation; immune response _____

37. ___ Part of enzyme system needed for protein and energy metabolism _____

38. ___ Cofactor for insulin; proper glucose metabolism _____

Match the terms listed in Part A with their definition listed in Part B.

PART A

a. Nutrition
b. Nutrients
c. Macronutrients
d. Micronutrients

e. Calories

f. Basal metabolism

g. RDA

h. Cholesterol

i. MyPyramid Food Guide

PART B

39. ___ The measurement of energy in the diet

40. ___ The study of nutrients and how they are handled by the body

41. ___ The recommendation for average daily amounts that healthy population groups should consume over time

42. ___ Specific biochemical substances used by the body for growth, development, activity, reproduction, lactation, health maintenance, and recovery from injury or illness

43. ___ A graphic device designed to represent a total diet and provide a firm foundation for health

44. ___ Essential nutrients that supply energy and build tissue

45. ___ The amount of energy required to carry on the involuntary activities of the body at rest

46. ___ Vitamins and minerals that are required in much smaller amounts to regulate and control body processes

SHORT ANSWER

1. Briefly explain the body's state of nitrogen balance.

_____

_____

_____

2. Explain the difference between the following fatty acids, and give an example of each. Note which of the two lowers serum cholesterol levels.

a. Saturated fatty acids: _____

_____

_____

b. Unsaturated fatty acids: _____

_____

_____

3. List four conditions that may predispose a person to mild or subclinical deficiencies of vitamin A, vitamin C, folate, and vitamin B_6.

a. _____

b. _____

c. _____

d. _____

4. Briefly describe the nutritional needs of the following age groups:

a. Infancy: _____

_____

b. Toddlers and preschoolers: _____

_____

c. School-aged children: _____

_____

d. Adolescents: _____

_____

e. Adults: _____

_____

f. Pregnant women: _____

_____

g. Older adults: _____

_____

5. Complete the table on page 239 that depicts the function and recommended percentage of the diet for the energy nutrients.

Nutrient	Function	Recommended %
a. Carbohydrates		
b. Proteins		
c. Fats		
d. Vitamins		
e. Minerals		
f. Water		

6. List four interventions to increase fiber in a patient's diet.

   a. _____

   b. _____

   c. _____

   d. _____

7. Briefly describe the following eating disorders and the typical characteristics of individuals affected by them.

   a. Anorexia nervosa: _____

   _____

   b. Bulimia: _____

   _____

8. Give an example of how the following variables may affect a patient's nutritional needs.

   a. Sex: _____

   _____

   b. State of health: _____

   _____

   c. Alcohol abuse: _____

   _____

   d. Medications: _____

   _____

   e. Megadoses of nutrient supplements: _____

   _____

f. Religion: _____
_____

g. Economics: _____
_____

9. Describe the following methods of collecting dietary data.

a. Food diaries: _____
_____

b. Diet history: _____
_____
_____

10. Describe how you would assess a patient you are caring for at home for adequate nourishment.
_____
_____
_____

11. List three teaching strategies a nurse may use to achieve compliance with diet instructions.

a. _____

b. _____

c. _____

12. Describe the following types of diets, noting their nutritional value, and give an example of the types of food provided in each.

a. Clear liquid diet: _____
_____

b. Full liquid diet: _____
_____

c. Soft diet: _____
_____

13. Briefly describe the following types of enteral feedings, noting their advantages and disadvantages.

a. Nasogastric feeding tube: _____
_____

b. Nasointestinal feeding tube: _____
_____
_____

14. List five areas that need to be evaluated for a patient at home who is receiving TPN.

a. _____

b. _____

c. _____

d. _____

e. _____

APPLYING YOUR KNOWLEDGE

CRITICAL THINKING QUESTIONS

1. Develop a nutritional assessment for the following patients. What developmental factors influence their nutritional needs?

a. An 18-month-old healthy infant

b. A 5-year-old who is extremely active

c. A 12-year-old who is 50 pounds overweight

d. A teenager who is concerned about body image and borders on being anorexic

e. A middle-aged adult with high blood pressure

f. A senior citizen who is anemic

2. Keep a diary of all the foods you eat in a week. Does your diet follow the USDA's dietary guidelines for a healthy diet? Does your diet include the recommended number of servings of foods from the food pyramid? Is your diet high or low in fat? Perform a nutritional nursing assessment of your dietary habits. Develop a plan of care to improve your nutritional intake, if necessary. What personal factors might interfere with your making the necessary changes? How might this self-knowledge influence your nursing care?

REFLECTIVE PRACTICE USING CRITICAL THINKING SKILLS

Use the following expanded scenario from Chapter 36 in your textbook to answer the questions below.

Scenario: William Johnston, a 42-year-old executive, is newly diagnosed with high blood pressure and high cholesterol. He confides that his health has been the last thing on his mind and that his health habits are less than admirable. "I usually eat on the run, often fast food, or big dinners with lots of alcohol. I can't

remember the last time I worked out or did any exercise, unless running from my car to the train counts! I guess it's no wonder I've gained a few pounds over the years!"

1. What patient teaching might the nurse provide to help Mr. Johnston meet his nutritional and exercise needs?

_____

_____

_____

2. What would be a successful outcome for this patient?

_____

_____

_____

3. What intellectual, technical, interpersonal, and/or ethical/legal competencies are most likely to bring about the desired outcome?

_____

_____

_____

4. What resources might be helpful for Mr. Johnston?

_____

_____

_____

PATIENT CARE STUDY

Read the following case study and use your nursing process skills to answer the questions below.

Scenario: Mr. Church, a 74-year-old white man, is being admitted to the geriatric unit of the hospital for a diagnostic workup. He was diagnosed with Alzheimer's disease 4 years ago, and 1 year ago, he was admitted to a long-term care facility. His wife of 49 years is

extremely devoted and informs the nurse taking the admission history that she instigated his admission to the hospital because she was alarmed by the amount of weight he was losing. Assessment reveals a 6-foot, 1-inch tall, emaciated man who weighs 149 pounds. His wife reports that he has lost 20 pounds in the past 2 months. The staff at the long-term care facility report that he was eating his meals and his wife validated that this was the case. No one seems sure, however, of the caloric content of his diet. Mrs. Church nods her head vigorously when asked if her husband had seemed more agitated and hyperactive recently. Mr. Church has dull, sparse hair; pale, dry skin; and dry mucous membranes.

1. Identify pertinent patient data by placing a single underline beneath the objective data in the case study and a double underline beneath the subjective data.

2. Complete the Nursing Process Worksheet on page 242 to develop a three-part diagnostic statement and related plan of care for this patient.

3. Write down the patient and personal nursing strengths you hope to draw on as you assist this patient to better health.

Patient strengths: _____

_____

_____

Personal strengths: _____

_____

_____

4. Pretend that you are performing a nursing assessment of this patient after the plan of care is implemented. Document your findings.

_____

_____

_____

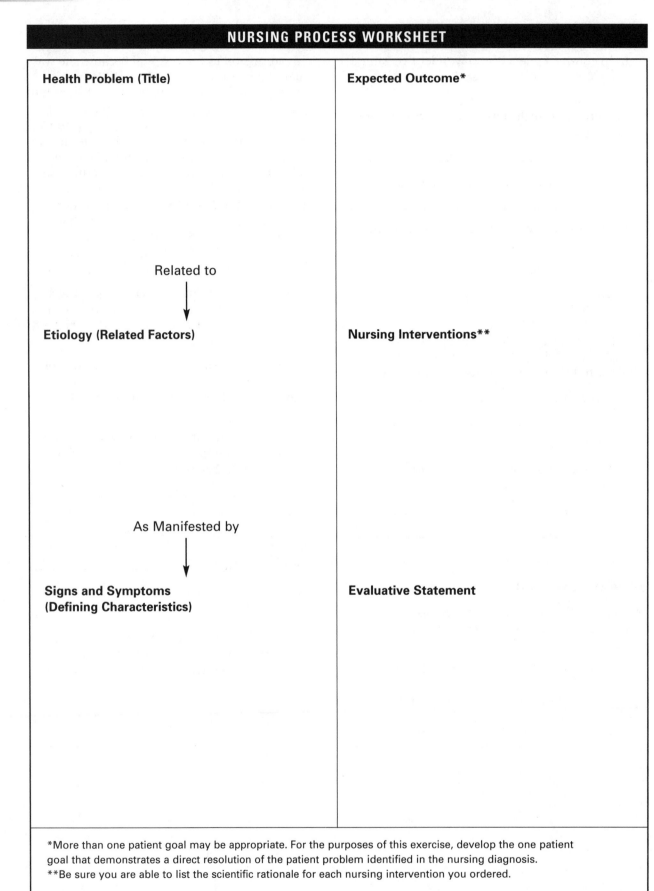

NURSING PROCESS WORKSHEET

Health Problem (Title)

Expected Outcome*

Related to
↓

Etiology (Related Factors)

Nursing Interventions**

As Manifested by
↓

**Signs and Symptoms
(Defining Characteristics)**

Evaluative Statement

*More than one patient goal may be appropriate. For the purposes of this exercise, develop the one patient goal that demonstrates a direct resolution of the patient problem identified in the nursing diagnosis.
**Be sure you are able to list the scientific rationale for each nursing intervention you ordered.

CHAPTER 37

Urinary Elimination

PRACTICING FOR NCLEX

MULTIPLE CHOICE QUESTIONS

Circle the letter that corresponds to the best answer for each question.

1. A woman who notices an involuntary loss of urine following a coughing episode is most likely experiencing which of the following types of incontinence?
   a. Stress incontinence
   b. Urge incontinence
   c. Overflow incontinence
   d. Functional incontinence

2. Measurement of residual urine by catheterization after voiding verifies which of the following conditions?
   a. Urinary tract infection
   b. Urinary retention
   c. Urinary incontinence
   d. Urinary suppression

3. Which of the following catheters should be used to drain a patient's bladder for short periods (5 to 10 minutes)?
   a. Foley catheter
   b. Suprapubic catheter
   c. Indwelling urethral catheter
   d. Straight catheter

4. Which of the following facts about the lower urinary tract system should be kept in mind when considering catheterization?

a. The bladder normally is a sterile cavity.
b. The external opening to the urethra should always be sterilized.
c. Pathogens introduced into the bladder remain in the bladder.
d. A normal bladder is as susceptible to infection as an injured one.

5. Which of the following events occurs when micturition is initiated?
   a. The detrusor muscle expands.
   b. The internal sphincter contracts.
   c. Urine enters the posterior urethra.
   d. The muscles of the perineum and external sphincter contract.

6. Which of the following collection devices is a nurse's best option when collecting urine from a nonambulatory male patient?
   a. Specimen hat
   b. Large urine collection bag
   c. Bedpan
   d. Urinal

7. Mr. Gonos is being transferred to the hospital from a nursing home with a diagnosis of dehydration and urinary bladder infection. His skin is also excoriated from urinary incontinence. Which of the following is the most appropriate nursing diagnosis for Mr. Gonos?
   a. Impaired Skin Integrity related to functional incontinence
   b. Urinary Incontinence related to urinary tract infection

c. Impaired Skin Integrity related to urinary tract infection and dehydration

d. Risk for Urinary Tract Infection related to dehydration

8. Which of the following nursing interventions would be least effective when trying to maintain safety for the patient with an indwelling catheter?

a. Maintain a closed drainage system.

b. Restrict fluid intake.

c. Apply a topical antibiotic ointment to urinary meatus.

d. Report signs of infection immediately.

9. A nurse determines that her patient has costovertebral tenderness. Which of the following conditions is indicated by this physical finding?

a. A bladder infection

b. A bladder obstruction

c. An inflamed kidney

d. The presence of a kidney stone

10. Mrs. Babb has had four urinary tract infections in the past year. Which physiologic change of aging is likely causing Mrs. Babb's problem?

a. Decreased bladder contractility

b. Diminished ability to concentrate urine

c. Decreased bladder muscle tone

d. Neurologic weakness

11. The doctor has ordered the collection of a fresh urine sample for a particular examination. Which urine sample would the nurse discard?

a. The sample collected immediately after lunch

b. The bedtime voiding

c. The voiding collected at 4 p.m.

d. The first voiding of the day

12. Mr. Morris has a urinary obstruction and is not a candidate for surgery. Which of the following would be an appropriate intervention for this patient?

a. Insertion of an indwelling urethral catheter

b. Insertion of a suprapubic catheter

c. Insertion of a straight catheter

d. Insertion of a urologic stent

ALTERNATE-FORMAT QUESTIONS

Multiple Response Questions

Circle the letters that correspond to the best answers for each question.

1. Which of the following statements accurately describe kidney function? *(Select all that apply.)*

a. It is estimated that the total blood volume passes through the kidneys for waste removal about every 2 hours.

b. One of the most significant functions of the kidneys is to maintain the composition and volume of body fluids.

c. Urine from the nephrons empties into the urinary bladder.

d. There are approximately 1,000 nephrons in each kidney.

e. The kidneys filter and excrete blood constituents that are not needed and retain those that are.

f. The basic unit of the kidney is the nephron, which removes the end products of metabolism.

2. When collecting a urine specimen for urinalysis, the nurse should be aware of which of the following facts? *(Select all that apply.)*

a. Sterile urine specimens may be obtained by catheterizing the patient's bladder.

b. A sterile urine specimen is required for a routine urinalysis.

c. If a woman is menstruating, a urine specimen cannot be obtained for urinalysis.

d. Strict aseptic technique must be used when collecting and handling urine specimens.

e. Urine should be left standing at room temperature for a 24-hour period before being sent to the laboratory.

f. A clean-catch specimen of urine may be collected in midstream.

3. You are preparing a female patient for catheterization. Which of the following are appropriate steps in this procedure? *(Select all that apply.)*

a. Place the patient in the dorsal recumbent position.

b. Explain to the patient that the procedure is painless and should cause no discomfort.

c. Place the patient on a soft surface, preferably a soft mattress or pillow.

d. Clean the genital and perineal area with antiseptic solution.

e. Place a fenestrated sterile drape over the perineal area, exposing the labia.

f. Insert the catheter tip into the meatus 7 to 10 cm or until the urine flows.

4. Which of the following actions are appropriate when conducting a physical assessment of a patient's urinary function? *(Select all that apply.)*

a. The nurse palpates the right kidney by pushing down on it when the patient exhales.

b. The nurse should palpate the kidney only under supervision.

c. The nurse checks for costovertebral tenderness by placing one palm flat over the costovertebral angle and striking the back of the hand with the other fist.

d. When percussing the bladder, a dull sound indicates an empty bladder

e. To examine the meatus, the female patient should be placed in a dorsal recumbent position.

f. The nurse may use a bedside scanner to assess the bladder.

5. Which of the following statements accurately describe the function and composition of the urinary bladder? *(Select all that apply.)*

a. The urinary bladder serves as a reservoir for urine.

b. The urinary bladder is composed of two layers of muscle tissue, the inner and outer longitudinal layer.

c. The urinary bladder muscle is innervated by the autonomic nervous system.

d. The autonomic nervous system carries inhibitory impulses to the bladder and motor impulses to the internal sphincter.

e. Inhibitory impulses to the bladder cause the detrusor muscle to relax and the internal sphincter to constrict, retaining urine in the bladder.

f. Motor impulses to the bladder and inhibitory impulses to the internal sphincter cause the detrusor muscle to contract and the sphincter to relax.

6. Which of the following statements accurately describe the function of the urethra? *(Select all that apply.)*

a. The anatomy of the urethra is the same in males and females.

b. The urethra's function is to convey urine from the bladder to the exterior.

c. The external sphincter is under involuntary control.

d. No portion of the female urethra is external to the body.

e. The male urethra functions in both the excretory system and the reproductive system.

f. The muscle at the meatus of the female is usually called the internal sphincter.

7. Which of the following is a normal characteristic of urine? *(Select all that apply.)*

a. A freshly voided specimen is pale yellow, straw-colored, or amber, depending on its concentration.

b. Freshly voided urine smells like ammonia.

c. Fresh urine should be clear or translucent.

d. The normal pH of urine is about 3.2, with a range of 2.6 to 5.

e. The normal range of the specific gravity of urine is 1.010 to 1.025.

f. Organic constituents of urine include ammonia, sodium, chloride, and potassium.

8. Which of the following actions would a nurse perform when measuring a patient's urinary output? *(Select all that apply.)*

a. The nurse asks the patient to void into a bedpan, urinal, or specimen hat, either in bed or in the bathroom.

b. The nurse pours the urine from the collection device into the appropriate measuring device.

c. The nurse places the calibrated container on a flat surface for an accurate reading and reads the amount by looking down into the specimen.

d. The nurse records the total amount voided during each shift and the 24-hour period on the patient's permanent record.

e. The nurse discards the urine into the toilet unless a specimen is required.

f. The nurse informs a patient that due to legal considerations he cannot measure and record his own output.

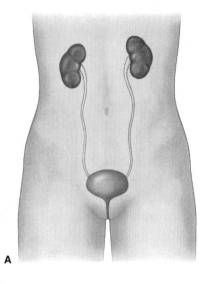

A

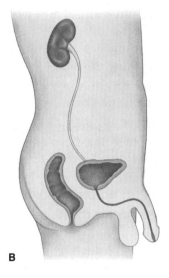

B

Hot Spot Questions

1. Place an X on figures A and B above to identify the female and male urethras.

2. Place an X on the figure below to identify the location of the external sphincter.

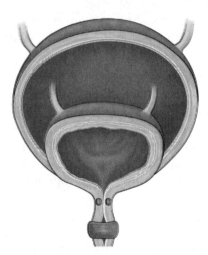

3. Place an X on the figure below to identify the urinary bladder.

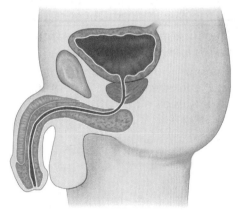

4. Place an X on the figure below to mark the spot where a suprapubic catheter would be inserted into the bladder.

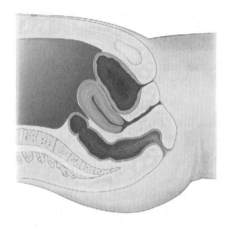

DEVELOPING YOUR KNOWLEDGE BASE

MATCHING EXERCISES

Match the terms associated with micturition in Part A with their definitions listed in Part B.

PART A

a. Micturition

b. Frequency

c. Urinary retention

d. Enuresis

e. Autonomic bladder

f. Hesitancy

g. Stress incontinence

h. Urge incontinence

i. Mixed incontinence

j. Overflow incontinence

k. Functional incontinence

l. Total incontinence

PART B

1. _____ A delay or difficulty in initiating voiding

2. _____ The involuntary loss of urine associated with an abrupt and strong desire to void

3. _____ Urine loss caused by factors outside the lower urinary tract, such as chronic impairments of physical or cognitive functioning

4. _____ The process of emptying the bladder

5. _____ Involuntary urination that occurs after an age when continence should be present

6. _____ Occurs when urine is produced normally but not appropriately excreted from the bladder

7. _____ The involuntary loss of urine associated with overdistention and overflow of the bladder

8. _____ Continuous and unpredictable loss of urine resulting from surgery, trauma, or physical malformation

9. _____ Voiding by reflex only

10. _____ Occurs when there is an involuntary loss of urine related to an increase in intra-abdominal pressure during coughing, sneezing, laughing, or other physical activities

11. _____ Symptoms of urge and stress incontinence are present, although one type may predominate.

Match the color of urine listed in Part A with the medication that produces that color listed in Part B. Answers may be used more than once.

PART A

a. Pale yellow

b. Orange, orange-red, or pink

c. Green or green-blue

d. Brown or black

e. Red

PART B

12. _____ Levodopa

13. _____ Diuretics

14. _____ Elavil

15. _____ B-complex vitamins

16. _____ Pyridium

17. _____ Injectable iron compounds

18. _____ Anticoagulants

SHORT ANSWER

1. Describe how the following factors affect micturition.

   a. Developmental considerations: _____

   _____

   b. Food and fluid: _____

   _____

   c. Psychological variables: _____

   _____

   d. Activity and muscle tone: _____

   _____

   e. Pathologic conditions: _____

   _____

   f. Medications: _____

   _____

2. List three factors that indicate a child is ready for toilet training.

   a. _____

   b. _____

   c. _____

3. Describe special urinary considerations that should be included in the nursing history for the following patients.

   a. Infants and young children: _____

   _____

   b. Older adults: _____

   _____

   c. Patients with limited or no bladder control or urinary diversions: _____

   _____

4. Describe how you would examine the following areas of the urinary system when performing a physical assessment.

   a. Kidneys: _____

   _____

   b. Bladder: _____

   _____

   c. Urethral orifice: _____

   _____

   d. Skin integrity and hydration: _____

   _____

   e. Urine: _____

   _____

5. Briefly describe the procedure for determining the specific gravity of urine with a urinometer or hydrometer.

   _____

   _____

6. List four expected outcomes that denote normal voiding in a patient.

   a. _____

   b. _____

   c. _____

   d. _____

7. Explain how the following factors influence a patient's voiding patterns.

   a. Schedule: _____

   _____

   b. Privacy: _____

   _____

   c. Position: _____

   _____

   d. Hygiene: _____

   _____

8. List three reasons for catheterization.

   a. _____

   b. _____

   c. _____

9. List two expected outcomes for a patient with a urinary appliance.

   a. _____

   b. _____

APPLYING YOUR KNOWLEDGE

CRITICAL THINKING QUESTIONS

1. Develop a teaching plan to teach a postsurgical patient and his wife how to insert and care for a Foley catheter in a home setting. What factors are likely to influence the success of your teaching plan?

2. Keep a record of your fluid intake and output for 3 days. Note how your intake influenced urinary elimination. Write down the factors that could affect urine elimination. Are you at risk for urinary problems? If possible, perform routine tests on a sample of your urine and record the results.

REFLECTIVE PRACTICE USING CRITICAL THINKING SKILLS

Use the following expanded scenario from Chapter 37 in your textbook to answer the questions below.

Scenario: Midori Morita, age 69, is taking care of her 70-year-old husband at home. She states, "I'd like to talk with my husband's doctor about getting him a urinary catheter. Ever since he came back from the hospital this last time, he seems unable to use the urinal. He dribbles constantly and I can't keep up with the laundry. He had a catheter in the hospital and I'm going to request that he has one at home."

1. How might the nurse respond to Mrs. Morita's remarks regarding her husband's home care?

   _____

   _____

   _____

2. What would be a successful outcome for this patient?

   _____

   _____

   _____

3. What intellectual, technical, interpersonal, and/or ethical/legal competencies are most likely to bring about the desired outcome?

_____

_____

_____

4. What resources might be helpful for the Morita family?

_____

_____

_____

PATIENT CARE STUDY

Read the following case study and use your nursing process skills to answer the questions below.

Scenario: Mr. Eisenberg, age 84, was admitted to a nursing home when his wife of 62 years died. He has two adult children, neither of whom feels prepared to care for him the way his wife did. "We don't know how Mom did it year after year," his son says. "After he retired from his law practice, he was terribly demanding, and it just seemed nothing she did for him pleased him. His Parkinson's disease does make it a bit difficult for him to get around, but he's able to do a whole lot more than he is letting on. He's always been this way." The aides have reported to you that Mr. Eisenberg is frequently incontinent of both urine and stool during the day as well as during the night. He is alert and appears capable of recognizing the need to void or defecate and signaling for any assistance. His son and daughter report that this was never a problem at home and that he was able to go into the bathroom with assistance. He has been depressed about his admission to the home and seldom speaks, even when directly approached. He has refused to participate in any of the floor social events since his arrival.

1. Identify pertinent patient data by placing a single underline beneath the objective data in the case study and a double underline beneath the subjective data.

2. Complete the Nursing Process Worksheet on page 250 to develop a three-part diagnostic statement and related plan of care for this patient.

3. Write down the patient and personal nursing strengths you hope to draw on as you assist this patient to better health.

   Patient strengths: _____

   _____

   _____

   Personal strengths: _____

   _____

   _____

4. Pretend that you are performing a nursing assessment of this patient after the plan of care is implemented. Document your findings.

   _____

   _____

   _____

NURSING PROCESS WORKSHEET

Health Problem (Title)

Expected Outcome*

Related to

↓

Etiology (Related Factors)

Nursing Interventions**

As Manifested by

↓

Signs and Symptoms (Defining Characteristics)

Evaluative Statement

*More than one patient goal may be appropriate. For the purposes of this exercise, develop the one patient goal that demonstrates a direct resolution of the patient problem identified in the nursing diagnosis.
**Be sure you are able to list the scientific rationale for each nursing intervention you ordered.

CHAPTER 38

Bowel Elimination

PRACTICING FOR NCLEX

MULTIPLE CHOICE QUESTIONS

Circle the letter that corresponds to the best answer for each question.

1. Which of the following statements concerning peristalsis is accurate?

   a. The sympathetic nervous system inhibits movement.

   b. Peristalsis occurs every 25 to 30 minutes.

   c. One half to three fourths of ingested food waste products normally are excreted in the stool within 24 hours.

   d. Mass peristaltic sweeps occur one to four times every 24 hours in most people.

2. A patient who is experiencing constipation should avoid which of the following foods?

   a. Beans

   b. Chocolate

   c. Cheese

   d. Onions

3. Which of the following is the correct procedure when using a rectal tube?

   a. Position the patient on his/her back and drape properly.

   b. Introduce the rectal tube beyond the anal canal into the rectum 7 to 10 cm for an adult.

   c. Leave the tube in place for 45 to 60 minutes.

   d. Have the patient lie still in a side-lying position when the tube is in place.

4. Tympany, the normal sound percussed over the abdomen, is caused by which of the following?

   a. Excess flatus

   b. Hollow organs

   c. Intestinal fluid

   d. Fecal contents

5. Which of the following is the barrier between the large intestine and the ileum of the small intestine?

   a. Ileocecal junction

   b. Sphincter

   c. Splenic flexure

   d. Hepatic flexure

6. Approximately how much water is absorbed daily by the intestinal tract?

   a. 300 to 400 mL

   b. 400 to 600 mL

   c. 600 to 800 mL

   d. 800 to 1,000 mL

7. Which of the following indicates the most logical sequence of tests to ensure an accurate diagnosis?

   a. Barium studies, endoscopic examination, fecal occult blood test

   b. Fecal occult blood test, barium studies, endoscopic examination

   c. Barium studies, fecal occult blood test, endoscopic examination

   d. Endoscopic examination, barium studies, fecal occult blood test

8. Which of the following drugs acts by increasing intestinal bulk to enhance mechanical stimulation of the intestine?

   a. Cascara

   b. Bisacodyl

   c. Magnesium sulfate

   d. Phenolphthalein

ALTERNATE-FORMAT QUESTIONS

Multiple Response Questions

Circle the letters that correspond to the best answers for each question.

1. Which of the following statements regarding the internal and external sphincter are accurate? *(Select all that apply.)*

   a. Both sphincters control the discharge of feces and intestinal gas.

   b. The internal sphincter consists of voluntary smooth muscle tissue.

   c. The internal sphincter is innervated by the autonomic nervous system.

   d. Motor impulses are carried by the sympathetic system and inhibitory impulses by the parasympathetic system.

   e. The external sphincter at the anus has striated muscle tissue and is not under voluntary control.

   f. The levator ani muscle reinforces the actions of the external sphincter.

2. Which of the following statements accurately describe the elimination patterns of the age group specified? *(Select all that apply.)*

   a. Voluntary control of defecation becomes possible between the ages of 12 and 18 months.

   b. The number of stools that infants pass varies greatly.

   c. Some children have bowel movements only every 2 or 3 days.

   d. Parents should be taught that a child who has not had a bowel movement daily is most likely constipated.

   e. In an infant, a liquid stool signifies diarrhea.

   f. Constipation is often a chronic problem for older adults.

3. Which of the following statements accurately describe the effect of foods and fluids on bowel elimination? *(Select all that apply.)*

   a. People who lack the enzyme lactase may experience diarrhea or gas when consuming starchy foods.

   b. A person who is constipated should eat eggs and pasta to relieve the condition.

   c. Fruits and vegetables have a laxative effect.

   d. Gas-producing foods include cauliflower and onions.

   e. Alcohol and coffee tend to have a constipating effect.

   f. Food intolerances may alter bowel elimination.

4. Which of the following actions would be performed when assessing bowel elimination? *(Select all that apply.)*

   a. The nurse palpates the abdomen before inspection and auscultation are performed.

   b. The nurse places the patient in the supine position with the abdomen exposed.

   c. The nurse drapes the patient's chest and pubic area and extends the patient's legs flat against the bed.

   d. The nurse encourages the patient to drink fluids before the assessment so that the bladder is full and can be examined.

   e. The nurse uses a warmed stethoscope to listen for bowel sounds in all abdominal quadrants.

   f. The nurse notes the character of bowel sounds, which are normally high-pitched, gurgling, and soft.

5. Which of the following measures are appropriate when a nurse collects a stool specimen? *(Select all that apply.)*

   a. The patient should be asked to void first because the lab study may be inaccurate if the stool contains urine.

   b. The patient should be asked to defecate into a clean bedpan or toilet bowl, depending on the nature of the study.

   c. The patient should be instructed not to place toilet tissue in the bedpan or specimen container.

d. Medical aseptic techniques are always followed.

e. Handwashing is performed before and after glove use when handling a stool specimen.

f. Generally, 2 inches of formed stool or 20 to 30 mL of liquid stool is sufficient for a stool specimen.

6. Which of the following statements accurately describe the normal characteristics of stool and special considerations for observation? *(Select all that apply.)*

a. Consistently large diarrheal stools suggest a disorder of the left colon or rectum.

b. The rapid rate of peristalsis in the breastfed infant causes the stool to be yellow.

c. The absence of bile may cause the stool to appear black.

d. Antacids in the diet cause the stool to be whitish.

e. A gastrointestinal obstruction may result in a narrow, pencil-shaped stool.

f. The odor of the stool is influenced by its pH value, which normally is slightly acidic.

7. Which of the following statements accurately describe the action of specific antidiarrheal medications? *(Select all that apply.)*

a. Kaopectate does not interfere with the absorption of other oral medications.

b. Imodium is an antimicrobial against bacterial and viral pathogens.

c. Imodium is a nonaddictive antidiarrheal medication that has a longer duration of action than Lomotil.

d. Pepto-Bismol contains salicylates; a physician should be consulted before giving it to children or patients taking aspirin.

e. Paregoric contains morphine and may be addictive.

f. Lomotil has a longer duration of action than Imodium.

8. Which of the following commonly used enema solutions distend the intestine and increase peristalsis? *(Select all that apply.)*

a. Tap water

b. Soap

c. Normal saline

d. Mineral oil

e. Hypertonic

f. Olive oil

9. Which of the following is an accurate guideline for inserting a rectal suppository? *(Select all that apply.)*

a. Have the patient lie on his/her stomach and pie-fold top linens over him.

b. Separate the buttocks and have the patient relax by breathing through his mouth while the suppository is being inserted.

c. Introduce the suppository just to the internal sphincter (4 inches for adults and 2 inches for children and infants).

d. Avoid embedding the suppository in the fecal mass.

e. Encourage the patient to lie flat in order to retain the suppository for 30 to 45 minutes.

f. Lubricate the suppository and fingertips to reduce irritation to intestinal mucosa while inserting the suppository.

Prioritization Questions

1. Place the following guidelines for testing for fecal occult blood in the order in which they would normally occur:

a. Follow instructions based on the type of test. Hemoccult slide test requires placing 2 drops of developer solution on the back side of the specimen paper. The tablet test directions include placing 2 to 3 drops of tap water on the tablet, which is centered on the stool specimen.

b. Instruct the patient about food and drug restrictions at least 2 to 3 days before the test if they apply.

c. Use tongue blades to transfer the stool to the test tape or folder.

d. Document the test results according to agency policy. A blue color is a positive result and needs to be reported. Inform the patient of the test results.

e. Collect the amount recommended for the particular test (usually only a small amount is required).

f. Inform the patient that multiple or serial specimens are usually collected from different bowel movements to verify results.

g. Wear gloves and perform hand hygiene if collecting a specimen from a bedpan, commode, or plastic receptacle.

h. Review manufacturer's directions for collecting the specimen and avoid mixing the specimen with urine or water.

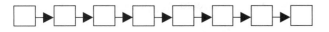

2. Place the following steps for digital removal of stool in the order in which they would normally occur:

a. Work the finger around and into the hardened mass to break it up and then remove pieces of it. Instruct the patient to bear down if possible while extracting feces to ease in removal.

b. Place the patient in a side-lying position and place a bedpan on the bed for depositing removed feces.

c. Use an oil-retention enema if necessary.

d. Remove the impaction at intervals if it is severe. This helps to avoid discomfort as well as irritation, which can injure intestinal mucosa.

e. Drape the patient to provide privacy, yet provide easy access.

f. Lubricate the forefinger generously to reduce irritation of the rectum and insert the finger gently into the anal canal. The presence of the finger added to the mass tends to cause discomfort for the patient if the work is not done slowly and gently.

g. Use clean gloves for the procedure because the intestinal tract is not sterile.

h. Have a second person assist with the procedure to reassure and comfort the patient while the first person breaks up the mass.

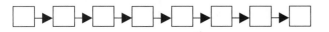

DEVELOPING YOUR KNOWLEDGE BASE

IDENTIFICATION

1. Locate the internal anal sphincter, the external anal sphincter, the anal canal, the rectum, and the anal valve on the figure below and write the appropriate body part on the lines provided.

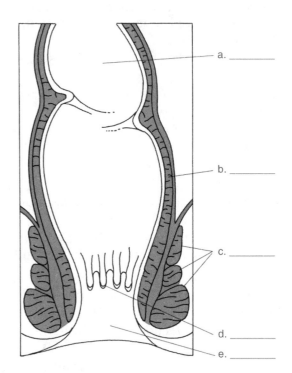

a. _____

b. _____

c. _____

d. _____

e. _____

2. Name the type of ostomy depicted in the figures below by writing your answers on the lines provided. Indicate the type of stool that would be expected with each ostomy.

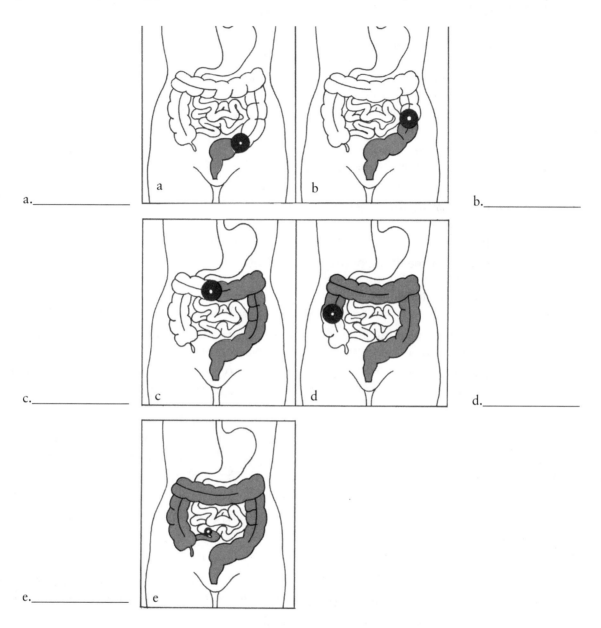

a._____

b._____

c._____

d._____

e._____

MATCHING EXERCISES

Match the bowel studies listed in Part A with their definition listed in Part B.

PART A

a. Endoscopy

b. Esophagogastroduodenoscopy

c. Colonoscopy

d. Sigmoidoscopy

e. Upper gastrointestinal examination

f. Lower gastrointestinal examination

g. Fecal occult blood test

h. Timed specimens

i. Pinworm test

PART B

1. ___ The collection of a specimen of every stool passed within a designated time period

2. ___ The direct visualization of the lining of a hollow body organ using a long flexible tube containing glass fibers that transmit light into the organ, allowing the return of an image that can be viewed

3. ____ The visual examination of the lining of the distal sigmoid colon, the rectum, and the anal canal using either a flexible or rigid instrument

4. ____ Barium sulfate is instilled into the large intestine through a rectal tube inserted through the anus. Fluoroscopy projects consecutive x-ray images onto a screen for continuous observation of the flow of the barium.

5. ____ Visual examination of the lining of the large intestine with a flexible, fiber-optic endoscope

6. ____ The patient drinks barium sulfate, which coats the esophagus, stomach, and small intestine to produce better visualization.

7. ____ Visual examination of the lining of the esophagus, the stomach, and the upper duodenum with a flexible, fiber-optic endoscope

8. ____ Use of a commercial tape, dipstick, or solution to test for pH or blood in the stool

Match the type of enema in Part A with its use listed in Part B. Some questions may have more than one answer.

PART A

a. Oil-retention enemas
b. Carminative enemas
c. Medicated enemas
d. Anthelmintic enemas
e. Nutritive enemas
f. Return flow or Harris flush enemas

PART B

9. ____ Used to lubricate the stool and intestinal mucosa, making defecation easier

10. ____ Administered to destroy intestinal parasites

11. ____ Used to administer medications that are absorbed through the rectal mucosa

12. ____ Used to administer fluids and nutrition rectally

13. ____ Used to help expel flatus from the rectum and provide relief from gaseous distention

Match the term in Part A with its definition listed in Part B.

PART A

a. Chyme
b. Feces
c. Stool
d. Flatus
e. Bowel movement
f. Hemorrhoids
g. Constipation
h. Diarrhea
i. Incontinence
j. Valsalva maneuver
k. Peristalsis

PART B

14. ____ The passage of dry, hard stools

15. ____ Waste product of digestion

16. ____ The passage of excessively liquid and unformed stools

17. ____ Waste product that reaches the distal end of the colon

18. ____ Intestinal gas

19. ____ The inability of the anal sphincter to control the discharge of fecal and gaseous material

20. ____ Excreted feces

21. ____ The emptying of the intestines

22. ____ The contraction of the circular and longitudinal muscles of the intestine

Match the organs of the gastrointestinal system listed in Part A with the illustration in Part B.

PART A

a. Splenic flexure
b. Sigmoid colon
c. Cecum
d. Hepatic flexure
e. Common bile duct
f. Stomach
g. Esophagus

h. Descending colon

i. Ileum

j. Hepatic duct

k. Gallbladder

l. Duodenum

m. Jejunum

n. Rectum

o. Ascending colon

p. Pancreatic duct

q. Ileocecal junction

r. Transverse colon

PART B

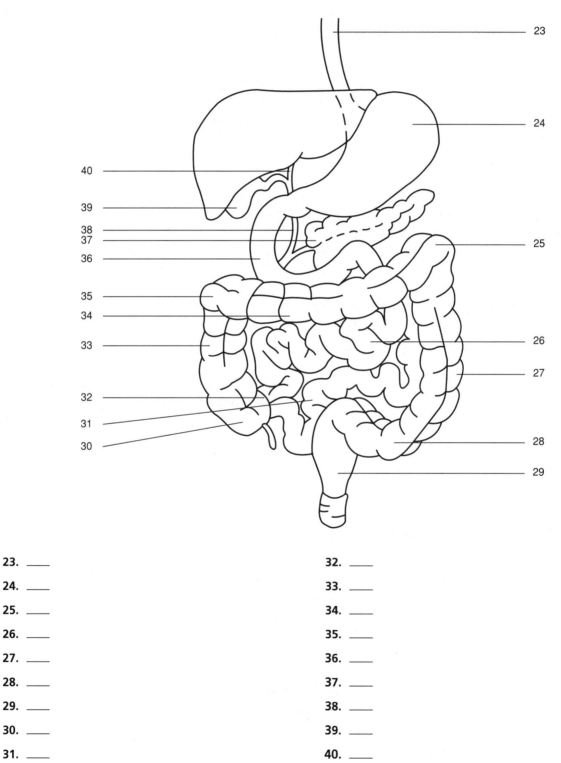

23. ____

24. ____

25. ____

26. ____

27. ____

28. ____

29. ____

30. ____

31. ____

32. ____

33. ____

34. ____

35. ____

36. ____

37. ____

38. ____

39. ____

40. ____

SHORT ANSWER

1. List four functions of the large intestine.

a. _____

b. _____

c. _____

d. _____

2. List the two centers of the nervous system that govern the reflex to defecate.

a. _____

b. _____

3. Describe two effects the following surgical procedures may have on peristalsis.

a. Direct manipulation of the bowel: _____

_____

_____

b. Inhalation of general anesthetic agents: ___

_____

_____

4. List the characteristics of the abdomen the nurse would assess by the following methods.

a. Inspection: _____

_____

b. Auscultation: _____

_____

c. Percussion: _____

_____

d. Palpation: _____

_____

5. Give an example of how the following factors might affect a patient's bowel elimination.

a. Developmental considerations: _____

_____

b. Daily patterns: _____

_____

c. Food and fluids: _____

_____

d. Activity and muscle tone: _____

_____

e. Lifestyle: _____

_____

f. Psychological variables: _____

_____

g. Medications: _____

_____

h. Diagnostic studies: _____

_____

6. Mrs. Manganello is a 52-year-old patient with acute stomach pain related to diverticular disease. Prepare an interview to assess Mrs. Manganello's bowel elimination.

_____

_____

_____

_____

7. List four factors that promote healthy elimination patterns.

a. _____

b. _____

c. _____

d. _____

8. Give three examples of foods that have the following effects on elimination.

a. Constipating: _____

_____

b. Laxative: _____

_____

c. Gas-producing: _____

_____

9. Mrs. Azhner is a 65-year-old postsurgical patient complaining of painful defecation due to hard, dry stools. List three expected outcomes for this patient.

a. _____

b. _____

c. _____

10. Specify dietary measures to alleviate the following gastrointestinal problems.

  a. Constipation: _____

  _____

  b. Diarrhea: _____

  _____

  c. Flatulence: _____

  _____

  d. Ostomies: _____

  _____

11. Describe the following exercises designed for patients with weak abdominal and perineal muscles who are using a bedpan.

  a. Abdominal settings: _____

  _____

  b. Thigh strengthening: _____

  _____

12. List four reasons for prescribing cleansing enemas.

  a. _____

  b. _____

  c. _____

  d. _____

13. Briefly describe the following types of ostomies.

  a. Ileostomy: _____

  _____

  b. Colostomy: _____

  _____

14. Describe how the following factors help promote healthy bowel habits in patients.

  a. Timing: _____

  _____

  b. Positioning: _____

  _____

  c. Privacy: _____

  _____

  d. Nutrition: _____

  _____

  e. Exercise: _____

  _____

APPLYING YOUR KNOWLEDGE

CRITICAL THINKING QUESTIONS

1. Develop a list of preferred foods to ensure healthy bowel elimination for the following patients.

  a. A woman complains of constipation following a cesarean section.

  b. A 40-year-old man who is under stress in his job complains of frequent diarrhea.

  c. A toddler's stools are hard and dry, and he complains of frequent stomachaches.

  What other factors are likely to promote healthy bowel elimination in these patients?

2. Perform a physical assessment and write a nursing diagnosis for a patient who has just had a colostomy performed. What changes will this patient face in his life, and what can be done to help him cope with them? How can you best learn this? Be sure to assess this patient's physical and psychological factors, body image, coping mechanisms, and support system. Develop a nursing care plan to provide postoperative care, hospital care, and follow-up care for this patient.

REFLECTIVE PRACTICE USING CRITICAL THINKING SKILLS

Use the following expanded scenario from Chapter 38 in your textbook to answer the questions below.

  Scenario: Leroy Cobbs, age 56, was recently diagnosed with prostate cancer. He is taking acetaminophen (Tylenol) with codeine for pain and is hospitalized for fecal impaction. During the physical examination, Mr. Cobbs says, "Nobody told me I would get so constipated. It's been almost a week and I'm still not moving my bowels normally. I didn't know anything could hurt so bad!" Mr. Cobbs reports that he had regular, pain-free bowel movements, once daily, before taking the pain medication. He appears frustrated and says, "I'll take my chances with the cancer pain in the future rather than take more pain medicine and have this happen again."

1. What nursing interventions might the nurse implement for this patient?

_____

_____

_____

2. What would be a successful outcome for Mr. Cobbs?

_____

_____

_____

3. What intellectual, technical, interpersonal, and/or ethical/legal competencies are most likely to bring about the desired outcome?

_____

_____

_____

4. What resources might be helpful for Mr. Cobbs?

_____

_____

_____

PATIENT CARE STUDY

Read the following patient care study and use your nursing process skills to answer the questions below.

Scenario: Ms. Elgaresta, age 54, a single Hispanic woman, is being followed by a cardiologist who monitors her arrhythmia. Last month, she started taking a new heart medication. At this visit, she says to the nurse practitioner who works with the cardiologist: "Right after I started taking that medication, I got terribly constipated, and nothing seems to help. I'm desperate and about ready to try dynamite unless you can think of something else!" She reports a change in her bowel movements from one soft stool daily to one or two hard stools weekly, stools that cause much straining. The nurse practitioner realizes that

regulating Ms. Elgaresta's heart is difficult and that her best cardiac response to date has been with the medication that is now causing constipation. Reluctant to suggest substituting another medication too quickly, she asks more questions and Ms. Elgaresta responds, "I've never been much of a drinker, 2 cups of coffee in the morning and maybe a glass of wine at night. Water? Almost never. And I don't drink juices or soft drinks." Analysis of her diet reveals a diet low in fiber: "I never was one much for vegetables, and they can just keep all this bran stuff that's out on the market! Coffee and a cigarette. That's for me!" Ms. Elgaresta is a workaholic computer programmer and spends what little spare time she has watching TV. She reports tiring after walking one flight of stairs and says she avoids all forms of vigorous exercise.

1. Identify pertinent patient data by placing a single underline beneath the objective data in the case study and a double underline beneath the subjective data.

2. Complete the Nursing Process Worksheet on page 261 to develop a three-part diagnostic statement and related plan of care for this patient.

3. Write down the patient and personal nursing strengths you hope to draw upon as you assist this patient to better health.

   Patient strengths: _____

   _____

   _____

   Personal strengths: _____

   _____

   _____

4. Pretend that you are performing a nursing assessment of this patient after the plan of care is implemented. Document your findings.

   _____

   _____

   _____

NURSING PROCESS WORKSHEET

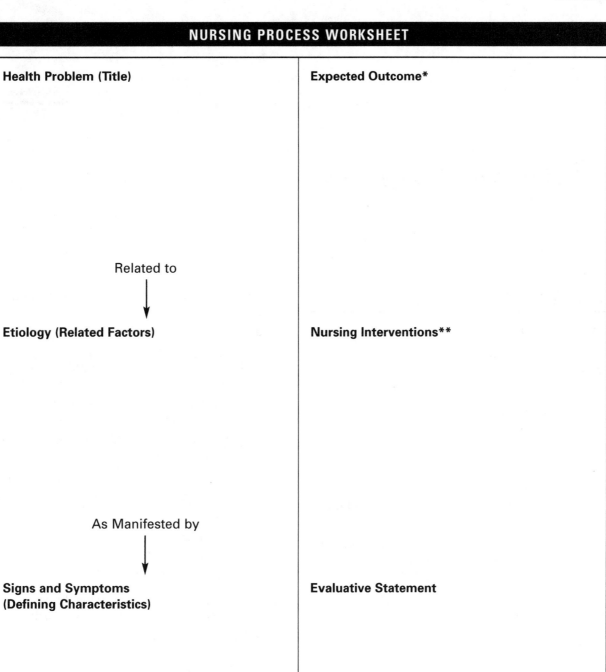

Health Problem (Title)

Expected Outcome*

Related to

↓

Etiology (Related Factors)

Nursing Interventions**

As Manifested by

↓

**Signs and Symptoms
(Defining Characteristics)**

Evaluative Statement

*More than one patient goal may be appropriate. For the purposes of this exercise, develop the one patient goal that demonstrates a direct resolution of the patient problem identified in the nursing diagnosis.
**Be sure you are able to list the scientific rationale for each nursing intervention you ordered.

39

Oxygenation

PRACTICING FOR NCLEX

MULTIPLE CHOICE QUESTIONS

Circle the letter that corresponds to the best answer for each question.

1. Which of the following is the primary purpose of surfactant?
   a. To propel sheets of mucus toward the upper airway
   b. To warm inspired air
   c. To produce watery mucus
   d. To reduce surface tension of the fluid lining the alveoli

2. The small air sacs at the end of the terminal bronchioles that are the sites of gas exchange are known as which of the following?
   a. Alveoli
   b. Pleurae
   c. Lobules
   d. Bronchioles

3. A patient who has difficulty breathing, increased respiratory and pulse rates, and pale skin with regions of cyanosis may be suffering from which of the following?
   a. Hyperventilation
   b. Hypoxia
   c. Perfusion
   d. Atelectasis

4. When inspecting a patient's chest to assess respiratory status, the nurse should be aware of which of the following normal findings?
   a. The contour of the intercostal spaces should be rounded.
   b. The skin at the thorax should be cool and moist.
   c. The anteroposterior diameter should be greater than the transverse diameter.
   d. The chest should be slightly convex with no sternal depression.

5. When percussing a normal lung, which of the following sounds should be heard?
   a. Tympany
   b. Resonance
   c. Dullness
   d. Hyperresonance

6. Which of the following normal breath sounds should be heard over the trachea?
   a. Vesicular
   b. Bronchovesicular
   c. Bronchial
   d. Tympanic

7. A patient who develops air in the pleural space is experiencing which of the following conditions?
   a. Pleural effusion
   b. Hemothorax
   c. Pneumothorax
   d. Pleura thorax

8. Which of the following cough suppressants is generally preferred, despite its addictive quality?
   a. Cough syrup with codeine
   b. Benylin
   c. Balminil DM
   d. Benadryl

9. A patient who complains of difficulty breathing should be placed in which of the following positions?
   a. Prone position
   b. Lateral position
   c. Supine position
   d. Fowler's position

10. To drain the apical sections of the upper lobes of the lungs, the nurse should place the patient in which of the following positions?
    a. Left side with a pillow under the chest wall
    b. Side-lying position, half on the abdomen and half on the side
    c. High Fowler's position
    d. Trendelenburg position

11. Which of the following inhalers is used to liquefy or loosen thick secretions?
    a. Bronchodilators
    b. Mucolytic agents
    c. Corticosteroids
    d. Metered-dose inhalers

12. The brain is sensitive to hypoxia and will sustain irreversible brain damage after how many minutes?
    a. 2 to 4 minutes
    b. 4 to 6 minutes
    c. 6 to 8 minutes
    d. 8 to 10 minutes

13. Mr. Parks has chronic obstructive pulmonary disease. His nurse has taught him pursed-lip breathing, which helps him in which of the following ways?
    a. Increases carbon dioxide, which stimulates breathing
    b. Teaches him to prolong inspiration and shorten expiration
    c. Helps liquefy his secretions
    d. Decreases the amount of air trapping and resistance

14. A nurse suctioning a patient through a tracheostomy tube should be careful not to occlude the Y-port when inserting the suction catheter because it would cause which of the following to occur?
    a. Trauma to the tracheal mucosa
    b. Prevention of suctioning
    c. Loss of sterile field
    d. Suctioning of carbon dioxide

15. When caring for a patient with a tracheotomy, the nurse should be aware of which of the following?
    a. The wound around the tube and inner cannula, if one is present, should be cleaned at least every 24 hours.
    b. The patient has no impairment of speaking function.
    c. A newly inserted tracheostomy tube requires no immediate attention.
    d. Suctioning of the tracheostomy tube must be done using sterile technique.

16. When percussing the lungs of a patient with emphysema, the nurse would probably hear which of the following sounds?
    a. Resonance
    b. Hyperresonance
    c. Tympany
    d. Dullness

17. Which of the following is a function of the upper airway?
    a. Conduction of air
    b. Mucociliary clearance
    c. Production of pulmonary surfactant
    d. Purification of inspired air

ALTERNATE-FORMAT QUESTIONS

Multiple Response Questions

Circle the letters that correspond to the best answers for each question.

1. Which of the following are components of the upper airway? *(Select all that apply.)*
   a. Nose
   b. Larynx
   c. Trachea
   d. Bronchi
   e. Epiglottis
   f. Bronchioles

2. Which of the following statements regarding the physiology of the lungs are accurate? *(Select all that apply.)*

   a. The right lung has two lobes.

   b. Each lobe in the lung is further divided into lobules.

   c. The right lung consists of 10 bronchopulmonary segments.

   d. The left lung consists of 12 bronchopulmonary segments.

   e. The lung is composed of alveoli.

   f. Surfactant in the lungs increases the surface tension of the fluid lining the alveoli.

3. Which of the following statements accurately describe how respirations are controlled in the body? *(Select all that apply.)*

   a. The medulla in the brain stem is the respiratory center.

   b. The medulla is stimulated by a decrease in the concentration of carbon dioxide and hydrogen ions and by the decreased amount of oxygen in the arterial blood.

   c. Chemoreceptors in the aortic arch and carotid bodies can shut down the medulla.

   d. Stimulation of the medulla increases the rate and depth of ventilation to blow off carbon dioxide and hydrogen and increase oxygen levels.

   e. The medulla sends an impulse down the spinal cord to the respiratory muscles to stimulate a contraction leading to inhalation.

   f. The lungs contract in response to pressure changes in the intrapleural space and lungs.

4. Which of the following statements describe the developmental variations that occur in the respiratory process? *(Select all that apply.)*

   a. The normal infant's chest is small, although the airways are comparatively long, and aspiration is a potential problem.

   b. The respiratory rate is slower in infants than at any other age.

   c. Respiratory rate stabilizes in young adulthood.

   d. Surfactant is formed in utero at about 34 to 36 weeks.

   e. Respiratory activity is primarily abdominal in infants.

   f. Infants have a rounded chest wall in which the anteroposterior diameter is greater than the transverse diameter.

5. Which of the following normal conditions would a nurse expect to find when performing a physical assessment of a patient's respiratory system? *(Select all that apply.)*

   a. The chest contour is slightly convex with no sternal depression.

   b. The anteroposterior diameter of the chest should be less than the transverse diameter.

   c. The contour of the intercostal spaces should be rounded, and the movement of the chest should be symmetric.

   d. When palpating the trachea, the nurse should note a slightly higher skin temperature.

   e. When assessing tactile fremitus by placing a palm to the patient's chest wall, the vibrations from the patient's repeated word should be equal bilaterally in different areas on the chest wall.

   f. Hyperresonance, a loud, hollow, low-pitched sound, should be heard over normal lungs when they are percussed.

6. Which of the following actions should a nurse perform when inserting an oropharyngeal airway? *(Select all that apply.)*

   a. Use an airway that is the correct size (size 60 mm is appropriate for the average adult).

   b. Wash hands and don gloves. Wear a mask and goggles if the patient is coughing.

   c. Position patient on his/her back with the head turned to one side, resting on the cheekbone.

   d. Insert the airway with the curved tip pointing down toward the base of the mouth.

   e. Slide the airway across the tongue to the back of the mouth and rotate it 180 degrees as it passes the uvula.

   f. Remove airway for a brief period every 4 hours.

7. Which of the following actions would a nurse perform when correctly providing postural drainage? *(Select all that apply.)*

   a. Place the patient in a high Fowler's position to drain the apical sections of the upper lobes of the lungs.

b. Place the patient in the Trendelenburg position to drain the right lobe of the lung.

c. Carry out postural drainage two to four times a day for 20 to 30 minutes.

d. Perform postural drainage 15 minutes after meals to aid digestion.

e. Place the patient in a lying position, half on the abdomen and half on the side, right and left, to drain the posterior sections of the upper lobes of the lungs.

f. Place the patient lying on the right side with a pillow under the chest wall to drain the right lobe of the lung.

8. Which of the following statements describes the proper use of inhaled medications? *(Select all that apply.)*

a. Bronchodilators are used to liquefy or loosen thick secretions or reduce inflammation in airways.

b. Nebulizers are used to deliver a controlled dose of medication with each compression of the canister.

c. When using an MDI, the patient must activate the device before and after inhaling.

d. DPIs are actuated by the patient's inspiration, so there is no need to coordinate the delivery of puffs with inhalation.

e. Metered-dose inhalers deliver a controlled dose of medications with each compression of the canister.

f. Inhalers can be used safely without serious side effects whenever they are needed by the patient.

9. Which of the following nutritional guidelines are recommended for a patient with COPD? *(Select all that apply.)*

a. The patient should follow a high-protein and low-calorie diet.

b. The diet should consist of 40% to 55% carbohydrates.

c. The diet should be rich in antioxidants and vitamin A, C, and B.

d. The diet should contain 45% to 50% fat to counter malnutrition.

e. The diet should contain 12% to 20% protein.

f. Obese patients should not be encouraged to try to lose weight to prevent malnutrition from occurring as the disease progresses.

Prioritization Questions

1. Place the following steps for teaching a patient to use an incentive spirometer in the order in which they should occur.

a. Instruct the patient to exhale normally and then place lips securely around mouthpiece and not to breathe through his or her nose.

b. Medicate with ordered pain medication if needed.

c. Tell patient to hold breath and count to three. Check position of gauge to determine progress and level attained.

d. Tell patient to complete breathing exercises about 10 times every hour, if possible, and to rest between breaths as necessary.

e. Assist patient to upright position if possible and remove dentures if they fit poorly.

f. Demonstrate how to steady device with one hand and hold mouthpiece with other hand.

g. Instruct the patient to inhale slowly and as deeply as possible through the mouthpiece.

h. Instruct the patient to remove lips from mouthpiece and exhale normally.

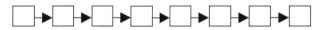

2. Place the following steps for inserting a nasopharyngeal airway in the order in which they should occur.

a. Remove the airway and place it in the other naris at least every 24 hours; assess for skin breakdown.

b. Perform hand hygiene and don gloves (wear mask and goggles if patient is coughing).

c. Explain the procedure to the patient.

d. Gently insert the airway into the naris. If resistance is met, stop and try inserting it into the other naris.

e. Lubricate the airway with the water-soluble lubricant; position the patient on his/her back or in a side-lying position.

f. Use an airway that is the correct size (size 28 French is an average adult size).

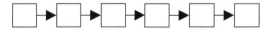

DEVELOPING YOUR KNOWLEDGE BASE

IDENTIFICATION

1. Identify the location of the organs of the respiratory tract listed here by writing the appropriate organ on the lines provided on the figure below.

Diaphragm

Epiglottis

Esophagus

Frontal sinus

Laryngeal pharynx

Larynx and vocal cords

Left lung

Mediastinum

Nasal cavity

Nasopharynx

Oropharynx

Right bronchus

Right lung

Sphenoidal sinus

Terminal bronchiole

Trachea

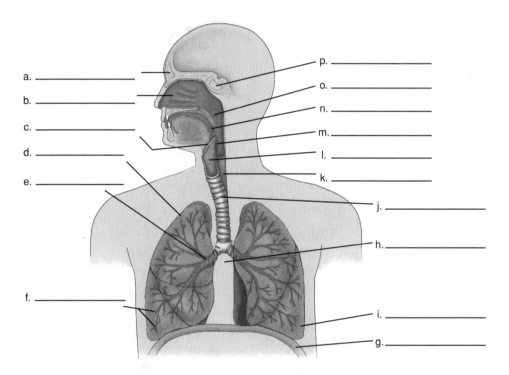

a. _____

b. _____

c. _____

d. _____

e. _____

f. _____

p. _____

o. _____

n. _____

m. _____

l. _____

k. _____

j. _____

h. _____

i. _____

g. _____

2. Identify the equipment illustrated below by placing your answer on the line provided.

_____

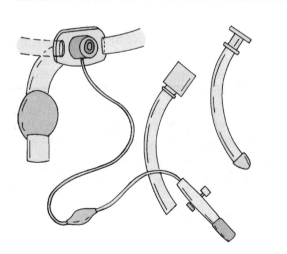

MATCHING EXERCISES

Match the definition in Part B with the term listed in Part A.

PART A

a. Ventilation

b. Inspiration

c. Expiration

d. Lung compliance

e. Airway resistance

f. Diffusion

g. Perfusion

h. Hypoventilation

i. Atelectasis

j. Hyperventilation

k. Hypoxia

PART B

1. ___ Movement of muscles and thorax to bring air into the lungs

2. ___ Movement of oxygen and carbon dioxide between the air and the blood

3. ___ Incomplete lung expansion or lung collapse

4. ___ An inadequate amount of oxygen in the cells

5. ___ Movement of air in and out of the lungs

6. ___ Any impediment or obstruction that air meets as it moves through the airway

7. ___ Stretchability of the lungs or the ease with which the lungs can be inflated

8. ___ Process in which the oxygenated capillary blood passes through tissue

9. ___ A decreased rate of air movement into the lungs

10. ___ An increased rate and depth of ventilation above the body's normal metabolic requirements

Match the type of oxygen delivery system listed in Part A with its description listed in Part B.

PART A

a. Nasal cannula
b. Nasopharyngeal catheter
c. Simple facemask
d. Partial rebreather mask
e. Nonrebreather mask
f. Venturi mask
g. Oxygen tent
h. Transtracheal oxygen delivery

PART B

11. ___ Connects to oxygen tubing, a humidifier, and flow meter and uses a delivery flow rate greater than 5 liters/minute; it should be comfortably snug over face but not tight; it has vents in sides to allow room air to leak in at many places, diluting the source oxygen

12. ___ Produces the highest concentration of oxygen with a mask; contains two one-way valves that prevent conservation of exhaled air, which escapes through side vents

13. ___ A tube is inserted into the throat through one nostril and must be changed to the other nostril every 12 to 24 hours. Gastric distention often occurs.

14. ___ This mask delivers the most precise concentration of oxygen and has a large tube with an oxygen inlet. As the tube narrows, pressure drops, causing air to be sucked in through the side ports.

15. ___ Probably the most commonly used respiratory aid, this consists of a disposable, plastic device with two protruding prongs for insertion into the nostrils; it is connected to an oxygen source with a humidifier and a flow meter.

16. ___ A small catheter is inserted into the trachea under local anesthesia and the catheter is attached to the oxygen source.

17. ___ This mask is equipped with a reservoir bag for the collection of the first part of the patient's exhaled air. The air is mixed with 100% oxygen for the next inhalation.

SHORT ANSWER

1. List three factors upon which normal respiratory functioning depends.

a. _____
b. _____
c. _____

2. Briefly describe the functions of the upper and lower airway, listing their main components.

a. Upper airway: _____

b. Lower airway: _____

3. Define Boyle's law.

_____

4. List four factors that influence the diffusion of gas in the lungs.

a. _____

_____

b. _____

_____

c. _____

_____

d. _____

_____

5. Describe the two ways that oxygen is carried in the body.

a. _____

b. _____

6. Briefly describe the variations in respiration experienced by the following age groups.

a. Infant: _____

_____

b. Preschool and school-aged child: _____

_____

c. Older adult: _____

_____

7. Explain how you would assess a patient for the following respiratory conditions.

a. Thoracic excursion: _____

_____

b. Tactile fremitus: _____

_____

_____

8. Describe nursing responsibilities before, during, and after a thoracentesis.

_____

_____

_____

9. How would you describe the effects of smoking on the lungs to a patient who smokes a pack of cigarettes a day? _____

_____

_____

10. Briefly describe the following techniques designed to promote proper breathing.

a. Deep breathing: _____

_____

b. Incentive spirometry: _____

_____

c. Abdominal or diaphragmatic breathing: ___

_____

11. You are the visiting nurse for a patient with emphysema who is receiving oxygen therapy. List five precautions you would take to prevent fire and injury to this patient.

a. _____

b. _____

c. _____

d. _____

e. _____

12. Briefly describe the following types of airways and their uses.

a. Oropharyngeal/nasopharyngeal airway:

_____

_____

b. Endotracheal tube: _____

_____

c. Tracheostomy tube: _____

_____

13. Describe the ABCs of basic life support.

a. _____

b. _____

c. _____

14. What is the nurse's responsibility when aspirating a patient's pleural cavity?

_____

_____

_____

_____

15. Describe seven comfort measures for patients with impaired respiratory functioning.

a. _____

b. _____

c. _____

d. _____

e. _____

f. _____

g. _____

APPLYING YOUR KNOWLEDGE

CRITICAL THINKING QUESTIONS

1. Develop a set of nursing strategies to promote adequate respiratory functioning in the following patients.

a. A patient with lung cancer presents with blood in his sputum.

b. A child with cystic fibrosis is having difficulty breathing.

c. A young woman with asthma develops pneumonia.

d. A 48-year-old man who smokes a pack of cigarettes a day presents with emphysema.

What is it that makes the strategies you selected appropriate/effective?

2. Interview young people who are smokers to find out their opinions about the health risks associated with smoking. See if they would be willing to quit with your help. Is the knowledge of health risk sufficient to motivate lifestyle

modifications? What are the implications for your practice?

REFLECTIVE PRACTICE USING CRITICAL THINKING SKILLS

Use the following expanded scenario from Chapter 39 in your textbook to answer the questions below.

Scenario: Joan McIntyre, age 72, is in the medical intensive care unit, diagnosed with severe COPD. Unable to breathe on her own, she has a tracheostomy and is receiving mechanical ventilation. Efforts are being made to wean her from the ventilator, but she has been unable to breathe on her own for any length of time. She has written notes asking the staff to "let me go" the next time she fails to be weaned. Her only daughter is by her side and asks that all measures to save her mother's life be initiated.

1. How might the nurse respond to Ms. McIntyre's request for a DNR order while taking into consideration the wishes of her daughter?

_____

_____

_____

2. What would be a successful outcome for this patient?

_____

_____

_____

3. What intellectual, technical, interpersonal, and/or ethical/legal competencies are most likely to bring about the desired outcome?

_____

_____

_____

4. What resources might be helpful for Ms. McIntyre?

_____

_____

_____

PATIENT CARE STUDY

Read the following case study and use your nursing process skills to answer the questions below.

Scenario: Toni is a 14-year-old girl who is in the adolescent mental health unit following a suicide attempt. Her chart reveals that on several occasions when her mother was visiting, she began hyperventilating (respiratory rate of 42 and increased depth). Gasping for breath on these occasions, she nevertheless pushed away all who approached her to assist. Her mother confided that she and her husband are in the midst of a divorce and that it hasn't been easy for Toni at home: "I know she's been having a rough time at school, and I guess I've been too caught up in my own troubles to be there for her." When you attempt to discuss this with Toni and mention her mother's concern, she begins hyperventilating again.

1. Identify pertinent patient data by placing a single underline beneath the objective data in the case study and a double underline beneath the subjective data.

2. Complete the Nursing Process Worksheet on page 271 to develop a three-part diagnostic statement and related plan of care for this patient.

3. Write down the patient and personal nursing strengths you hope to draw on as you assist this patient to better health.

   Patient strengths: _____

   _____

   _____

   Personal strengths: _____

   _____

   _____

4. Pretend that you are performing a nursing assessment of this patient after the plan of care is implemented. Document your findings.

   _____

   _____

   _____

NURSING PROCESS WORKSHEET

Health Problem (Title)	**Expected Outcome***
Related to ↓	
Etiology (Related Factors)	**Nursing Interventions****
As Manifested by ↓	
Signs and Symptoms (Defining Characteristics)	**Evaluative Statement**

*More than one patient goal may be appropriate. For the purposes of this exercise, develop the one patient goal that demonstrates a direct resolution of the patient problem identified in the nursing diagnosis.

**Be sure you are able to list the scientific rationale for each nursing intervention you ordered.

Fluid, Electrolyte, and Acid–Base Balance

PRACTICING FOR NCLEX

MULTIPLE CHOICE QUESTIONS

Circle the letter that corresponds to the best answer for each question.

1. Which of the following short- or long-term venous access devices is usually introduced into the subclavian or internal jugular veins and passed to the superior vena cava just above the right atrium?
   a. Peripherally inserted central catheter
   b. Implanted port
   c. Central venous catheter
   d. Electronic infusion device

2. When teaching a patient about foods that affect his fluid balance, the nurse will keep in mind that the electrolyte that primarily controls water distribution throughout the body is which of the following?
   a. Na^+
   b. K^+
   c. Ca^{++}
   d. Mg^{++}

3. A healthy patient eats a regular, balanced diet and drinks 3,000 mL of liquids during a 24-hour period. In evaluating this patient's urine output for the same 24-hour period, the nurse realizes that it should total approximately how many mL?
   a. 3,750
   b. 3,000

   c. 1,000
   d. 500

4. For the patient with "hyperkalemia related to decreased renal excretion secondary to potassium-conserving diuretic therapy," an appropriate expected outcome would be which of the following?
   a. Bowel motility will be restored within 24 hours after beginning supplemental K^+.
   b. ECG will show no cardiac arrhythmias within 48 hours after removing salt substitutes, coffee, tea, and other K^+-rich foods from diet.
   c. ECG will show no cardiac arrhythmias within 24 hours after beginning supplemental K^+.
   d. Bowel motility will be restored within 24 hours after eliminating salt substitutes, coffee, tea, and other K^+-rich foods from the diet.

5. Which of the following nursing diagnoses would you expect to be based on the effects of fluid and electrolyte imbalance on human functioning?
   a. Constipation related to immobility
   b. Pain related to surgical incision
   c. Altered Thought Processes related to cerebral edema, including mental confusion and disorientation
   d. Health Risk for Infection related to inadequate personal hygiene

6. Which of the following is the liquid constituent of blood?
   a. Intracellular fluid
   b. Extracellular fluid
   c. Interstitial fluid
   d. Intravascular fluid

7. The body eliminates excess sodium through which of the following organs?
   a. Kidneys
   b. Bowels
   c. Skin
   d. Heart

8. Which of the following food items is a leading source of potassium?
   a. Canned vegetables
   b. Cheese
   c. Bread
   d. Bananas

9. Which of the following is the most abundant electrolyte in the body?
   a. Sodium
   b. Calcium
   c. Potassium
   d. Magnesium

10. "Pumping uphill" would describe which of the following means of transporting materials to and from intracellular compartments?
    a. Osmosis
    b. Diffusion
    c. Filtration
    d. Active transport

11. When determining a site for an IV infusion, the nurse should consider which of the following guidelines?
    a. Scalp veins should be selected for infants because of their accessibility.
    b. Antecubital veins should be used for long-term infusions.
    c. Veins in the leg should be used to keep the arms free for the patient's use.
    d. Veins in surgical areas should be used to increase the potency of medication.

12. Individuals with which of the following blood types are often called universal donors?
    a. Type A
    b. Type O
    c. Type B
    d. Type AB

13. A nurse who has diagnosed a patient as having "fluid volume excess" related to compromised regulatory mechanism (kidneys) may have been alerted by which of the following symptoms?
    a. Muscle twitching
    b. Distended neck veins
    c. Fingerprinting over sternum
    d. Nausea and vomiting

ALTERNATE-FORMAT QUESTIONS

Multiple Response Questions

Circle the letters that correspond to the best answers for each question.

1. Which of the following accurately reflect the role of water in the human body? *(Select all that apply.)*
   a. A person can live for many days without water.
   b. Water provides a medium for transporting wastes to cells for elimination.
   c. Water facilitates cellular metabolism and proper chemical functioning.
   d. Water acts as a solvent for electrolytes and nonelectrolytes.
   e. The desirable amount of fluid intake and loss in the normal adult averages about 1,000 mL per day.
   f. Water helps maintain normal body temperature.

2. Which of the following are proper actions for preparing an IV solution and tubing when starting an IV infusion? *(Select all that apply.)*
   a. Maintain aseptic technique when opening sterile packages and IV solution.
   b. Clamp tubing, uncap spike, and insert into entry site on bag as manufacturer directs.
   c. Squeeze drip chamber and allow it to fill one-fourth full.
   d. Remove cap at end of tubing, release clamp, and allow fluid to move through tubing.
   e. Allow fluid to flow and cap at end of tubing before all air bubbles have disappeared.

f. Apply label if medication was added to the container, if not done by the pharmacy.

3. Following preparation of the IV solution and tubing, which of the following actions would be performed by the nurse when selecting a site and palpating a vein to start an IV infusion? *(Select all that apply.)*

   a. Place the patient in a high Fowler's position in bed.

   b. Select an appropriate site and palpate accessible veins.

   c. Apply a tourniquet 2 to 3 inches above the venipuncture site to obstruct venous flow and distend the vein.

   d. Direct the ends of the tourniquet away from the site and check that the radial pulse is still present.

   e. Ask the patient to keep a tightly closed fist while observing and palpating for a suitable vein.

   f. If a vein cannot be felt, release the tourniquet and have the patient lower the arm below the level of the heart to fill the veins.

4. Which of the following are recommended actions for a nurse to perform after selecting a site and palpating accessible veins in order to start an IV infusion? *(Select all that apply.)*

   a. Clean the entry site with saline, followed by an alcohol swab according to agency policy.

   b. Place the dominant hand about 4 inches below the entry site to hold the skin taut against the vein.

   c. Enter the skin gently with the catheter held by the hub in the nondominant hand, bevel side down, at a 10- to 30-degree angle.

   d. Advance the needle or catheter into the vein. A sensation of "give" can be felt when the needle enters the vein.

   e. When blood returns through the lumen of the needle or the flashback chamber of the catheter, advance either device ⅛ to ¼ inch farther into the vein.

   f. Release the tourniquet and quickly remove the protective cap from the IV tubing and attach the tubing to the catheter or needle.

5. Which of the following are signs of complications and their probable causes that may occur when administering an IV solution to a patient? *(Select all that apply.)*

   a. Swelling, pain, coolness, or pallor at the insertion site may indicate infiltration of the IV.

   b. Redness, swelling, heat, and pain at the site may indicate phlebitis.

   c. Local or systemic manifestations may indicate an infection is present at the site.

   d. A pounding headache, fainting, rapid pulse rate, increased blood pressure, chills, back pains, and dyspnea occur when an air embolus is present.

   e. Bleeding at the site when the IV is discontinued indicates an infection is present.

   f. Engorged neck veins, increased blood pressure, and dyspnea occur when a thrombus is present.

6. Which of the following statements accurately describe the function or regulation of sodium in the human body? *(Select all that apply.)*

   a. Sodium does not influence ICF volume.

   b. Sodium is the primary regulator of ECF volume.

   c. The daily value of sodium cited on nutrition facts labels is 1,200 mg.

   d. Sodium is normally maintained in the body within a relatively narrow range, and deviations quickly result in serious health problems.

   e. The normal extracellular concentration of sodium is 85 to 95 mEq/L.

   f. Sodium participates in the generation and transmission of nerve impulses.

7. Which of the following statements accurately describe the function or regulation of potassium in the body? *(Select all that apply.)*

   a. Potassium is the major cation of ICF and works reciprocally with sodium.

   b. Potassium is the chief regulator of cellular enzyme activity and cellular water content.

   c. Potassium is needed for vitamin B_{12} absorption and for its use by body cells.

   d. Potassium determines the thickness and strength of cell membranes.

e. The kidneys conserve potassium when cellular potassium is decreased.

f. The normal range for serum potassium is 6.5 to 8.0 mEq/L.

8. Which of the following statements accurately describe fluid and electrolyte movement? *(Select all that apply.)*

a. Cell membranes are impermeable, making it impossible for water to be transported through cell walls.

b. Active transport is the major method of transporting body fluids.

c. Through the process of osmosis, the solvent water passes from an area of lesser solute concentration to an area of greater solute concentration until equilibrium is established.

d. A hypertonic solution has a greater concentration of particles in solution, causing water to move out of the cells and into the intravascular compartment in which the fluid is hypertonic, causing the cells to shrink.

e. In the process of diffusion, the solute moves from an area of higher concentration to an area of lower concentration until equilibrium is established.

f. Active transport is the passage of fluid through a permeable membrane from an area of high pressure to one of lower pressure.

9. Which of the following statements accurately describe the functions of the organs to maintain fluid homeostasis? *(Select all that apply.)*

a. The kidneys normally filter 210 L of plasma daily in the adult while excreting only 1.5 L of urine.

b. The cardiovascular system is responsible for pumping and carrying nutrients and water throughout the body.

c. The regulation of the carbon dioxide level by the lungs is crucial in maintaining acid–base balance.

d. The thyroid gland secretes aldosterone, a hormone that helps the body conserve sodium, saves chloride and water, and causes potassium to be excreted.

e. Thyroxine, released by the thyroid gland, increases blood flow in the body, leading to increased renal circulation and resulting in increased glomerular filtration and urinary output.

f. The adrenal glands secrete parathyroid hormone, which regulates the level of calcium in ECF.

Chart/Exhibit Questions

Determine the acid–base imbalance in the cases appearing on page 276 and circle the letter that corresponds to the best answer for each scenario. Refer to the Rules of ABG Interpretation table below for your answers.

Rules of ABG Interpretation		
pH	**$PaCO_2$**	**HCO_3**
<7.35 = acidosis	>45 mm Hg = respiratory acidosis	<22 mEq/L = metabolic acidosis
>7.45 = alkalosis	>35 mm Hg = respiratory alkalosis	>26 mEq/L = metabolic alkalosis

- It is OK to use what you know about your patient.
- The body responds to acid–base imbalances by activating compensatory mechanisms that minimize pH changes; a metabolic disturbance is compensated by the lungs, and a respiratory system disturbance is compensated by the kidneys.
- Any pH less than 7.35 = state of acidosis. Any pH greater than 7.45 = state of alkalosis.
- CO_2 is an acid; HCO_3 is a base. Any change in CO_2 reflects a respiratory change. Any change in HCO_3 reflects a metabolic change.
- If the pH has returned to *normal*, compensation has taken place.
- If the primary event is a *fall* in pH, whether respiratory or metabolic in origin, the arterial pH stays on the *acid* side after compensation.
- If the primary event is an *increase* in pH, whether respiratory or metabolic in origin, the arterial pH stays on the *base* side after compensation.

1. Mr. W. is a 90-year-old man who had a successful cardiopulmonary resuscitation a few hours ago. He received bicarbonate during that resuscitation.

   ABGs: pH = 7.55; $PaCO_2$ = 43; HCO_3 = 36

   a. Respiratory acidosis
   b. Metabolic acidosis
   c. Metabolic alkalosis
   d. Respiratory alkalosis

2. Mr. F. is a 56-year-old man with a history of COPD.

   ABGs: pH = 7.36; $PaCO_2$ = 60; HCO_3 = 35

   a. Respiratory acidosis with renal compensation
   b. Metabolic acidosis with partial respiratory compensation
   c. Respiratory alkalosis
   d. Respiratory acidosis

3. A 55-year-old woman is admitted with chronic renal failure. She is weak and tired.

   ABGs: pH = 7.24; $PaCO_2$ = 30; HCO_3 = 12

   a. Respiratory acidosis
   b. Respiratory alkalosis
   c. Metabolic alkalosis with partial respiratory compensation
   d. Metabolic acidosis with partial respiratory compensation

4. Mrs. S. is a 55-year-old woman with heart failure and dyspnea. She complains of pleuritic pain.

   ABGs: pH = 7.56; $PaCO_2$ = 22; HCO_3 = 24

   a. Respiratory alkalosis
   b. Respiratory acidosis
   c. Metabolic acidosis
   d. Metabolic alkalosis

5. Ms. S. is a 21-year-old woman who was found by her friends on the floor of her room. She is "out of it."

   ABGs: pH = 7.18; $PaCO_2$ = 79; HCO_3 = 26

   a. Respiratory alkalosis
   b. Respiratory acidosis
   c. Metabolic alkalosis with partial respiratory compensation
   d. Metabolic acidosis with partial respiratory compensation

6. Indicate on the chart below the nature of the acid–base disturbance, whether compensation is present or not, and if present, whether compensation is renal or respiratory, and partial or complete.

				Comp. Present?		If Yes		If Yes	
pH	$PaCO_2$	HCO_3^-	Nature of Disturbance	Yes	No	Renal	Respiratory	Partial	Complete
7.28	63	25							
7.20	40	14							
7.52	40	35							
7.16	82	30							
7.36	68	35							
7.56	23	26							
7.40	40	26							
7.56	23	26							
7.26	70	25							
7.52	44	38							
7.32	30	18							
7.49	34	26							

Hot Spot Questions

1. Place an "X" on the figure below to indicate the spot where a peripherally inserted central catheter (PICC) would be inserted.

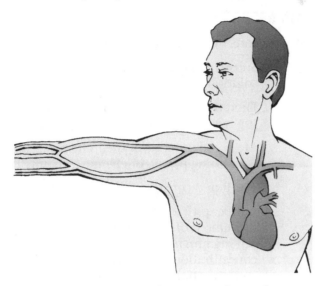

2. Indicate the proper placement of a triple-lumen nontunneled percutaneous central venous catheter by placing an "X" on the figure below where it would be inserted.

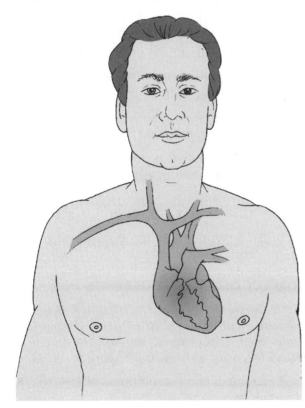

DEVELOPING YOUR KNOWLEDGE BASE

MATCHING EXERCISES

Match the cation in Part A with its function listed in Part B. Some answers may be used more than once.

PART A

a. Sodium

b. Potassium

c. Calcium

d. Magnesium

PART B

1. _____ It is the chief regulator of cellular enzyme activity and cellular water content.

2. _____ It is necessary for nerve impulse transmission and blood clotting.

3. _____ It controls and regulates the volume of body fluids.

4. _____ It is the primary regulator of ECF volume.

5. _____ It is important for the metabolism of carbohydrates and proteins.

6. _____ It is a catalyst for muscle contraction.

7. _____ It assists in the regulation of acid–base balance by cellular exchange with H^+.

8. _____ It is necessary for protein and DNA synthesis, DNA and RNA transcription, and translation of RNA.

Match the anion in Part A with its function listed in Part B. Some answers may be used more than once.

PART A

a. Chloride

b. Bicarbonate

c. Phosphate

d. Sulfate

PART B

9. _____ It acts with sodium to maintain the osmotic pressure of the blood.

10. _____ It is important for cell division and for the transmission of hereditary traits.

11. ____ It is important in the buffering system that is activated by the exchange of oxygen and carbon dioxide between body tissues and red blood cells.

12. ____ It is found primarily within cells and is associated with intracellular protein.

13. ____ It is essential for acid–base balance and, in combination with carbonic acid, constitutes the body's primary buffer system.

14. ____ It participates in many important chemical reactions in the body; for example, it is necessary for many B vitamins to be effective and plays a role in carbohydrate metabolism.

15. ____ It is essential for the production of hydrochloric acid in gastric cells.

Match the equations in Part B with the type of imbalance listed in Part A.

PART A

a. Respiratory acidosis

b. Metabolic acidosis

c. Respiratory alkalosis

d. Metabolic alkalosis

PART B

16. ____ Low pH, normal $PaCO_2$, low HCO_3

17. ____ Low pH, high $PaCO_2$, normal HCO_3

18. ____ High pH, normal $PaCO_2$, high HCO_3

19. ____ High pH, low $PaCO_2$, normal HCO_3

Match the term in Part A with its definition listed in Part B.

PART A

a. Ion

b. Electrolyte

c. Cation

d. Anion

e. Solvents

f. Solutes

g. Osmolarity

h. Filtration

i. Oncotic pressure

j. Hydrostatic pressure

k. Diffusion

l. Active transport

m. Filtration pressure

n. Buffer

o. Intravascular fluid

p. Interstitial fluid

PART B

20. ____ Ions that develop a positive charge

21. ____ Substances that are dissolved in a solution

22. ____ Fluid that surrounds tissue cells, including lymph

23. ____ Measured in terms of their chemical combining power, or chemical activity

24. ____ The liquid constituent of blood

25. ____ A process that requires energy for the movement of substances through a cell membrane from an area of lesser concentration to an area of higher concentration

26. ____ The passage of a fluid through a permeable membrane

27. ____ An atom or molecule carrying an electric charge

28. ____ An ion with a negative charge

29. ____ Liquids that hold a substance in solution

30. ____ A force exerted by a fluid against the container wall

31. ____ The difference between colloid osmotic pressure and blood hydrostatic pressure

32. ____ A substance that prevents body fluids from becoming overly acidic or alkaline

33. ____ The concentration of particles in a solution, or its pulling power

34. ____ The tendency of solutes to move freely throughout a solvent

CORRECT THE FALSE STATEMENTS

Circle the word "true" or "false" that follows the statement. If you circled "false," change the underlined word or words to make the statement true. Place your answer in the space provided.

1. The human body is composed of 50% to 60% water by weight.

   True   False _____

2. Substances capable of breaking into electrically charged ions when dissolved in a solution are called <u>solutes</u>.

True False _____

3. A <u>hypertonic solution</u> has less osmolarity than plasma.

True False _____

4. <u>Ingested liquids</u> make up the largest amount of water normally taken into the body.

True False _____

5. The acidity or alkalinity of a solution is determined by its concentration of <u>oxygen</u> ions.

True False _____

6. An <u>acid</u> is a substance that can accept or trap hydrogen ions.

True False _____

7. Normal blood plasma is slightly <u>acidic</u> and has a normal pH of 7.35 to 7.45.

True False _____

8. The <u>kidneys</u> are the primary controller of the body's carbonic acid supply.

True False _____

9. Excessive retention of water and sodium in ECF results in a condition termed fluid volume excess or <u>hypervolemia</u>.

True False _____

10. <u>Hypokalemia</u> refers to a surplus of sodium in ECF that can result from excess water loss or an overall excess of sodium.

True False _____

11. Acid–base imbalances occur when the ECF and ICF carbonic acid or bicarbonate levels become <u>equal</u>.

True False _____

12. <u>Arterial blood gases</u> are most commonly used to assess and treat acid–base imbalances.

True False _____

SHORT ANSWER

1. Briefly describe how the following processes transport materials to and from intracellular compartments.

a. Osmosis: _____
_____

b. Diffusion: _____
_____

c. Active transport: _____
_____

2. Give an example of how water is derived from the following sources.

a. Ingested liquids: _____
_____

b. Food: _____
_____

c. Metabolic oxidation: _____
_____

3. List three mechanisms for water loss in the body.

a. _____
b. _____
c. _____

4. Explain how the following organs/systems of the body maintain fluid homeostasis.

a. Kidneys: _____
_____

b. Cardiovascular system: _____
_____

c. Lungs: _____
_____

d. Thyroid: _____
_____

e. Parathyroid glands: _____
_____

f. Gastrointestinal tract: _____
_____

g. Nervous system: _____
_____

5. Give a brief description of the following conditions.

a. Acidosis: _____
_____

b. Alkalosis: _____

_____

6. Describe the following acid–base imbalances and their effect on the body.

a. Respiratory acidosis: _____

_____

_____

b. Respiratory alkalosis: _____

_____

_____

c. Metabolic acidosis: _____

_____

_____

d. Metabolic alkalosis: _____

_____

_____

7. Describe the causes of the following changes in hemoglobin and hematocrit.

a. Increased hematocrit: _____

_____

b. Decreased hematocrit: _____

_____

c. Increased hemoglobin: _____

_____

d. Decreased hemoglobin: _____

_____

8. Briefly describe the following screening tests.

a. Urine pH and specific gravity: _____

_____

b. Serum electrolytes: _____

_____

c. Arterial blood gases: _____

_____

9. You are the visiting nurse for an elderly patient with diabetes. List four factors you should consider to prevent fluid imbalance for this patient.

a. _____

_____

b. _____

_____

c. _____

_____

d. _____

_____

10. List four guidelines for selecting a vein for an IV.

a. _____

b. _____

c. _____

d. _____

11. List the important points a home healthcare nurse should address when caring for a patient on home infusion therapy.

_____

_____

_____

APPLYING YOUR KNOWLEDGE

CRITICAL THINKING QUESTIONS

1. Assess the following patients for fluid, electrolyte, and acid–base balance. What knowledge of the factors that influence fluid and electrolyte and acid–base balance would you draw on to develop a plan to prevent recurrence of these patient problems?

a. A long-distance runner who is practicing on a hot day experiences dizziness and shows signs of dehydration

b. An older man with persistent heartburn ingests a large amount of sodium bicarbonate in 1 day

c. An infant is brought to the ER severely dehydrated after an extended bout of diarrhea.

2. Plan a low-salt diet for a patient who has high blood pressure. List healthy foods that are low in salt, as well as foods that are high in salt and that should be avoided. Check the sodium content of fast food in restaurants to see if any of these foods could be included on the diet.

REFLECTIVE PRACTICE USING CRITICAL THINKING SKILLS

Use the following expanded scenario from Chapter 40 in your textbook to answer the questions below.

Scenario: Jack Soo Park, a 78-year-old man receiving intravenous (IV) therapy with antibiotics, states, "I'm having trouble breathing. It just started a little while ago." Physical examination reveals a bounding pulse, distended neck veins, shallow, rapid respirations, and crackles and wheezes in the lungs. Excess fluid volume is suspected. Further checking reveals an IV fluid-administration error that has resulted in overhydration.

1. Based on the data in this scenario, what body systems are involved in Mr. Park's fluid volume excess? What interventions would be appropriate?

_____

_____

_____

2. What would be a successful outcome for Mr. Park?

_____

_____

_____

3. What intellectual, technical, interpersonal, and/or ethical/legal competencies are most likely to bring about the desired outcome?

_____

_____

_____

4. What resources might be helpful for Mr. Park?

_____

_____

_____

PATIENT CARE STUDY

Read the following patient care study and use your nursing process skills to answer the questions below.

Scenario: Rebecca is a college freshman who had her wisdom teeth removed yesterday morning. She had a sore throat several days before the extraction but did not mention this to the oral surgeon. Because of her sore throat, she had greatly decreased her food and fluid intake. The night of the surgery, she had an oral temperature of 39.5°C (103.1°F). Friends gave her some Tylenol, which brought her temperature down, and encouraged her to drink more fluids. When they checked on her this morning, her temperature was elevated again and she said she had felt too weak during the night to drink. They took her to the student health service, where the admitting nurse noticed her dry mucous membranes, decreased skin turgor, and rapid pulse. At 5 feet 2 inches and 98 pounds, Rebecca had lost 4 pounds in the past week.

1. Identify pertinent patient data by placing a single underline beneath the objective data in the case study and a double underline beneath the subjective data.

2. Complete the Nursing Process Worksheet on page 282 to develop a three-part diagnostic statement and related plan of care for this patient.

3. Write down the patient and personal nursing strengths you hope to draw on as you assist this patient to better health.

Patient strengths: _____

_____

_____

Personal strengths: _____

_____

_____

4. Pretend that you are performing a nursing assessment of this patient after the plan of care has been implemented. Document your findings.

_____

_____

_____

NURSING PROCESS WORKSHEET

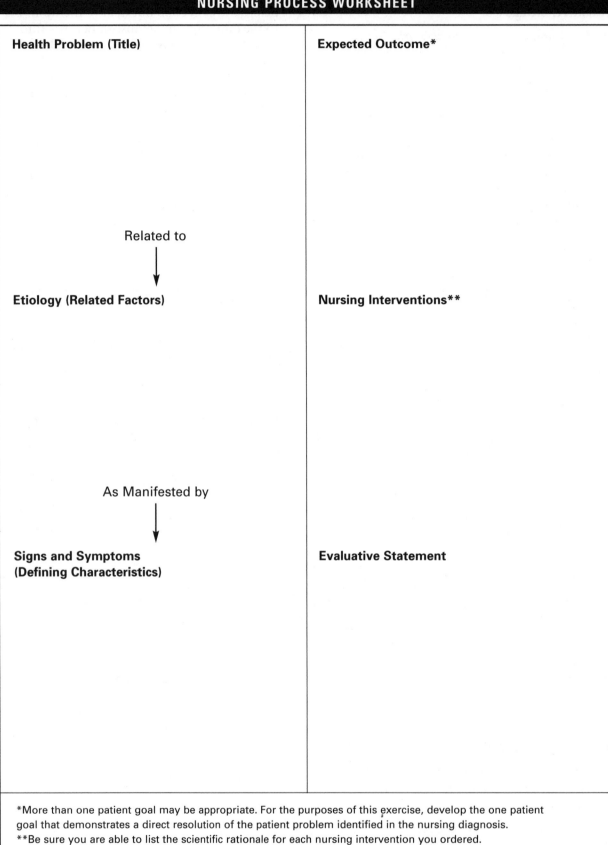

Health Problem (Title)

Expected Outcome*

Related to

↓

Etiology (Related Factors)

Nursing Interventions**

As Manifested by

↓

**Signs and Symptoms
(Defining Characteristics)**

Evaluative Statement

*More than one patient goal may be appropriate. For the purposes of this exercise, develop the one patient
goal that demonstrates a direct resolution of the patient problem identified in the nursing diagnosis.
**Be sure you are able to list the scientific rationale for each nursing intervention you ordered.

Self-Concept

PRACTICING FOR NCLEX

MULTIPLE CHOICE QUESTIONS

Circle the letter that corresponds to the best choice for each question.

1. When children identify sports figures as their heroes, they are experiencing which of the following aspects of self-concept?
   a. Self-knowledge
   b. Self-expectations
   c. Self-evaluation
   d. Self-actualization

2. The need to reach one's potential through full development of one's unique capability is known as which of the following?
   a. Self-actualization
   b. Self-concept
   c. Self-esteem
   d. Ideal self

3. A child is able to learn self-recognition in which of the following stages of childhood?
   a. Infancy
   b. 18 months
   c. 3 years
   d. 6 to 7 years

4. A student nurse who has not maintained healthy relationships with his/her peers would be at risk for which of the following self-concept disturbances?
   a. Personal identity disturbance
   b. Body image disturbance
   c. Self-esteem disturbance
   d. Altered role performance

5. When a nurse asks a patient to describe her personal characteristics and traits, the nurse is most likely assessing the patient for which of the following self-concept factors?
   a. Body image
   b. Role performance
   c. Self-esteem
   d. Personal identity

6. Which of the following questions would you expect to find on a self-concept assessment related to body image?
   a. Do you like who you are?
   b. Who influenced you the most growing up?
   c. How do you feel about any physical changes you noticed recently?
   d. Who would you most like to be?

7. Which of the following questions would best relate to self-identity on a focused self-concept assessment?
   a. Who would you like to be?
   b. What do you like most about your body?
   c. What are your personal strengths?
   d. Do you like being a teacher?

8. Which of the following nursing diagnoses lacks a self-concept disturbance etiology?
   a. Self-Care Deficit related to dysfunctional grieving
   b. Noncompliance related to low self-esteem

c. Posttrauma Response related to disturbance in personal identity

d. Altered Health Maintenance related to altered role performance

9. Which of the following questions would provide the healthcare worker with the information needed first when assessing self-concept?

a. How would you describe yourself to others?

b. Do you like yourself?

c. What do you see yourself doing 5 years from now?

d. What are some of your personal strengths?

ALTERNATE-FORMAT QUESTIONS

Multiple Response Questions

Circle the letters that correspond to the best answers for each question.

1. Which of the following are bases of self-esteem as identified by Coopersmith (1967)? *(Select all that apply.)*

a. Consequence

b. Significance

c. Competence

d. Importance

e. Capacity

f. Power

2. Which of the following are major self-evaluation feelings or effects in children as described by Harter (1999)? *(Select all that apply.)*

a. Pride

b. Anger

c. Honesty

d. Guilt

e. Shame

f. Fear

3. Which of the following psychological conditions foster healthy development of self in children (according to McClowry, 2003)? *(Select all that apply.)*

a. Emotional warmth and acceptance

b. Helping children meet challenges

c. Loosely defined structure and discipline

d. Clearly defined standards and limits

e. No specific roles for members of the family

f. No set methods of handling children to produce desired behavior

DEVELOPING YOUR KNOWLEDGE BASE

FILL-IN-THE-BLANKS

1. When a man strives to reach his full potential, he is fulfilling the need for _____.

2. The dimensions of self-knowledge, self-expectations, and self-evaluation describe _____.

3. The composite of all the basic facts, qualities, traits, images, and feelings one holds about oneself is known as _____.

4. The self one wants to be that developed in childhood and was based on the image of role models is known as the _____.

5. When a teenager attempts to please his parents by attending church, although he doesn't believe in organized religion, he is displaying his _____.

6. _____ describes an individual's conscious sense of who he/she is.

MATCHING EXERCISES

Match the definition in Part B with the term listed in Part A.

PART A

a. Self-esteem

b. Self-actualization

c. Self-concept

d. Body image

e. Self-knowledge

f. Self-expectations

g. Self-evaluation

h. Personal identity

PART B

1. ___ The need to feel good about oneself and believe others also hold one in high regard

2. ___ How I experience my body

3. ___ Describes an individual's conscious sense of who he/she is

4. ___ Includes basic facts, which place that person in social groups, and a listing of qualities or traits, which describe typical behaviors, feelings, moods, and other characteristics

5. ____ These flow from the ideal self, the self one wants to be or thinks one should be

6. ____ The mental image or picture of self

7. ____ The assessment of how well I like myself

Match the examples of risk factors for self-concept disturbances in Part B with the factors listed in Part A. Some answers may be used more than once.

PART A

a. Personal identity disturbances

b. Body image disturbances

c. Self-esteem disturbances

d. Altered role performance

PART B

8. ____ A 55-year-old executive is laid off from his job due to cutbacks

9. ____ A 45-year-old woman undergoes a radical mastectomy

10. ____ A 30-year-old woman finds herself in a relationship with an abusive husband

11. ____ An exchange student from France attends high school in America to learn a new language and customs

12. ____ A new mother discovers she is terrified of taking care of her newborn son on her own

13. ____ An 11-year-old girl starts menstruating and developing earlier than her peers

14. ____ A 65-year-old retired lawyer regrets that he was unable to become a judge as he had always dreamed of doing

15. ____ An athlete loses his pitching arm to cancer

16. ____ A 38-year-old woman who is recently divorced is lost without her husband

SHORT ANSWER

1. What measures could you, as a nurse, employ to promote self-esteem in older adults?

_____

_____

_____

2. Reflect on your personal self-concept and how it affects the way you live your life. Keeping this in mind, answer the following questions.

   a. Who am I? _____

   _____

   b. Who or what do I want to be? _____

   _____

   c. How well do I like me? _____

   _____

3. Give an example of a question you might use to assess a patient for the following concepts.

   a. Significance: _____

   _____

   b. Competence: _____

   _____

   c. Virtue: _____

   _____

   d. Power: _____

   _____

4. Give an example of how each of the following factors might influence an individual's self-concept.

   a. Developmental considerations: _____

   _____

   b. Culture: _____

   _____

   c. Internal and external resources: _____

   _____

   d. History of success or failure: _____

   _____

   e. Stressors: _____

   _____

   f. Aging, illness, or trauma: _____

5. List one example from your experience as a nurse that exemplifies the use of the following strategies for developing self-esteem into your practice.

   a. Dispel the myth that it is necessary to know all there is to know about nursing to be a good nurse: _____

   _____

   b. Realistically evaluate strengths and weaknesses: _____

   _____

   c. Accentuate the positive: _____

   _____

   d. Develop a conscious plan for changing weaknesses into strengths: _____

   _____

   e. Work to develop team self-esteem: _____

   _____

   f. Actively demonstrate your commitment to nursing and concern about the nursing profession's public image: _____

   _____

6. Describe how you would record a self-concept assessment, using your own personal strengths as an example. _____

   _____

   _____

7. Give an example of an interview question you could use to assess self-concept in the following areas. _____

   a. Personal identity: _____

   _____

   b. Patient strengths: _____

   _____

   c. Body image: _____

   _____

   d. Self-esteem: _____

   _____

   e. Role performance: _____

   _____

8. Write a sample nursing diagnosis and goal for the following disturbances in self-concept.

   a. A 42-year-old woman is anxious about disfigurement from her mastectomy.

   Diagnosis: _____

   _____

   Patient goal: _____

   _____

   b. A teen is anxious about being able to cope with pregnancy.

   Diagnosis: _____

   _____

   Patient goal: _____

   _____

   c. A 76-year-old man stops taking care of his physical needs because he doesn't want to go on with life without his recently deceased spouse.

   Diagnosis: _____

   _____

   Patient goal: _____

   _____

   d. A parent doesn't know how to teach a child who is being ridiculed by his peers in school how to establish self-esteem.

   Diagnosis: _____

   _____

   Patient goal: _____

   _____

   e. A battered woman feels her situation is hopeless and believes she deserves to be abused because she is so weak.

   Diagnosis: _____

   _____

   Patient goal: _____

   _____

f. A woman who underwent a hysterectomy feels she can no longer have a sexual relationship with her husband.

Diagnosis: _____

_____

Patient goal: _____

_____

9. Describe three strategies nurses can use to help patients identify and use personal strengths.

a. _____

b. _____

c. _____

10. Give three examples of how nurses can help patients maintain a sense of self-worth.

a. _____

_____

b. _____

_____

c. _____

_____

11. Describe nursing strategies to develop self-esteem that you might use to meet the needs of the following elderly patients with disturbances in self-concept.

a. An 88-year-old woman, newly admitted to a nursing home, says she has lost all sense of self (Self-Identity Disturbance): _____

_____

_____

b. A 75-year-old man with crippling arthritis tells you he no longer recognizes himself when he looks in the mirror (Body Image Disturbance): _____

_____

_____

c. A 62-year-old man who is recovering from a stroke that has paralyzed his right side says, "I don't know if I can live like this." (Self-Esteem Disturbance): _____

_____

_____

d. A 67-year-old woman complains that she no longer has the patience to babysit for her grandchildren, whom she loves (Role Performance Disturbance): _____

_____

_____

_____

APPLYING YOUR KNOWLEDGE

CRITICAL THINKING QUESTIONS

1. There are many factors that influence the self-concept of patients, including developmental considerations, culture, internal or external resources, history of success or failure, stressors, and aging, illness, or trauma. Interview several patients to find out how these factors have influenced their self-concept. Once you've identified these factors, write a nursing diagnosis for each patient and develop patient health goals where appropriate.

2. Would you describe yourself as having high or low self-concept? Ask your friends if they agree with your assessment. How might your self-concept influence the relationship you establish with patients and colleagues?

REFLECTIVE PRACTICE AND BLENDED SKILLS

Use the following expanded scenario from Chapter 41 in your textbook to answer the questions below.

Scenario: Anthony Santorini is a middle-aged man with a history of diabetes. He recently underwent a below-the-knee amputation due to complications resulting from poor glucose control. One morning, he states, "I feel like damaged goods. I'm not a whole man anymore." When the nurse attempts to initiate an assessment of his self-concept, he turns his back on her and states: "Just leave me alone, I don't want to talk about it."

1. What interventions might the nurse employ to try to resolve Mr. Santorini's self-image disturbance?

_____

_____

_____

2. What would be a successful outcome for Mr. Santorini?

_____

_____

_____

3. What intellectual, technical, interpersonal, and/or ethical/legal competencies are most likely to bring about the desired outcome?

_____

_____

_____

4. What resources might be helpful for Mr. Santorini?

_____

_____

_____

PATIENT CARE STUDY

Read the following patient care study and use your nursing process skills to answer the questions below.

Scenario: An English teacher asks you, the school nurse, to see one of her students, Julie, whose grades have recently dropped and who no longer seems to be interested in school or anything else. "She was one of my best students, and I can't figure out what's going on," the teacher says. "She seems reluctant to talk about this change." When Julie, a 16-year-old junior, walks into your office, you are immediately struck by her stooped posture, unstyled hair, and sloppy appearance. Julie is attractive, but at 5 feet 3 inches and 150 pounds, she is overweight. Julie is initially reluctant to talk, but she breaks down at one point and confides that for the first time in her life she feels "absolutely awful" about herself. "I've always concentrated on getting good grades and achieved this easily. But now, this doesn't seem so important. I don't have any friends.

All I hear the girls talking about is boys, and I was never even asked out by a boy, which I guess isn't surprising. Look at me!" After a few questions, it becomes clear that Julie has new expectations for herself based on what she observes in her peers, and she finds herself falling far short of her new, ideal self. Julie admits that in the past, once she set a goal for herself, she was always able to achieve it because she is strongly self-motivated. Although she has withdrawn from her parents and teachers, she admits that she does know adults she can trust who have been a big support to her in the past. She says, "If only I could become the kind of teenager other kids like and have lots of friends!"

1. Identify pertinent patient data by placing a single underline beneath the objective data in the case study and a double underline beneath the subjective data.

2. Complete the Nursing Process Worksheet on page 289 to develop a three-part diagnostic statement and related plan of care for this patient.

3. Write down the patient and personal nursing strengths you hope to draw upon as you assist this patient to better health.

Patient strengths: _____

_____

_____

Personal strengths: _____

_____

_____

4. Pretend you are performing a nursing assessment of this patient after the plan of care has been implemented. Document your findings.

_____

_____

_____

NURSING PROCESS WORKSHEET

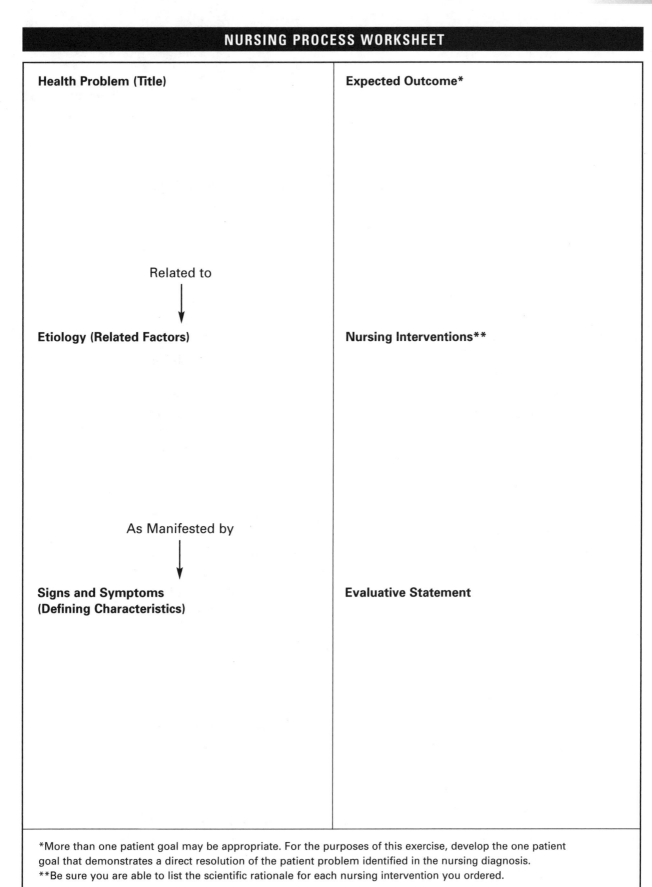

Health Problem (Title)

Expected Outcome*

Related to
↓

Etiology (Related Factors)

Nursing Interventions**

As Manifested by
↓

**Signs and Symptoms
(Defining Characteristics)**

Evaluative Statement

*More than one patient goal may be appropriate. For the purposes of this exercise, develop the one patient goal that demonstrates a direct resolution of the patient problem identified in the nursing diagnosis.
**Be sure you are able to list the scientific rationale for each nursing intervention you ordered.

CHAPTER 42

Stress and Adaptation

PRACTICING FOR NCLEX

MULTIPLE CHOICE QUESTIONS

Circle the letter that corresponds to the best answer for each question.

1. Which of the following describes the change that takes place as a result of a response to a stressor?
   a. Adaptation
   b. Stress
   c. Defense mechanism
   d. Anxiety

2. The primary controller of homeostatic mechanisms is which of the following systems?
   a. Respiratory
   b. Cardiovascular
   c. Autonomic
   d. Gastrointestinal

3. In which of the stages of the GAS does the body attempt to adapt to the stressor?
   a. Alarm reaction
   b. Resistance
   c. Exhaustion
   d. Homeostasis

4. A patient who responds to bad news concerning his lab reports by crying uncontrollably is handling stress by using which of the following?
   a. Adaptation technique
   b. Coping mechanism
   c. Withdrawal behavior
   d. Defense mechanism

5. Which of the following statements concerning interactions with basic human needs is accurate?
   a. As a person strives to meet basic human needs at each level, stress can serve as either a stimulus or barrier.
   b. Basic human needs and responses to stress are generalized.
   c. Basic human needs and responses to stress are unaffected by sociocultural backgrounds, priorities, and past experiences.
   d. Stress affects all people in their attainment of basic human needs in the same manner.

6. A withdrawn and isolated patient is most likely suffering from which of the following stressors on basic human needs?
   a. Physiologic needs
   b. Safety and security needs
   c. Self-esteem needs
   d. Love and belonging needs

7. Which of the following reactions would be considered anxiety due to a psychological response?
   a. Tremors
   b. Sleep disturbances
   c. Expressions of anger
   d. Withdrawal from interactions with others

8. When physiologic mechanisms within the body respond to internal changes to maintain an essential balance, which of the following processes has occurred?

   a. Stress

   b. Self-regulation

   c. Homeostasis

   d. Fight-or-flight response

9. You respond to an approaching examination with a rapidly beating heart and shaking hands. This is the result of what type of response?

   a. Coping mechanism

   b. Stress adaptation

   c. Defense mechanism

   d. Withdrawal behavior

10. Which of the following phrases best illustrates the panic level of anxiety?

    a. Loss of control and rational thought

    b. Increased alertness and motivated learning

    c. Narrow focus on specific detail

    d. Narrow perception field

11. When nurses become overwhelmed in their jobs and develop symptoms of anxiety and stress, they are experiencing which of the following conditions?

    a. Culture shock

    b. Adaptation syndrome

    c. Ineffective coping

    d. Burnout

12. Which of the following best illustrates a general task for a patient adapting to acute and chronic illness?

    a. Maintain self-esteem

    b. Handle pain

    c. Carry out medical treatment

    d. Confront family problems

13. Which of the following is the most common response to stress?

    a. Anger

    b. Anxiety

    c. Despair

    d. Depression

ALTERNATE-FORMAT QUESTIONS

Multiple Response Questions

Circle the letters that correspond to the best answers for each question.

1. Which of the following statements accurately describe the four levels of anxiety? *(Select all that apply.)*

   a. Moderate anxiety is present in day-to-day living, and it increases alertness and perceptual fields.

   b. Although mild anxiety may interfere with sleep, it also facilitates problem solving.

   c. Mild anxiety is manifested by a quivering voice, tremors, increased muscle tension, and a slight increase in respirations and pulse.

   d. Severe anxiety creates a very narrow focus on specific detail, causing all behavior to be geared toward getting relief.

   e. Severe anxiety causes a person to lose control and experience dread and terror.

   f. During the panic stage, the person cannot learn, concentrates only on the present situation, and often experiences feelings of impending doom.

2. Which of the following statements accurately describe the body's defense mechanisms against stressors? *(Select all that apply.)*

   a. Withdrawal behavior involves physical withdrawal from the threat or emotional reactions such as admitting defeat, becoming apathetic, or feeling guilty and isolated.

   b. Defense mechanisms are conscious reactions to stressors.

   c. Displacement occurs when a person refuses to acknowledge the presence of a condition that is disturbing.

   d. Projection occurs when a person's thoughts or impulses are attributed to another person.

   e. Repression occurs when a person involuntarily excludes an anxiety-producing event from conscious awareness.

   f. Reaction formation occurs when a person tries to give questionable behavior a logical or socially acceptable explanation.

3. Which of the following are effects of stress on the body? *(Select all that apply.)*

   a. Stress has a negative impact on a person as he/she strives to meet basic human needs at each level.

   b. People react to stress in a consistent and predictable manner.

   c. The health–illness continuum is affected by stress.

   d. The effects of stress on a sick or injured person are usually positive.

   e. As the duration, intensity, or number of stressors increases, a person's ability to adapt is lessened.

   f. Recovery from illness and return to normal function are compromised by prolonged stress.

4. Which of the following would be considered situational stress? *(Select all that apply.)*

   a. A toddler learning to control elimination

   b. A school-aged child attending her first party

   c. A man getting married to his high school sweetheart

   d. A woman recovering from a car accident

   e. A teenager being offered a cigarette by a friend

   f. A high school graduate enrolling in the armed services

5. Which of the following are considered psychosocial stressors? *(Select all that apply.)*

   a. News reports on television about a war

   b. Being caught in a blizzard

   c. Acquiring a nosocomial infection

   d. Being diagnosed with HIV

   e. Fearing a terrorist attack

   f. Being involved in an accident

Prioritization Question

1. Place the following steps of the General Adaptation Syndrome (GAS) in the order in which they would normally occur:

   a. Rest and recovery or death occur.

   b. Alarm reaction begins.

   c. Fight-or-flight response occurs.

   d. Neuroendocrine activity increases vital signs.

e. Stage of resistance begins.

f. Panic, crisis, and exhaustion occur.

g. Neuroendocrine activity returns to normal.

h. Stage of exhaustion begins.

i. Threat occurs.

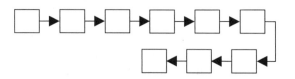

DEVELOPING YOUR KNOWLEDGE BASE

FILL-IN-THE-BLANKS

1. A(n) _____ is anything that is perceived as challenging, threatening, or demanding.

2. The _____ syndrome is a localized response of the body to stress.

3. The _____ response is a local response to injury or infection.

4. The _____ response is the body's method of preparing the body to either fight off a stressor or run away from it.

5. A person who develops diarrhea while under prolonged stress is said to be experiencing a(n) _____ disorder.

6. The most common human response to stress is _____.

7. Behaviors used to decrease stress and anxiety are called _____.

8. The prolonged stress experienced by family members caring for a loved one at home is known as _____.

MATCHING EXERCISES

Match the type of defense mechanism listed in Part A with its example listed in Part B.

PART A

a. Compensation

b. Denial

c. Displacement

d. Introjection

e. Projection

f. Rationalization

g. Reaction formation

h. Regression

i. Repression

j. Sublimation

k. Suppression

l. Undoing

PART B

1. ____ A patient bangs his hand on the bed tray in frustration over his rehabilitation progress.

2. ____ A patient doesn't remember striking a nurse during a painful procedure.

3. ____ A patient who screamed at a nurse in anger over a lack of privacy gives the nurse a box of candy.

4. ____ A patient who continually forgets to take his medications complains, "There are too many pills to take."

5. ____ A patient refuses to accept her diagnosis of cancer.

6. ____ A patient who has sexual feelings for a nurse accuses her of sexual harassment.

7. ____ A patient who cannot stop smoking becomes a fitness fanatic.

8. ____ A patient adopts his spiritual director's philosophy of life.

9. ____ A patient who actually admires her doctor's medical ability questions his competency.

10. ____ A nursing home patient who is depressed becomes incontinent.

11. ____ A wheelchair-bound patient becomes involved in wheelchair races.

Match the homeostatic regulators of the body listed in Part A with their action listed in Part B.

PART A

a. Parasympathetic

b. Sympathetic

c. Pituitary

d. Adrenals

e. Thyroid

f. Cardiovascular

g. Renal

h. Respiratory

i. Gastrointestinal

PART B

12. ____ Secretes adrenocorticotropic hormone and thyroid-stimulating hormone

13. ____ Takes in food and fluids and eliminates waste products

14. ____ Functions under stress conditions to bring about the fight-or-flight response

15. ____ Regulates intake and output of oxygen and carbon dioxide

16. ____ Functions under normal conditions and at rest

17. ____ Secretes thyroid hormone and calcitonin

18. ____ Serves as a transport system and pump

19. ____ Filters, excretes, and reabsorbs metabolic products and water

SHORT ANSWER

1. Briefly describe the following adaptive responses to stress, and give an example of each response.

   a. Mind–body interaction: _____

   _____

   b. Local adaptation syndrome: _____

   _____

   c. General adaptation syndrome: _____

   _____

2. Describe the three stages of the inflammatory response.

   a. _____

   _____

   b. _____

   _____

   c. _____

   _____

3. List three variables affecting the length of the alarm stage.

a. _____
_____

b. _____
_____

c. _____
_____

4. Describe the following types of anxiety. In your practice, have you experienced any of these levels of anxiety?

a. Mild anxiety: _____
_____
_____

b. Moderate anxiety: _____
_____
_____

c. Severe anxiety: _____
_____
_____

d. Panic: _____
_____
_____

5. Give an example of a situation in which you experienced the following coping mechanisms personally or witnessed them in a friend, relative, or patient.

a. Attack behavior: _____
_____

b. Withdrawal behavior: _____
_____

c. Compromise behavior: _____
_____

6. List three examples of situations in which stress may have a positive impact on an individual.

a. _____
b. _____
c. _____

7. Give three examples of the following sources of stress.

a. Developmental stress: _____
_____
_____

b. Situational stress: _____
_____
_____

8. An 18-year-old boy is admitted to your unit with a broken leg and facial lacerations from an automobile accident. List two remarks a nurse might make during the nursing history to assess this patient for anxiety.

a. _____
b. _____

9. You are a visiting nurse for a patient recovering from a stroke who is being taken care of by her daughter-in-law, who is also the mother of 2-year-old twins. During your visit, you notice that your patient's daughter is restless and unfocused. She tells you she has resumed her smoking habit. You suspect she is suffering from caregiver burden. How would you plan and implement care to help relieve her stress?

_____
_____
_____
_____

10. Briefly describe how the following components can help reduce stress.

a. Exercise: _____
_____

b. Rest and sleep: _____
_____

c. Nutrition: _____
_____

11. List the five steps of the problem-solving technique used in crisis intervention.

a. _____
b. _____
c. _____

d. _____

e. _____

12. List four personal factors that affect stress.

    a. _____

    b. _____

    c. _____

    d. _____

13. Give three examples of how a family can help a patient manage stress.

    a. _____

    b. _____

    c. _____

APPLYING YOUR KNOWLEDGE

CRITICAL THINKING QUESTIONS

1. Describe the nursing interventions you would use to relieve the stress of the following patients:

   a. A 42-year-old man with a wife and three children is being treated for an ulcer. He recently lost his job and is having a hard time finding a new one. He doesn't know if he can make his mortgage and school payments.

   b. A 16-year-old boy is admitted to a unit for drug rehabilitation. He put pressure on himself to be "the best" in sports and schoolwork and says he couldn't handle the stress without getting high.

   How would you use your knowledge of the patients to individualize the plan of care?

2. Think of a period in your life when you were under a considerable amount of stress, such as during exams, following a death, or during an illness. How did the stress affect you physically? Did it alter your health state? What did you do to compensate for the effects of stress on your body? How can you use this information in caring for patients?

REFLECTIVE PRACTICE USING CRITICAL THINKING SKILLS

Use the following expanded scenario from Chapter 42 in your textbook to answer the questions below.

Scenario: Joan Rogerrio is a middle-aged woman with a history of inflammatory bowel disease. She comes to the outpatient clinic with complaints of increasing episodes of diarrhea. She says, "I think my bowel disease is flaring up again." Further assessment reveals that she started a new job 1 month ago after being out of the workforce for the past 15 years. She tells the nurse, "Since the children are in school most of the day, my husband and I decided it was time for me to go back to work to help out financially." She says her skills are rusty and she is having a difficult time adapting to her new work schedule.

1. What might be the cause of the flare-up of Ms. Rogerrios's inflammatory bowel disease? What nursing interventions would be beneficial for this patient?

   _____

   _____

   _____

2. What would be a successful outcome for this patient?

   _____

   _____

   _____

3. What intellectual, technical, interpersonal, and/or ethical/legal competencies are most likely to bring about the desired outcome?

   _____

   _____

   _____

4. What resources might be helpful for Ms. Rogerrio?

   _____

   _____

   _____

PATIENT CARE STUDY

Read the following patient care study and use your nursing process skills to answer the questions below.

Scenario: Tisha Brent, age 52, comes to the clinic complaining of feelings of nervousness and an inability to sleep. During the health history, she says, "This past year has been almost more than I could stand." She tells you that in 1 year, her grandmother and father died, her husband was diagnosed with cancer, her daughter got a divorce, and her son became depressed and unable to work. She believes herself to be, "the strong person in the family; the one who always takes care of everyone else."

Mrs. Brent works full time as a social worker but is finding it more and more difficult to help others because of her own worries. She tells you that she rarely sees her friends anymore because she must care for her husband. She also says that she has no appetite, cries often, and sometimes has trouble catching her breath. Findings from the physical assessment included a weight loss of 10 pounds in the past 3 months (with weight 5% below normal for height), tachycardia, slightly elevated blood pressure, and hand tremors.

1. What additional questions might you ask to complete the health history?

   _____

   _____

   _____

2. What physical manifestations of stress might be elicited during the health history and physical assessment?

   _____

   _____

   _____

3. List the nursing diagnoses obtained from your data.

   _____

   _____

   _____

4. List the expected outcomes for Mrs. Brent.

   _____

   _____

5. Mrs. Brent is diagnosed as being in crisis. What does this mean?

   _____

   _____

   _____

6. What are the steps of crisis intervention that may be used with Mrs. Brent?

   _____

   _____

   _____

7. What would you teach Mrs. Brent about reducing stress through healthy activities of daily living?
   a. Exercise
   b. Rest and sleep
   c. Nutrition

8. How would you know if Mrs. Brent had decreased her level of stress and increased her ability to cope with stressors?

   _____

   _____

   _____

Loss, Grief, and Dying

PRACTICING FOR NCLEX

MULTIPLE CHOICE QUESTIONS

Circle the letter that corresponds to the best answer for each question.

1. Which of the following stages of grief, according to Engel, involve the rituals surrounding loss, including funeral services?

   a. Shock and disbelief

   b. Developing awareness

   c. Restitution

   d. Resolving the loss

2. The husband of a patient who has died cannot express his feelings of loss and at times denies them. His bereavement has extended over a lengthy period. Which of the following types of grief would the husband be experiencing?

   a. Anticipatory grief

   b. Inhibited grief

   c. Normal grief

   d. Unresolved grief

3. A patient who was brought to the emergency room for gunshot wounds dies in intensive care 15 hours later. Which of the following statements concerning the need for an autopsy would apply to this patient?

   a. The closest surviving family member should be consulted to determine whether an autopsy should be performed.

   b. The coroner must be notified to determine the need for an autopsy.

   c. The physician should be present to prepare the patient for an autopsy.

   d. An autopsy should not be performed because the nature of death has been established.

4. Mr. Cooney, age 85, is in advanced stages of pneumonia with a no-code order in his chart. Which of the following nursing care actions will help establish a trusting nurse–patient relationship?

   a. The nurse should not express his/her own fears about death in order to better concentrate on the patient's needs.

   b. The nurse should reduce verbal and nonverbal contact with the patient to avoid confusing him.

   c. The nurse should encourage family members to assist in his nursing care.

   d. The nurse should arrange a visit from a spiritual advisor, regardless of the patient's wishes, to provide hope in the face of death.

5. A nurse informs a woman that there is nothing more that can be done medically for her premature infant, who is expected to die. Which of the following types of grief might the mother be experiencing?

   a. Anticipatory grief

   b. Inhibited grief

   c. Unresolved grief

   d. Dysfunctional grief

6. According to Engel (1964), the exaggeration of the good qualities of the person or object lost, followed by acceptance of the loss, is which of the following?

   a. Restitution

   b. Awareness

c. Outcome

d. Idealization

7. Before the death of her husband, Mrs. Sardi complained of frequent headaches and loss of appetite. No medical cause was found. Mrs. Sardi probably was experiencing which type of grief?

   a. Abbreviated grief

   b. Anticipatory grief

   c. Unresolved grief

   d. Inhibited grief

8. Which of the following diagnoses specifically addresses human response to loss and impending death in the problem statement?

   a. Dysfunctional Grieving related to loss of partner

   b. Anxiety related to unknown reaction to stages of death

   c. Self-Care Deficit related to weakness

   d. Altered Comfort related to complications of chemotherapy for end-stage liver cancer

ALTERNATE-FORMAT QUESTIONS

Multiple Response Questions

Circle the letters that correspond to the best answers for each question.

1. Which of the following are stages of grieving according to Engel? *(Select all that apply.)*

   a. Shock and disbelief

   b. Developing awareness

   c. Anger and denial

   d. Resolving the loss

   e. Moralization

   f. Prioritizing

2. Which of the following are impending signs of death? *(Select all that apply.)*

   a. Inability to swallow

   b. Increased gastrointestinal activity

   c. Pitting edema

   d. Decreased temperature

   e. Warm, flushed skin

   f. Lowered blood pressure

3. Which of the following are suggested guidelines when breaking bad news to a patient? *(Select all that apply.)*

   a. Explain the entire condition in detail regardless of what the patient may already know.

   b. Assume that the patient wants to know the entire truth about his/her condition.

   c. Give the information in "small chunks" and stop occasionally to see that the information is being understood.

   d. Do not allow emotional reactions to distract the patient from your goal of dispensing information.

   e. Summarize the information and ask for questions.

   f. Respond to the patient with sincerity and empathy when appropriate.

4. Which of the following statements regarding end-of-life decision making are accurate? *(Select all that apply.)*

   a. Living wills provide specific instructions about the kinds of healthcare that should be provided or foregone in particular situations.

   b. In a living will, a patient appoints an agent that he/she trusts to make decisions if he/she becomes incapacitated.

   c. The Patient Self-Determination Act of 1990 requires all hospitals to inform their patients about advance directives.

   d. The status of advance directives varies from state to state.

   e. Nurses are legally responsible for arranging for a durable power of attorney for all terminal patients.

   f. Legally, all attempts must be made by the healthcare team to resuscitate a terminal patient.

5. Which of the following statements accurately describe the process of preparing a death certificate? *(Select all that apply.)*

   a. U.S. law requires that a death certificate be prepared for each person who dies.

   b. Death certificates are sent to a national health department, which compiles many statistics from the information.

c. The nurse assumes responsibility for handling and filing the death certificate with the proper authorities.

d. A physician's signature is required on a death certificate.

e. It is the nurse's responsibility to ensure that the physician has signed a death certificate.

f. A death certificate is signed by the pathologist, the coroner, and others in special cases.

6. Which of the following are actions performed by the nurse when a patient dies? *(Select all that apply.)*

a. Washing the patient's body

b. Removing all tubes, unless an autopsy is to be performed

c. Placing identification on the shroud or garment and wrist

d. Placing identification tags on the patient's dentures or other prostheses

e. Arranging for family members to view the body before it is discharged to the mortician

f. Attending the funeral of a deceased patient and making follow-up visits to the family

DEVELOPING YOUR KNOWLEDGE BASE

FILL-IN-THE-BLANKS

1. When an older man grieves for the loss of his youth, this type of loss is known as _____ loss.

2. _____ is the state of grieving during which a person experiences grief reaction.

3. According to Engel, _____ is the final resolution of the grief process.

4. Abnormal or distorted grief that may be unresolved or inhibited is known as _____ grief.

5. According to the Uniform Definition of Death Act (1981), death is defined as present when an individual has sustained either irreversible cessation of circulation and respiratory functions or _____.

6. _____ care involves taking care of the whole person—body, mind, and spirit, heart and soul.

MATCHING EXERCISES

Match the term in Part A with the appropriate definition listed in Part B.

PART A

a. Actual loss
b. Perceived loss
c. Physical loss
d. Psychological loss
e. Anticipatory loss
f. Grief
g. Bereavement
h. Mourning

PART B

1. ____ The period of acceptance of loss during which the person learns to deal with the loss

2. ____ A type of loss in which a person displays loss and grief behaviors for a loss that has yet to take place

3. ____ A type of loss that can be recognized by others as well as by the person sustaining the loss

4. ____ The state of grieving during which a person experiences grief reaction

5. ____ A type of loss that is felt by the individual but is intangible to others, such as loss of youth or financial independence

6. ____ A type of loss that may be caused by an altered self-image and inability to return to work

7. ____ A type of loss that is tangible, such as the loss of a limb or organ

Match Engel's six stages of grief listed in Part A with the appropriate conversation that may occur during each stage listed in Part B.

PART A

a. Shock and disbelief
b. Developing awareness
c. Restitution
d. Resolving the loss

e. Idealization

f. Outcome

PART B

8. ____ "I know I won't be having Sunday dinner with my mother anymore. Maybe my husband and I can eat out this Sunday."

9. ____ "I can't believe my mother died of breast cancer! She was never seriously ill in her life."

10. ____ "My mother was the perfect parent. I wish I could be more like her with my kids."

11. ____ "Every time I think of my mother, I can't help but cry."

12. ____ "I've been attending Mass every morning to pray for my mother's soul and to help me get over her death."

13. ____ "I miss my mother, but at least now I can accept her death and try to get on with my life."

CORRECT THE FALSE STATEMENTS

Circle the word "true" or "false" that follows the statement. If you circled "false," change the underlined word or words to make the statement true. Place your answer in the space provided.

1. A person experiencing <u>abbreviated grief</u> may have trouble expressing feelings of loss or may deny them.

   True   False _____

2. In the <u>denial and isolation</u> stage of dying, the patient expresses rage and hostility and adopts a "why me?" attitude.

   True   False _____

3. In the case of a terminal illness, the <u>physician</u> is usually responsible for deciding what and how much the patient should be told.

   True   False _____

4. In a <u>living will</u>, the patient appoints an agent he/she trusts to make decisions if he/she becomes incapacitated.

   True   False _____

5. The <u>Patient Self-Determination Act of 1990</u> requires all hospitals to inform their patients of advance directives.

   True   False _____

6. A <u>slow-code</u> order may be written on the chart of a terminally ill patient if the patient or family has expressed a wish that there be no attempts to resuscitate the patient in the event of cardiopulmonary failure.

   True   False _____

7. <u>Terminal weaning</u> is the gradual withdrawal of mechanical ventilation from a patient with a terminal illness or an irreversible condition with a poor prognosis.

   True   False _____

8. The <u>nurse</u> assumes responsibility for handling and filing the death certificate with proper authorities.

   True   False _____

9. After the patient has been pronounced dead, the <u>physician</u> is responsible for preparing the body for discharge.

   True   False _____

SHORT ANSWER

1. List two nursing responsibilities that should be carried out after the death of a patient in each of the following areas.

   a. Care of the body: _____

   _____

   b. Care of the family: _____

   _____

   c. Discharging legal responsibilities: _____

   _____

2. Briefly describe the following stages of dying, according to Kübler-Ross.

   a. Denial and isolation: _____

   _____

   b. Anger: _____

   _____

c. Bargaining: _____

_____

d. Depression: _____

_____

e. Acceptance: _____

_____

3. Your patient is a 50-year-old woman newly diagnosed with terminal uterine cancer. What information should be provided to her regarding her condition?

_____

_____

4. How would you respond to a patient dying of AIDS who says: "Nurse, please help me die"?

_____

_____

_____

5. Describe the role of the nurse in terminal weaning.

_____

_____

_____

6. List three goals for nurses who wish to become effective in caring for patients experiencing loss, grief, or dying and death.

a. _____

_____

b. _____

_____

c. _____

_____

7. Your patient is a 62-year-old man dying of liver cancer at home with his family. List three patient goals or outcomes for this patient and his family.

a. _____

b. _____

c. _____

8. List three arguments in favor of and against assisted suicide and direct voluntary euthanasia.

a. In favor of: _____

_____

_____

b. Against: _____

_____

_____

9. What is the role of the nurse during the following code situations?

a. No-code: _____

_____

_____

b. Comfort measures only: _____

_____

_____

c. Do-not-hospitalize order: _____

_____

_____

d. Terminal weaning: _____

_____

_____

10. Explain the role of the nurse in obtaining the following advance directives for a patient.

a. Durable power of attorney: _____

_____

_____

b. Living will: _____

_____

_____

APPLYING YOUR KNOWLEDGE

CRITICAL THINKING QUESTIONS

1. Develop nursing plans to help the following patients deal with their grief.

   a. A 22-year-old male athlete has his left leg amputated after it was crushed in a car accident.

   b. You find a 30-year-old woman crying softly in her bed after undergoing a hysterectomy.

   c. A 50-year-old woman has just been told she has an inoperable brain tumor.

   What knowledge and skills would you need to meet their needs?

2. Think of a time when you lost someone dear to you. How did you cope with your loss? Were you aware of going through Engel's six stages of grief? How long did it take you to resolve the loss and get back to normal life activities? Interview some friends about coping with losing a loved one, and compare their experiences to yours. How can you use this knowledge in your care of patients?

REFLECTIVE PRACTICE USING CRITICAL THINKING SKILLS

Use the following expanded scenario from Chapter 43 in your textbook to answer the questions below.

Scenario: Yvonne Malic, age 20, is admitted to the hospital after her water broke, and labor begins 7 weeks early. She delivers a female infant who is immediately transported to the neonatal intensive care unit. Yvonne is single and desperately wants to be a mother. She had a normal pregnancy up to this point and was expecting a healthy baby girl. The nurse informs Ms. Malic that her baby has less than a 50% chance of surviving the next 24 hours. Ms. Malic tearfully tells the nurse, "Leave me alone!" and turns her body to face the wall.

1. How might the nurse react to Ms. Malic in a manner that respects her right to privacy while at the same time helping her through the grief process?

   _____

   _____

   _____

2. What would be a successful outcome for this patient?

   _____

   _____

   _____

3. What intellectual, technical, interpersonal, and/or ethical/legal competencies are most likely to bring about the desired outcome?

   _____

   _____

   _____

4. What resources might be helpful for Ms. Malic?

   _____

   _____

   _____

PATIENT CARE STUDY

Read the following patient care study and use your nursing process skills to answer the questions on page 303.

Scenario: LeRoy is a 40-year-old architect whose life partner, Michael, is dying of AIDS. Although both LeRoy and Michael "did the bathhouse scene" in the early 1980s and had multiple unprotected sexual encounters, they have been in a monogamous relationship for the past 14 years. Michael has been in and out of the hospital during the past 3 years and is now dying of end-stage AIDS at home. He is enrolled in a hospice program. LeRoy has been very supportive of Michael throughout the different phases of his illness but at present seems to be "losing it." Michael noticed that LeRoy is sleeping at odd times and seems to be losing weight. He suspects that LeRoy may be drinking more than usual and using recreational drugs. He also says that LeRoy is "acting strangely"; he seems emotionally withdrawn and unusually uncommunicative. "I don't think he's able to deal with the fact that I'm dying," Michael tells you. "He won't let me talk about it at all." The hospice nurse notes that LeRoy is now rarely home when he comes to visit. When the hospice nurse calls to arrange a meeting with LeRoy, LeRoy informs him that he is "managing quite well, thank you" and that he has no concerns or problems to discuss.

1. Identify pertinent patient data by placing a single underline beneath the objective data in the patient care study and a double underline beneath the subjective data.

2. Complete the Nursing Process Worksheet on page 304 to develop a three-part diagnostic statement and related plan of care for this patient.

3. Write down the patient and personal nursing strengths you hope to draw on as you assist this patient to better health.

Patient strengths: _____

_____

_____

Personal strengths: _____

_____

_____

4. Pretend that you are performing a nursing assessment of LeRoy after the plan of care is implemented. Document your findings.

_____

_____

_____

NURSING PROCESS WORKSHEET

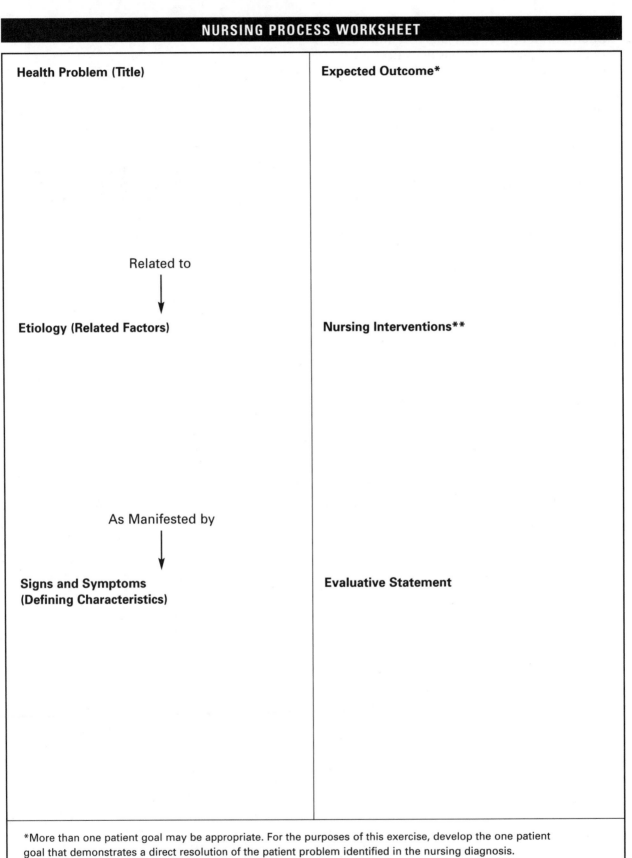

Health Problem (Title)

Expected Outcome*

Related to
↓

Etiology (Related Factors)

Nursing Interventions**

As Manifested by
↓

**Signs and Symptoms
(Defining Characteristics)**

Evaluative Statement

*More than one patient goal may be appropriate. For the purposes of this exercise, develop the one patient goal that demonstrates a direct resolution of the patient problem identified in the nursing diagnosis.
**Be sure you are able to list the scientific rationale for each nursing intervention you ordered.

CHAPTER 44

Sensory Functioning

PRACTICING FOR NCLEX

MULTIPLE CHOICE QUESTIONS

Circle the letter that corresponds to the best answer for each question.

1. A patient who has been living in a nursing home for the past 5 years no longer responds to the everyday noises outside his room. This ability to ignore continuing noise is known as which of the following?
   a. Sensoristasis
   b. Sensory overload
   c. Adaptation
   d. Stereognosis

2. Which of the following statements concerning sensory stimulation is accurate?
   a. Different personality types demand the same level of stimulation.
   b. Decreased sensory stimulation may be sought during periods of low stress.
   c. Illness does not affect the reception of sensory stimuli.
   d. An individual's culture may dictate the amount of sensory stimulation considered normal.

3. An unconscious patient is assigned to your unit. When caring for this patient, you should follow which of the following guidelines for communication?
   a. Hearing is the first sense lost in an unconscious patient; therefore, verbal communication is unnecessary.

   b. You should assume the patient can hear you, and talk with the person in a normal tone of voice.
   c. You should not touch the unconscious patient unnecessarily because it may confuse him/her.
   d. You should keep the environmental noise level high to help stimulate the patient.

4. Which of the following is the optimal arousal state of the RAS?
   a. Sensoristasis
   b. Presbycusis
   c. Kinesthesia
   d. Stereognosis

5. Which of the following conditions occurs when the RAS is no longer able to activate the brain at a normal level and the individual hallucinates simply to maintain an optimal level of arousal?
   a. Sensory overload
   b. Sensory deprivation
   c. Cultural care deprivation
   d. Sleep deprivation

6. Your patient in a nursing home cannot control the direction of thought content, has a decreased attention span, and cannot concentrate. Which of the following effects of sensory deprivation might he be experiencing?
   a. Perceptual response
   b. Emotional response
   c. Physical response
   d. Cognitive response

7. Which of the following refers to impaired or absent functioning in one or more senses?

   a. Sensory overload

   b. Sensory deficit

   c. Sensory deprivation

   d. Sensory overstimulation

ALTERNATE-FORMAT QUESTIONS

Multiple Response Questions

Circle the letters that correspond to the best answers for each question.

1. Which of the following conditions must be present for a person to receive the data necessary to experience the world? *(Select all that apply.)*

   a. A response

   b. A stimulus

   c. A receptor or sense organ

   d. An arousal mechanism

   e. An intact nerve pathway

   f. A functioning brain

2. Which of the following are factors contributing to severe sensory alteration? *(Select all that apply.)*

   a. Sensory saturation

   b. Sensory discrepancies

   c. Sensory overload

   d. Sensory deprivation

   e. Sleep deprivation

   f. Cultural overload

3. Which of the following statements accurately describe the effects of sensory deprivation? *(Select all that apply.)*

   a. Inaccurate perception of sights, sounds, tastes, and smells

   b. Increased coordination and equilibrium

   c. Inability to control direction of thought content

   d. Increased attention span and ability to concentrate

   e. Difficulty with memory, problem solving, and task performance

   f. Emotionally caring attitude and stable moods

4. Which of the following statements accurately describe factors that affect sensory stimulation? *(Select all that apply.)*

   a. The amount of stimuli different individuals consider optimal is constant.

   b. Sensory functioning is established at birth and is independent of stimulation received during childhood.

   c. It is recommended that medically fragile infants have greater light and visual and vestibular stimulation.

   d. Sensory functioning tends to decline progressively throughout adulthood.

   e. An individual's culture may dictate the amount of sensory stimulation considered normal.

   f. Different personality types demand different levels of stimulation.

5. Which of the following are characteristics of sensory deprivation or overload? *(Select all that apply.)*

   a. Boredom

   b. Decreased sleeping

   c. Quickness of thought

   d. Anxiety

   e. Dreamless sleep

   f. Thought disorganization

6. Which of the following are guidelines that should be followed when caring for visually impaired patients? *(Select all that apply.)*

   a. Wait for the person to sense your presence in the room before identifying yourself.

   b. Speak in a normal tone of voice.

   c. Explain the reason for touching the person after doing so.

   d. Orient the person to the arrangement of the room and its furnishings.

   e. Assist with ambulation by walking slightly behind the person.

   f. Sit in the person's field of vision if he or she has partial or reduced peripheral vision.

7. Which of the following are guidelines to follow when dealing with patients with hearing impairments? *(Select all that apply.)*

   a. Increase the noise level in the room.

   b. Clean ears on a daily basis.

c. Position yourself so that the light is on your face when you speak.

d. Talk to the person from a distance so that he/she may read your lips.

e. Demonstrate or pantomime ideas you wish to express.

f. Write any ideas that you cannot convey to the person in another manner.

DEVELOPING YOUR KNOWLEDGE BASE

FILL-IN-THE-BLANKS

1. _____ is the process of receiving data about the internal or external environment through the senses.

2. _____ refers to awareness of positioning of body parts and body movement.

3. _____ is the sense that perceives the solidity of objects and their size, shape, and texture.

4. The state in which an individual cannot remember bits of information is known as _____.

5. Impaired or absent functioning in one or more senses is termed _____.

MATCHING EXERCISES

Match the senses in Part A with their definition in Part B.

PART A

a. Visual

b. Auditory

c. Olfactory

d. Gustatory

e. Tactile

f. Kinesthesia

g. Visceral

h. Stereognosis

PART B

1. ____ The sense that perceives the solidity of objects and their size, shape, and texture

2. ____ The sense of taste

3. ____ The sense of sight

4. ____ The sense of smell

5. ____ The sense of hearing

6. ____ The awareness of positioning of body parts and body movement

7. ____ The sense of touch

Match the examples in Part B with the appropriate stimulation listed in Part A. Some answers may be used more than once.

PART A

a. Visual stimulation

b. Auditory stimulation

c. Gustatory/olfactory stimulation

d. Tactile stimulation

PART B

8. ____ A nurse wears a brightly colored top when caring for patients confined to bed.

9. ____ A nurse collaborates with the hospital nutritionist to prepare meals with varied seasonings and textures.

10. ____ A patient confined to bed is given daily massages.

11. ____ Soft music is played in the room of a patient who has eye patches following his surgery.

12. ____ In a long-term care facility, a nurse checks a patient for properly fitting dentures.

13. ____ A nurse hugs a depressed patient who has made the effort to bathe and dress herself.

14. ____ A nurse explains a procedure to a comatose patient.

15. ____ A nurse arranges a patient's cards in a heart shape on her wall.

SHORT ANSWER

1. List four conditions that must be present for a person to receive data necessary to experience the world.

a. _____

b. _____

c. _____

d. _____

2. Give an example of how the following factors may place a patient at high risk for sensory deprivation.

   a. Environment: _____

   _____

   b. Impaired ability to receive environmental stimuli: _____

   _____

   c. Inability to process environmental stimuli:

   _____

3. Briefly describe the following effects of sensory deprivation:

   a. Perceptual responses: _____

   _____

   b. Cognitive responses: _____

   _____

   c. Emotional responses: _____

   _____

4. List three examples of sensory overload you have observed when caring for patients on your nursing unit.

   a. _____

   b. _____

   c. _____

5. Describe the concept of cultural care deprivation, and list an example from your own experience of a patient who has experienced this alteration.

   _____

   _____

   _____

6. Give an example of sensory stimulation that could be provided for each of the following age groups.

   a. Infant: _____

   _____

   b. Adult: _____

   _____

   c. Elderly: _____

   _____

7. Give an example of two goals for patients with impaired sensory functioning.

   a. _____

   b. _____

8. You have been assigned to visit a home healthcare patient, a 75-year-old woman with diabetes living at home with her husband. When you arrive at their home, you notice the drapes are shut, the room is dark and bleak, and there are no pictures, flowers, or the like to visually stimulate the patient. The patient appears in good physical health but slightly disoriented and confused about the date and time of day. Develop a nursing care plan for this patient with emphasis on the need for sensory stimulation.

   _____

   _____

   _____

   _____

9. List four precautions you could teach a patient to avoid eye injury in the home.

   a. _____

   b. _____

   c. _____

   d. _____

10. Give two suggestions for increasing environmental stimulation and role model appropriate interactional behaviors for children in the following areas.

   a. Visual: _____

   _____

   b. Auditory: _____

   _____

   c. Olfactory: _____

   _____

   d. Gustatory: _____

   _____

   e. Tactile: _____

   _____

11. Give an example of how each of the following factors may influence the amount and quality of stimuli needed to maintain cortical arousal.

    a. Developmental considerations: _____

    _____

    b. Culture and lifestyle: _____

    _____

    c. Personality: _____

    _____

    d. Stress: _____

    _____

    e. Illness and medication: _____

    _____

12. Explain how you might assess a patient for the following sensory experiences.

    a. Stimulation: _____

    _____

    b. Reception: _____

    _____

    c. Transmission–perception–reaction: _____

    _____

13. Give three examples of how a nurse might communicate with the following patients.

    a. Visually impaired patients: _____

    _____

    b. Hearing-impaired patients: _____

    _____

    c. Unconscious patients: _____

    _____

APPLYING YOUR KNOWLEDGE

CRITICAL THINKING QUESTIONS

1. Test your friends' senses by trying out these tactile, gustatory, and olfactory exercises.

    a. Gather several items from your home/work area and place them in a paper bag. These items could include things such as a key, a cotton ball, a toothpick, a tongue depressor, and so on. Have your friends take turns feeling the objects in the bag and guessing what they are without looking at them. As an item is identified, remove it from the bag. Discuss the importance of tactile experiences to the vision-impaired patient.

    b. Gather several foods for your friends to taste and identify. You could use pudding, gelatin, mints, chocolate, and so on. Blind-fold your friends and give them a taste of each food. See how many they can identify correctly.

    c. Gather items with a pungent odor for your friends to smell and identify. You could use alcohol, lemon juice, pickle juice, cinnamon, mint, and so on. See how many odors they can identify correctly.

Reflect on the role different senses play. Do you believe using only one sense at a time heightens the awareness of that sense? Relate the exercises above to the special needs of hearing-impaired and vision-impaired patients.

2. Walk down a busy street in a city and try to pick out individual noises. How many noises were you able to identify? How many noises became indistinct due to sensory overload? Relate this experience to a patient in a critical care unit.

REFLECTIVE PRACTICE USING CRITICAL THINKING SKILLS

Use the following expanded scenario from Chapter 44 in your textbook to answer the questions below.

Scenario: Dolores Pirolla, age 74, comes to the older adult clinic with her 77-year-old husband, who was diagnosed with macular degeneration and progressive vision loss. She says, "Now I've noticed he's also having difficulty hearing me. I'm worried because he doesn't want to leave the house. We hardly see any of our friends anymore. We used to go out to the movies or dinner at least once a week, and lately if we get out once a month, that's a lot!" Mrs. Pirolla also expresses concerns about her husband's safety when moving about the house and neighborhood.

1. What nursing interventions might be appropriate for Mr. Pirolla?

    _____

    _____

    _____

2. What would be a successful outcome for this patient?

_____

_____

_____

3. What intellectual, technical, interpersonal, and/or ethical/legal competencies are most likely to bring about the desired outcome?

_____

_____

_____

4. What resources might be helpful for Mr. Pirolla?

_____

_____

_____

PATIENT CARE STUDY

Read the following patient care study and use your nursing process skills to answer the questions below.

Scenario: George Gibson, an 81-year-old, married, African American man, reluctantly reports, after much prodding from his wife, that he is not hearing as well as he used to be. "I don't know what the trouble is," he tells you. "I'm in perfect health, always have been. More and more, people just seem to be mumbling instead of talking." You notice he is seated on the edge of his chair and bends toward you when you speak to him. His wife reports that he has stopped going out and

pretty much stays in his room whenever people come to visit because he is embarrassed by his inability to hear. "This is really a shame, because George was always the life of the party," she says. You ask Mr. Gibson if he has ever had his hearing evaluated, and he tells you no, until now, he's been trying to convince himself that nothing's wrong with his hearing.

1. Identify pertinent patient data by placing a single underline beneath the objective data in the patient care study and a double underline beneath the subjective data.

2. Complete the Nursing Process Worksheet on page 311 to develop a three-part diagnostic statement and related plan of care for this patient.

3. Write down the patient and personal nursing strengths you hope to draw upon as you assist this patient to better health.

Patient strengths: _____

_____

_____

Personal strengths: _____

_____

_____

4. Pretend that you are performing a nursing assessment of this patient after the plan of care is implemented. Document your findings.

_____

_____

_____

NURSING PROCESS WORKSHEET

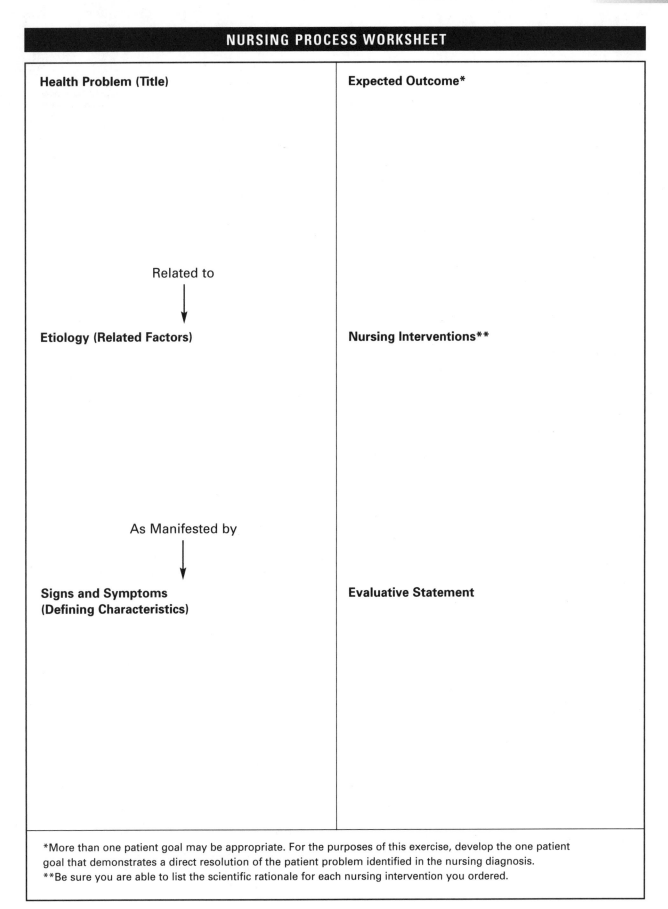

Health Problem (Title)

Expected Outcome*

Related to

↓

Etiology (Related Factors)

Nursing Interventions**

As Manifested by

↓

**Signs and Symptoms
(Defining Characteristics)**

Evaluative Statement

*More than one patient goal may be appropriate. For the purposes of this exercise, develop the one patient goal that demonstrates a direct resolution of the patient problem identified in the nursing diagnosis.
**Be sure you are able to list the scientific rationale for each nursing intervention you ordered.

Sexuality

PRACTICING FOR NCLEX

MULTIPLE CHOICE QUESTIONS

Circle the letter that corresponds to the best answer for each question.

1. The function of which of the following female organs is to transport a mature ovum from an ovary to the uterus?
   a. Fallopian tubes
   b. Ovaries
   c. Uterus
   d. Vagina

2. Which of the following parts of the uterus consists of tissue that thickens and sloughs off during menses?
   a. Perimetrium
   b. Myometrium
   c. Endometrium
   d. Cervix

3. During which stage of the menstrual cycle are hormones produced that encourage a fertilized egg to grow?
   a. Follicular phase
   b. Proliferation phase
   c. Luteal phase
   d. Secretory phase

4. Which of the following male organs produces the sperm?
   a. Scrotum
   b. Testes
   c. Vas deferens
   d. Penis

5. Which of the following organs is believed to act as a reservoir for sperm between ejaculations?
   a. Scrotum
   b. Testes
   c. Epididymis
   d. Vas deferens

6. What amount of sperm is released by a fertile man during an ejaculation?
   a. 60 to 100 million/mL
   b. 100 to 120 million/mL
   c. 120 to 160 million/mL
   d. 160 to 180 million/mL

7. The condom, cervical cap, and vaginal sponge are examples of which of the following types of contraceptives?
   a. Hormonal methods
   b. Barrier methods
   c. Natural family planning
   d. Sterilization

8. Which of the following statements about orgasm is accurate?
   a. Women who have multiple orgasms are promiscuous.
   b. A mature sexual relationship does not require a man and woman to achieve simultaneous orgasm.
   c. The larger the penis, the greater the potential for achieving orgasm.
   d. The ability to achieve orgasm is the only indicator of a person's sexual responsiveness.

9. Which of the following examples best supports the diagnosis of Sexual Dysfunction: Dyspareunia?
   a. A patient with a colostomy believes she cannot have a sexual relationship with her husband because he will be repulsed by her stoma.
   b. A 50-year-old woman with a history of stroke is afraid to have sex with her partner for fear it will elevate her blood pressure.
   c. A 50-year-old woman in the process of menopause has pain and burning during intercourse.
   d. A 39-year-old alcoholic woman is no longer interested in having sex with her partner.

ALTERNATE-FORMAT QUESTIONS

Multiple Response Questions

Circle the letters that correspond to the best answers for each question.

1. Which of the following statements accurately describe common sexual orientations? *(Select all that apply.)*
   a. A heterosexual is a person who experiences sexual fulfillment with a person of the opposite gender.
   b. A homosexual is a person who experiences sexual fulfillment with a person of the same gender.
   c. A bisexual is a person of a certain biologic gender with the feelings of the opposite sex.
   d. A transvestite is a person who finds pleasure with both opposite-sex and same-sex partners.
   e. Homosexual or heterosexual people may have bisexual relationships at times.
   f. A transsexual feels trapped within the body of the wrong sex.

2. Which of the following statements describe the physiology of the female genitalia? *(Select all that apply.)*
   a. The mons pubis consists of two rounded folds of fatty tissue.
   b. The clitoris is found above the urinary meatus at the joining of the labia minora.
   c. Women normally have two ovaries, one on each side of the body.

   d. The cervix is a pear-shaped organ about 3 inches long located between the urinary bladder and rectum.
   e. The uterus consists of three layers: the perimetrium, the myometrium, and the endometrium.
   f. The vagina is the structure at the lower portion of the uterus that connects the uterus and the cervix.

3. Which of the following statements regarding the menstrual cycle are true? *(Select all that apply.)*
   a. The first menstrual period, called menarche, is generally experienced at about 15 years of age.
   b. Menopause, the cessation of a woman's menstrual activity, occurs between the ages of 55 and 60 years.
   c. The menstrual cycle is controlled by a series of reactions that rely on feedback from the ovaries to the pituitary gland.
   d. In the ovaries, in a typical 28-day cycle, the phase from day 4 to 14 is called the luteal phase.
   e. In the luteal phase, the leftover empty follicle fills with a yellow pigment and is then called the corpus luteum, or yellow body.
   f. At day 28 of the menstrual cycle, menses begin as a result of the uterus shedding the useless portion of its endometrium.

4. Which of the following are structures of the male genitalia? *(Select all that apply.)*
   a. Testes
   b. Scrotum
   c. Fallopian tubes
   d. Mons pubis
   e. Cul-de-sac of Douglas
   f. Cowper's glands

5. Which of the following are phases of the sexual response cycle? *(Select all that apply.)*
   a. Stimulation
   b. Excitement
   c. Valley
   d. Plateau
   e. Orgasm
   f. Reinstatement

6. Which of the following statements accurately describe alternative forms of sexual expression? *(Select all that apply.)*

   a. Masochism refers to the practice of gaining sexual pleasure while inflicting abuse on another person.

   b. Sadism refers to gaining sexual pleasure from the humiliation of being abused.

   c. Voyeurism is the achievement of sexual arousal by looking at the body of another.

   d. Pedophilia is a term used to describe the practice of adults gaining sexual fulfillment by sexual acts with children.

   e. Sadomasochism is the act of practicing sadism and masochism together.

   f. Celibacy involves the use of inanimate objects to stimulate ejaculation.

7. Which of the following statements describe sexual dysfunction in males or females? *(Select all that apply.)*

   a. Premature ejaculation is a condition in which a man consistently reaches ejaculation or orgasm before or soon after entering the vagina.

   b. Retarded ejaculation refers to the man's inability to ejaculate into the vagina, or delayed intravaginal ejaculation.

   c. Vaginismus is painful intercourse.

   d. Dyspareunia is a condition in which the vaginal opening closes tightly and prevents penile penetration.

   e. Vulvodynia is a chronic vulvar discomfort or pain characterized by burning, stinging, irritation, or rawness of the female genitalia that interferes with sexual activity.

   f. Inhibited sexual desire refers to the inability of a woman to reach orgasm.

8. Which of the following are accurate descriptions of contraceptive methods? *(Select all that apply.)*

   a. Continuous abstinence depends on charting a woman's fertility pattern.

   b. The best approach to monitoring fertility is to use the calendar method along with the cervical mucus method, also known as the symptothermal method.

   c. Pregnancy cannot occur with coitus interruptus because sperm is kept out of the vagina.

   d. The diaphragm is a dome-shaped device made of latex rubber that mechanically prevents semen from coming into contact with the cervix.

   e. The cervical cap is a thimble-shaped rubber device placed over the cervix that may be left there for up to 3 days at a time.

   f. The vaginal sponge is a barrier method that contains a spermicide.

Prioritization Questions

1. Place the following series of reactions that control the menstrual cycle in the order in which they occur.

   a. The leftover empty follicle fills up with a yellow pigment and is then called the corpus luteum.

   b. A number of follicles mature, but only one produces a mature ovum.

   c. Ovulation occurs.

   d. If fertilization does not occur, the corpus luteum begins to disintegrate.

   e. Menstrual flow begins.

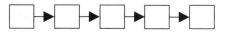

2. Place the following events in the order in which they occur in the sexual response cycle.

   a. The climax occurs.

   b. There is a heightened feeling of physical pleasure followed by overwhelming release and involuntary contraction of the genitals.

   c. The excitement phase is initiated by erotic stimulation and arousal.

   d. The women's breasts swell, and the nipples become erect. The penis becomes erect in the man.

   e. The intensity of the plateau phase builds and intensifies; the woman's clitoris retracts and disappears under the clitoral hood and secretions from Cowper's glands may appear at the glans of the penis.

   f. The body returns to normal functioning; the man experiences a refractory period.

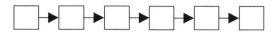

DEVELOPING YOUR KNOWLEDGE BASE

FILL-IN-THE-BLANKS

1. _____ is the degree to which a person exhibits and experiences maleness or femaleness physically, emotionally, and mentally.

2. _____ is the inner sense a person has of being male or female, which may be the same as or different from biologic gender.

3. _____ refers to the preferred gender of the partner of an individual.

4. A woman who experiences menstrual cycle–related distress is said to have _____.

5. Areas that when stimulated cause sexual arousal and desire are called _____.

6. The _____ system of contraception is a reversible, 5-year, low-dose progestin-only contraceptive consisting of six capsules placed under the skin of the woman's upper arm.

7. The _____ patch supplies continuous daily circulating levels of ethinyl estradiol and norelgestromin to prevent conception.

MATCHING EXERCISES

Match the terms listed in Part A with their definition listed in Part B.

PART A

a. Biologic sex
b. Gender role
c. Gender identity
d. Sexual orientation
e. Heterosexual
f. Homosexual
g. Bisexual
h. Transsexual
i. Transvestite

PART B

1. ____ Refers to the preferred gender of an individual's sexual partner

2. ____ Term used to denote chromosomal sexual development

3. ____ Person of a certain biologic gender with the feelings of the opposite sex

4. ____ The behavior a person displays about being male or female

5. ____ A person who finds pleasure with both same-sex and opposite-sex partners

6. ____ One who experiences sexual fulfillment with a person of the opposite gender

7. ____ The inner sense a person has of being male or female

8. ____ One who experiences sexual fulfillment with a person of the same gender

SHORT ANSWER

1. Give an example of an intervention for patients with the following health problems that could improve their sexual relations.

   a. Chronic pain: _____

   b. Diabetes: _____

   c. Cardiovascular disease: _____

   d. Loss of body part: _____

   e. Spinal cord injury: _____

   f. Mental illness: _____

   g. Sexually transmitted infections: _____

2. Briefly describe the four phases of the menstrual cycle.

   a. Follicular phase: _____

   b. Proliferation phase: _____

   c. Luteal phase: _____

   d. Secretory phase: _____

3. Briefly describe the male and female responses in the following phases of the sexual response cycle.

   a. Excitement phase—Female: _____

   _____

   Male: _____

   _____

   b. Plateau—Female: _____

   _____

   Male: _____

   _____

   c. Orgasm—Female: _____

   _____

   Male: _____

   _____

   d. Resolution—Female: _____

   _____

   Male: _____

   _____

4. List three general categories of patients who should have a sexual history recorded by the nurse.

   a. _____

   b. _____

   c. _____

5. List three interview questions a nurse may use during a sexual history when assessing a male for impotence.

   a. _____

   b. _____

   c. _____

6. List three major goals of patient teaching about sexuality and wellness.

   a. _____

   b. _____

   c. _____

7. Complete the following table, listing the advantages and disadvantages associated with contraceptive methods.

Method	Advantages	Disadvantages
a. Natural family planning		
b. Barrier methods		
c. Intrauterine devices		
d. Hormonal methods		
e. Sterilization		

APPLYING YOUR KNOWLEDGE

CRITICAL THINKING QUESTIONS

1. Write down the interview questions you would use to obtain a sexual history from the following patients.

   a. An 18-year-old female victim of date rape who is brought to the emergency room for testing and treatment

   b. A 48-year-old man diagnosed with prostate cancer who is seeking a prescription for Viagra

   c. An HIV-positive woman who has had multiple sexual partners and admits she probably infected other people through unsafe practices

   d. A 5-year-old girl who presents with soreness and redness in the genital area

   How comfortable would you be asking these patients the necessary questions, and how might you develop the skills necessary to perform the interview?

2. Describe the knowledge and skills you would need to care for patients experiencing the following sexual dysfunctions.

   a. A man undergoing radiation treatment for colon cancer complains of impotence.

   b. A menopausal woman complains of vaginal dryness and pain during intercourse.

   c. A sexually active teenager complains of a burning sensation during urination.

REFLECTIVE PRACTICE USING CRITICAL THINKING SKILLS

Use the following expanded scenario from Chapter 45 in your textbook to answer the questions below.

Scenario: Jefferson Smith is a middle-aged man who was recently married after the death of his first wife 10 years ago. He has a history of diabetes and hypertension and is receiving numerous medications as treatment. During a routine visit to his primary care physician, Mr. Smith confides that he has been having problems "in the bedroom." He reports difficulty attaining and maintaining an erection. He asks, "What about all those new drugs they keep advertising on TV? Would they work for me?"

1. What issues might the nurse address in the plan of care for Mr. Smith? What patient teaching should be incorporated into the plan of care?

_____

_____

_____

2. What would be a successful outcome for this patient?

_____

_____

_____

3. What intellectual, technical, interpersonal, and/or ethical/legal competencies are most likely to bring about the desired outcome?

_____

_____

_____

4. What resources might be helpful for Mr. Smith?

_____

_____

_____

PATIENT CARE STUDY

Read the following patient care study and use your nursing process skills to answer the questions on page 318.

Scenario: Anthony Piscatelli, a 6-foot tall, muscular, healthy 19-year-old college freshman in the School of Nursing, confides to his nursing advisor that "everything is great" about college life, with one exception: "All of a sudden, I find myself questioning the values I learned at home about sex and marriage. My mom was really insistent that each of her sons should respect women and that intercourse was something you saved until you were ready to get married. If she told us once, she told us a hundred times, that we'd save ourselves, the girls in our lives, and her and dad a lot of heartache if we could just learn to control ourselves sexually. Problem is that no one here seems to subscribe to this philosophy. I feel like I'm abnormal in some way to even think like this. There's a lot of sexual activity in the dorms, and no one even thinks you're serious if you talk about virginity positively. What do you think? Did my mom sell me a bill of goods? Is it true that if you take the proper precautions, no one gets hurt and everyone has a good time?" Tony reports that he is a virgin and that he really misses his close family back home: "I do get lonely at times and would love to just cuddle with someone or even give and get a big hug, but no one seems to understand this."

1. Identify pertinent patient data by placing a single underline beneath the objective data in the patient care study and a double underline beneath the subjective data.

2. Complete the Nursing Process Worksheet on page 319 to develop a three-part diagnostic statement and related plan of care for this patient.

3. Write down the patient and personal nursing strengths you hope to draw upon as you assist this patient to better health.

    Patient strengths: _____

    _____

    _____

    Personal strengths: _____

    _____

    _____

4. Pretend that you are performing a nursing assessment of this patient after the plan of care is implemented. Document your findings.

    _____

    _____

    _____

NURSING PROCESS WORKSHEET

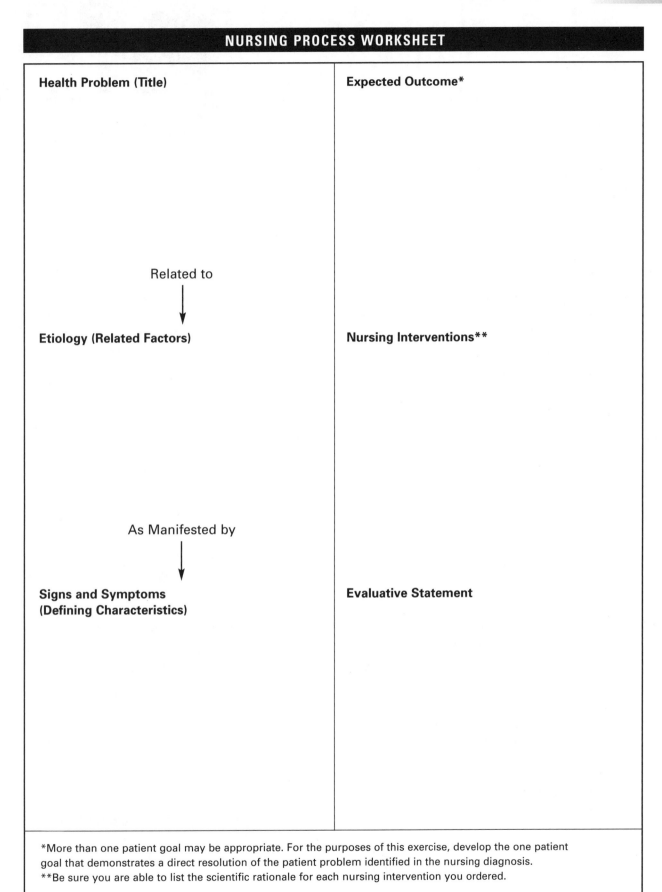

| Health Problem (Title) | Expected Outcome* |

Related to
↓

Etiology (Related Factors)   **Nursing Interventions****

As Manifested by
↓

Signs and Symptoms   **Evaluative Statement**
(Defining Characteristics)

*More than one patient goal may be appropriate. For the purposes of this exercise, develop the one patient goal that demonstrates a direct resolution of the patient problem identified in the nursing diagnosis.

**Be sure you are able to list the scientific rationale for each nursing intervention you ordered.

Spirituality

PRACTICING FOR NCLEX

MULTIPLE CHOICE QUESTIONS

Circle the letter that corresponds to the best answer for each question.

1. Which of the following terms describes anything that pertains to a person's relationship with a nonmaterial life force or higher power?
   a. Religion
   b. Spirituality
   c. Faith
   d. Belief

2. A terminally ill patient tells you that he does not belong to an organized religion. It is safe to assume which of the following?
   a. The patient is an atheist.
   b. The patient has no belief system.
   c. The patient is an agnostic.
   d. The patient may still be deeply spiritual.

3. Which of the following statements concerning atheists and agnostics is accurate?
   a. Both deny the existence of God.
   b. Nurses should attempt to change the views of these patients and offer religious counseling.
   c. Both are guided by a philosophy of living that does not include a religious faith.
   d. Both have religious influences that are life denying.

4. In which of the following religions are women not allowed to make independent decisions and husbands must be present when consent is sought?
   a. Islam
   b Judaism
   c. Roman Catholicism
   d. Protestantism

5. In which religion are members encouraged to obtain healthcare provided by members of the black community?
   a. Baha'i International Community
   b. American Muslim Mission
   c. Native American religion
   d. Islam

6. According to Shelly and Fish (1988), which of the following is a spiritual need underlying all religious traditions?
   a. Need for formal ceremony
   b. Need for power in relationship with God
   c. Need for justice
   d. Need for meaning and purpose

7. When assessing a child's spiritual dimension, a nurse should be aware of which of the following basic tenets?
   a. Children do not have a definite perception of God.
   b. Children attribute to God tremendous and expansive power.
   c. Children do not experience spiritual distress.
   d. Children view God as a person with divine powers.

8. In which religion do common therapeutic measures include sucking, blowing, and drawing out with a feather fan?

   a. Native American religion

   b. Islam

   c. Baha'i International Community

   d. Roman Catholicism

ALTERNATE-FORMAT QUESTIONS

Multiple Response Questions

Circle the letters that correspond to the best answers for each question.

1. Which of the following statements accurately describe the central themes in children's descriptions of God, according to David Heller's study? *(Select all that apply.)*

   a. Children have a notion of a God who works through human intimacy.

   b. Children believe in the interconnectedness of human lives.

   c. Children believe that God is a constant deity that limits self-change and transformation.

   d. Children believe that God's power is limited and has little effect on their lives.

   e. Children show considerable anxiety in the face of God's power.

   f. An image of darkness surrounds the spiritual world of the child.

2. Which of the following religions prohibit the use of alcohol? *(Select all that apply.)*

   a. Christian Science

   b. Church of Jesus Christ of Latter-Day Saints

   c. Roman Catholicism

   d. American Muslim Mission

   e. Hinduism

   f. Judaism

3. Which of the following are beliefs related to the religion Daoism? *(Select all that apply.)*

   a. Allah, who is all-seeing, all-hearing, all-speaking, all-knowing, all-willing, and all-powerful, is their one God.

   b. They oppose the "false teachings" of other sects.

   c. They worship one God revealed to the world through Jesus Christ.

   d. They believe that health is a manifestation of the harmony of the universe, obtained through the proper balancing of internal and external forces.

   e. The universal principle is the mysterious biologic and spiritual life rhythm or order of nature.

   f. Inherent in Daoism is the appreciation of life and the desire to keep the body from untimely or unnecessary death.

4. Which of the following is a healthcare practice of participants in the Hindu religion? *(Select all that apply.)*

   a. There are obligatory prayers, holy days, fasting, and almsgiving.

   b. Their medicine shows a surprising openness to new ideas, at least in respect to practical treatment.

   c. Women are not allowed to make independent decisions.

   d. There are many dietary restrictions, conforming to individual sect doctrine.

   e. The nurse administering medications should avoid touching the patient's lips.

   f. Rituals mark important life changes, birth, puberty, initiation rites, and death.

5. Which of the following religions regard Saturday as the Sabbath? *(Select all that apply.)*

   a. Roman Catholicism

   b. Buddhism

   c. Adventist

   d. Judaism

   e. Islam

   f. Hinduism

DEVELOPING YOUR KNOWLEDGE BASE

FILL-IN-THE-BLANKS

1. A patient recently diagnosed with prostate cancer tells the nurse that he believes God is far away and could not care less about his condition. This patient may be suffering from spiritual _____.

2. _____ is a disruption in the life principle that pervades a person's entire being and that integrates and transcends one's biologic and psychosocial nature.

3. A nurse who asks a patient how his religious beliefs help or hinder him to feel at peace is assessing the patient for the spiritual need for _____.

4. A patient who tells a nurse that she no longer goes to church on Sunday may be experiencing what form of spiritual distress? _____

5. A mother who refuses to sign a consent form for a blood transfusion for her daughter due to religious reasons is most likely practicing what faith? _____

MATCHING EXERCISES

Match the type of spiritual distress listed in Part A with the appropriate example listed in Part B.

PART A

a. Spiritual pain

b. Spiritual alienation

c. Spiritual anxiety

d. Spiritual guilt

e. Spiritual anger

f. Spiritual loss

g. Spiritual despair

PART B

1. ____ A Roman Catholic college student stops going to Mass on Sundays and moves in with her boyfriend; she tells you, "I really want to do this, but it still feels wrong."

2. ____ A woman cannot accept the death of her newborn and says, "How long will it hurt this bad?"

3. ____ A man with a terminal illness cannot accept his eventual death and asks, "What kind of God are you?"

4. ____ An elderly woman with a hip replacement is confined to her home and cannot get to her usual daily religious services.

5. ____ A man dying of AIDS has no friends or support system and believes that God and humanity have abandoned him.

6. ____ A young man challenges his faith and his own belief in God.

Match the examples of a nurse's supportive presence listed in Part B with the appropriate measure listed in Part A. Answers may be used more than once.

PART A

a. Facilitating the practice of religion

b. Promoting meaning and purpose

c. Promoting love and relatedness

d. Promoting forgiveness

PART B

7. ____ A nurse attempts to meet a patient's religious dietary restrictions.

8. ____ A nurse explores with a patient the importance of learning to accept himself, even with his faults.

9. ____ A nurse treats her patient with respect, empathy, and genuine caring.

10. ____ A nurse explores with a patient spiritual practices from which he might derive strength and hope.

11. ____ A nurse respects a patient's need for privacy during prayer.

12. ____ A nurse helps a patient explore his self-expectations and determine how realistic they are.

13. ____ A nurse encourages a patient to explore her relationship with her family and identify the origin of negative beliefs about people.

SHORT ANSWER

1. List three spiritual needs underlying all religious traditions that are common to all people.

   a. _____

   b. _____

   c. _____

2. List four methods nurses can use to assist patients in meeting their spiritual needs.

a. _____

b. _____

c. _____

d. _____

3. Explain how the following religious influences may affect an individual.

a. Life-affirming influences: _____
_____

b. Life-denying influences: _____
_____

4. Give two examples of practices associated with healthcare that may have religious significance to a patient.

a. _____

b. _____

5. Briefly describe how religious faith may affect a patient in the following areas.

a. As a guide to daily living: _____
_____

b. As a source of support: _____
_____

c. As a source of strength and healing: _____
_____

d. As a source of conflict: _____
_____

6. Give an example of how the following factors may influence a person's spirituality.

a. Developmental considerations: _____
_____

b. Family: _____
_____

c. Ethnic background: _____
_____

d. Formal religion: _____
_____

e. Life events: _____
_____

7. Describe how you would handle the following cases.

a. A family who insists on care deemed medically futile for a terminally ill patient because they believe that God is going to work a miracle:

_____

_____

_____

b. Christian Scientist parents of a child needing an appendectomy who refuse to sign a consent form for surgery:

_____

_____

_____

8. List six characteristics the religions discussed in this chapter have in common.

a. _____

b. _____

c. _____

d. _____

e. _____

f. _____

9. Give an example of an interview question or statement you might use to assess a patient for the following types of spiritual distress.

a. Spiritual pain: _____
_____

b. Spiritual alienation: _____
_____

c. Spiritual anxiety: _____
_____

d. Spiritual anger: _____
_____

e. Spiritual loss: _____
_____

f. Spiritual despair: _____
_____

10. You are visiting a patient at home who was paralyzed in a car accident. She tells you she believes God has abandoned her and her family, which includes two small children. Suggest a nursing diagnosis for this patient and develop a nursing care plan that includes at least two interventions to help her with her spiritual needs.

Diagnosis: _____

Nursing care plan: _____

_____

_____

11. Develop a prayer expressing a patient's needs that could be used for a patient facing surgery.

_____

_____

12. List four guidelines for preparing a patient's room to receive a spiritual counselor.

a. _____

b. _____

c. _____

d. _____

13. List three interventions to assist a patient with the following deficits.

a. Deficit: Meaning and purpose: _____

_____

b. Deficit: Love and relatedness: _____

_____

c. Deficit: Forgiveness: _____

_____

APPLYING YOUR KNOWLEDGE

CRITICAL THINKING QUESTIONS

1. How would you respond to parents who ask you to pray with them for their child's recovery from surgery? Would you feel comfortable praying with them? Do you believe nurses should pray aloud with patients and families? Write down a prayer for the sick that you can use in these situations.

2. Identify your own spiritual beliefs. How do these beliefs influence the way you carry on your daily routine in life? Do these beliefs affect the way you relate to others? In what ways might they affect the way you react to patients of different faiths?

REFLECTIVE PRACTICE USING CRITICAL THINKING SKILLS

Use the following expanded scenario from Chapter 46 in your textbook to answer the questions below.

Scenario: Margot Zeuner, a 75-year-old woman, is taking care of her 80-year-old husband with advanced Alzheimer's disease, who was just discharged from the hospital and requires constant supervision. When visited at home, she says, "I really miss going to church and seeing everyone. They're so supportive. That was the one thing that helped to keep me going." She further states that she no longer feels connected to her church or community.

1. How might the nurse use blended nursing skills to provide holistic, competent nursing care for Mrs. Zeuner?

_____

_____

_____

2. What would be a successful outcome for this patient?

_____

_____

_____

3. What intellectual, technical, interpersonal, and/or ethical/legal competencies are most likely to bring about the desired outcome?

_____

_____

_____

4. What resources might be helpful for Mrs. Zeuner?

_____

_____

_____

PATIENT CARE STUDY

Read the following patient care study and use your nursing process skills to answer the questions below.

Scenario: Jeffrey Stein, a 31-year-old attorney, is in a step-down unit following his transfer from the cardiac care unit, where he was treated for a massive heart attack. "Bad hearts run in my family, but I never thought it would happen to me," he says. "I jog several times a week and work out at the gym, eat a low-fat diet, and I don't smoke." Jeffrey is 5 feet 7 inches tall, weighs about 150 pounds, and is well built. During his second night in the step-down unit, he is unable to sleep and tells the nurse, "I've really got a lot on my mind tonight. I can't stop thinking about how close I was to death. If I wasn't with someone who knew how to do CPR when I keeled over, I probably wouldn't be here today." Gentle questioning reveals that Mr. Stein is worried about what would have happened had he died. "I don't think I've ever thought seriously about my mortality, and I sure don't think much about God. My parents were semiobservant Jews, but I don't go to synagogue myself. I celebrate the holidays, but that's about all. If there is a God, I wonder what He thinks about me." He asks if there is a rabbi or anyone he can talk with in the morning who could answer some questions for him and perhaps help him get himself back on track. "For the last couple of years, all I've been concerned about is paying off my school debts and making money. I guess there's a whole lot more to life, and maybe this was my invitation to sort out my priorities."

1. Identify pertinent patient data by placing a single underline beneath the objective data in the patient care study and a double underline beneath the subjective data.

2. Complete the Nursing Process Worksheet on page 326 to develop a three-part diagnostic statement and related plan of care for this patient.

3. Write down the patient and personal nursing strengths you hope to draw upon as you assist this patient to better health.

   Patient strengths: _____

   _____

   _____

   Personal strengths: _____

   _____

   _____

4. Pretend that you are performing a nursing assessment of this patient after the plan of care is implemented. Document your findings.

   _____

   _____

   _____

NURSING PROCESS WORKSHEET

Health Problem (Title)

Expected Outcome*

Related to

Etiology (Related Factors)

Nursing Interventions**

As Manifested by

Signs and Symptoms (Defining Characteristics)

Evaluative Statement

*More than one patient goal may be appropriate. For the purposes of this exercise, develop the one patient goal that demonstrates a direct resolution of the patient problem identified in the nursing diagnosis.

**Be sure you are able to list the scientific rationale for each nursing intervention you ordered.

Answer Key

CHAPTER 1

PRACTICING FOR NCLEX
MULTIPLE CHOICE QUESTIONS

1. b	**2.** d	**3.** c	**4.** b	**5.** a
6. a	**7.** b	**8.** c	**9.** b	**10.** d

ALTERNATE-FORMAT QUESTIONS
Multiple Response Questions

1. a, c, e
2. c, d, f
3. a, c, d, f
4. a, c, d
5. a, c, e
6. a, c, d

Prioritization Questions

1.

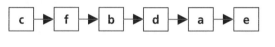

2.

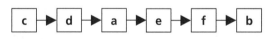

DEVELOPING YOUR KNOWLEDGE BASE

FILL-IN-THE-BLANKS

1. International Council of Nurses (ICN)
2. American Nurses Association (ANA)
3. Clinical Nursing Standards
4. Nurse Practice Acts
5. Nursing Process

CORRECT THE FALSE STATEMENTS

1. True
2. True
3. False—licensure
4. False—registered nurse
5. False—distinct and separate
6. False—ICN
7. False—the patient
8. True

9. False—the nurse facilitates coping with disability or death.
10. False—person-centered process

SHORT ANSWER

1. Nursing is the demonstration of nonpossessive caring for and about others.
2. Nursing is sharing self with patients, other health team members, and other nurses.
3. Nursing is touching to provide comfort and give care.
4. Nursing is feeling with patients the human feelings of sorrow, joy, frustration, and satisfaction.
5. Nursing is listening attentively to the verbal and nonverbal communication signals of others.
6. Nursing is accepting self in order to accept others.
7. Nursing is respecting individual differences through unconditional acceptance, ensuring confidence and privacy, and individualizing care.
8. Sample answers:
  a. Promoting health: The nurse prepares the patient for tests, explaining each test thoroughly to the patient and focusing on any questions the patient may have. The nurse also identifies the patient's strengths (e.g., healthy diet, daily exercise routine) and weaknesses (e.g., inability to quit smoking).
  b. Preventing illness: The nurse refers the patient to a smoking-cessation program and, if necessary, educates the patient about the nature and treatment of lung cancer.
  c. Restoring health: The nurse provides direct care for the patient, administers medications, and carries out procedures and treatments for the patient.
  d. Facilitating coping: The nurse facilitates patient and family coping by helping the patient to live with altered functioning or prepare for death.
9. **a.** Profession: A well-defined body of knowledge, strong service orientation, recognized authority as a professional group, code of ethics, professional organization that sets standards, ongoing research, and autonomy.
  b. Discipline: Nursing uses existing and new knowledge to solve problems creatively and meet human needs within ever-changing boundaries.

10. **a.** Rapid advances in technology require nurses to update their knowledge and skills to use the technology to give safe, individualized care.
   b. Nursing autonomy has increased the need for nurses to use critical thinking based on knowledge to provide safe care.

11. Sample answers:
   a. Cognitive skills: A nurse selects nursing interventions to promote wound healing.
   b. Technical skills: A nurse correctly administers medication to a patient via an IV infusion.
   c. Interpersonal skills: A nurse displays a caring attitude when interacting with a patient.
   d. Ethical/legal skills: A nurse explains an advance directives form to a patient.

12. See table below.

Title	Education/Preparation	Role Description
Example Nurse Researcher	Advanced degree	Conducts research relevant to nursing practice and education
Nurse Midwife	Certificate or advanced degree	Provides pre/postnatal care; delivers babies in uncomplicated pregnancies
Nurse Practitioner	Advanced degree, certification	Works in a variety of settings, providing health assessment and primary care
Nurse Anesthetist	Advanced degree	Administers and monitors anesthesia
Nurse Administrator	Advanced degree	Functions at various levels of management in healthcare settings
Nurse Entrepreneur	Advanced degree	Manages a clinic or health-related business, conducts research, provides education, or serves as an advisor or consultant to institutions, political agencies or businesses

REFLECTIVE PRACTICE USING CRITICAL THINKING SKILLS

Sample Answers

1. What might be causing Mr. Rowlings to respond negatively to patient teaching related to lifestyle modification and stress reduction?
   Fear of failure; inability to recognize the dangers of his lifestyle; possible loneliness or depression
2. What would be a successful outcome for this patient?
   Mr. Rowlings describes the effect of alcohol, cigarettes, stress, and inactivity on his cardiovascular system and makes an informed decision regarding lifestyle modification that is consistent with his beliefs and values.
3. What intellectual, technical, interpersonal, and/or ethical/legal competencies are most likely to bring about the desired outcome?
   Intellectual: knowledge of risk factors of heart disease and factors that can and cannot be modified
   Technical: ability to use the Internet to research appropriate teaching strategies and adapt these strategies as needed
   Interpersonal: ability to establish a trusting relationship with Mr. Rowlings that demonstrates respect for his human dignity throughout the patient care plan
   Ethical/Legal: empathy for the patient with commitment to getting him the help he needs to achieve health goals
4. What resources might be helpful for Mr. Rowling?
   Print or A/V teaching aids, counseling services, support groups

CHAPTER 2

PRACTICING FOR NCLEX
MULTIPLE CHOICE QUESTIONS

1. c   **2.** d   **3.** d   **4.** a   **5.** b
6. b   **7.** c   **8.** a   **9.** d

ALTERNATE-FORMAT QUESTIONS
Multiple Response Questions

1. a, d, e
2. a, d, e, f

3. b, d, e
4. a, b, f
5. a, c, d, e

DEVELOPING YOUR KNOWLEDGE BASE

FILL-IN-THE-BLANKS

1. Keloid formation
2. Subculture
3. Ethnicity
4. Ethnocentrism
5. Sickle cell anemia
6. Cultural blindness
7. Culture shock
8. Stereotyping

MATCHING EXERCISES

| **1.** b | **2.** c | **3.** g | **4.** a | **5.** a |
| **6.** c, d | **7.** e | **8.** c | **9.** f | **10.** d |

SHORT ANSWER

1. Sample answers:
   a. Investigate bus routes from patient's home; check if medical services are available within walking distance; see if insurance will cover transportation to and from medical services.
   b. Boil water before using it; check with social services to see if they can provide any necessary services for patient.
   c. Refer patient to drug and alcohol counseling service.
2. Sample answers:
   a. Reassure the patient that the "granny" woman is an important part of her recovery and attempt to contact this person. Include the "granny" woman's assessment in medical history of patient.
   b. Ask family members to allow patient to answer questions; reassure them that their input is also important and that they can add any information they feel is necessary at the end of the interview.
   c. Find out what herb the patient has been taking and its efficacy, and check with the physician to determine whether the patient can still take this herb. Explain the prescribed medications to the patient and how they will alleviate her symptoms.
3. Answers will vary with student's experiences.
4. Sample answers:
   a. The number of female-headed households is increasing as a result of divorce, abandonment, unmarried motherhood, and changes in abortion laws. Many households depend on two incomes for economic survival, and a single woman supporting a household is at a financial disadvantage.
   b. Most older adults live on fixed incomes, which often do not keep up with inflation. Many, particularly widows, are on the borderline of poverty or have already slipped into poverty.
   c. In many cases, poverty is passed from generation to generation. This is true in such groups as migrant farm workers, families living on welfare, and people who live in isolated areas of Appalachia.

REFLECTIVE PRACTICE USING CRITICAL THINKING SKILLS

Sample Answers

1. How might the nurse respond to Ms. Dorvall's request for a Haitian folk healer?
In order to provide culturally competent care, the nurse honors Ms. Dorvall's request and arranges a meeting with the folk healer. Prior to the meeting, the nurse researches the Haitian culture in order to properly prepare the room and patient for the visit. The nurse reassesses the patient following the visit and documents the findings in the patient record.
2. What would be a successful outcome for this patient?
Ms. Dorvall verbalizes that the folk healer relieved her anxiety regarding the healing of her leg and states her desire to continue with the nursing care plan.
3. What intellectual, technical, interpersonal, and/or ethical/legal competencies are most likely to bring about the desired outcome?
Intellectual: knowledge of Haitian cultural healthcare practices gained from research
Interpersonal: formation of a caring relationship with the patient that encompasses the patient's beliefs and values
Ethical/Legal: careful documentation of patient goals and outcomes
4. What resources might be helpful for Ms. Dorvall?
Research materials on the Haitian culture, community services

CHAPTER 3

PRACTICING FOR NCLEX

MULTIPLE CHOICE QUESTIONS

| **1.** a | **2.** c | **3.** c | **4.** d | **5.** a |
| **6.** b | | | | |

ALTERNATE-FORMAT QUESTIONS

Multiple Response Questions

1. a, b, d, f
2. b, c, e
3. c, f
4. a, b, e
5. b, d, e
6. c, d, e

Chart/Exhibit Questions

1. Physical dimension
2. Emotional dimension
3. Intellectual and spiritual dimension
4. Environmental dimension
5. Sociocultural dimension

6. Intellectual and spiritual dimension
7. Intellectual and spiritual dimension
8. Physical dimension

DEVELOPING YOUR KNOWLEDGE BASE

FILL-IN-THE-BLANKS

1. Disease
2. Chronic
3. Acute
4. Exacerbation
5. Environmental

MATCHING EXERCISES

1. f	**2.** a	**3.** e	**4.** b	**5.** c
6. d	**7.** b	**8.** d	**9.** a	**10.** c
11. b	**12.** a	**13.** c	**14.** d	**15.** a
16. b	**17.** e			

SHORT ANSWER

1. Answers will vary with student's experiences.
2. a. Acute: A temporary condition of illness in which patient goes through four stages: 1. symptoms, 2. assuming sick role, 3. dependent role—accepting diagnosis and following the treatment plan, and 4. recovery and rehabilitation—person gives up dependent role and resumes normal activities and responsibilities.
   b. Chronic: A permanent change caused by irreversible alterations in normal anatomy and physiology; requires patient education for rehabilitation; requires long period of care or support. Characteristics: slow onset, periods of remission.
3. Answers will vary with student's experiences.
4. Sample answers:
   a. Primary: Giving immunizations, providing dental care teaching
   b. Secondary: Providing physical therapy, giving medications
   c. Tertiary: Facilitating a support system, doing diabetic teaching
5. a. Being: Recognizing self as separate and individual
   b. Belonging: Being part of a whole
   c. Becoming: Growing and developing
   d. Befitting: Making personal choices to benefit the self for the future

REFLECTIVE PRACTICE USING CRITICAL THINKING SKILLS

Sample Answers

1. How might the nurse respond to Ms. Jacobi's stated desire for a higher level of wellness?
This is the perfect opportunity for patient teaching provided throughout Ms. Jacobi's hospital stay and incorporated into the discharge plan. The nurse should present information regarding a "heart healthy diet," the need for exercise, and reinforcement for smoking cessation.
2. What would be a successful outcome for this patient? Ms. Jacobi describes her condition and identifies three factors in her lifestyle (smoking, diet, exercise) that can be modified for stroke prevention.

3. What intellectual, technical, interpersonal, and/or ethical/legal competencies are most likely to bring about the desired outcome?
Intellectual: ability to integrate knowledge of preventive measures into the patient care plan
Interpersonal: ability to assess health-related beliefs, goals, and practices
Ethical/Legal: ability to participate as a trusted and effective patient advocate, including a commitment to securing the best possible care for Ms. Jacobi
4. What resources might be helpful for Ms. Jacobi? Smoking cessation materials, menu plans, support groups

CHAPTER 4

PRACTICING FOR NCLEX

MULTIPLE CHOICE QUESTIONS

1. d	**2.** a	**3.** d	**4.** c

ALTERNATE-FORMAT QUESTIONS

Multiple Response Questions

1. d, f
2. a, c, f
3. b, d, e
4. b, c

Prioritization Question

1.

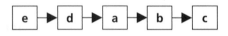

DEVELOPING YOUR KNOWLEDGE BASE

FILL-IN-THE-BLANKS

1. Oxygen
2. Physiologic
3. Extended
4. Affective and coping
5. Community

MATCHING EXERCISES

1. e	**2.** a	**3.** b	**4.** b	**5.** d
6. b	**7.** c	**8.** a	**9.** d	**10.** c
11. e	**12.** b	**13.** c	**14.** e	

SHORT ANSWER

1. Sample answers:
   a. Physical: A family lives in a comfortable home located in a safe neighborhood. This meets the family needs of safety and comfort and enhances growth and development of the children.
   b. Economic: A family is able to afford adequate housing, food, clothing, and community demands. This meets the family's need for nourishment, shelter, and acceptance in society.
   c. Reproductive: A family seeks family planning to limit their offspring to three children. This meets society's need for more members without putting

too heavy a demand on the family to care for their children.

   d. Affective and coping: Parents counsel their children to avoid drinking alcohol, smoking cigarettes, and using drugs. This meets the children's needs to be productive members of society and to avoid the pitfalls surrounding adolescence.

   e. Socialization: Parents seek expert counseling for a kindergarten child who is having difficulty adjusting to school and relating to other children. This meets the child's need to fit in with other schoolmates and helps correct a problem before it gets out of hand.

2. Sample answers:

   a. Physiologic needs: The nurse helps to prepare the mother for her cesarean birth and administers any medications prescribed.

   b. Safety and security needs: The nurse monitors the blood pressure of the mother and baby during the procedure.

   c. Love and belonging needs: The nurse helps the husband to cope with his fears and gets him ready to participate in the birth of his child.

   d. Self-esteem needs: The nurse reassures the mother that having a cesarean birth is a common procedure and that she should not feel guilty for not being able to have the baby vaginally.

   e. Self-actualization needs: The nurse helps the mother after surgery to continue with her original plan to breastfeed her infant.

3. Answers will vary with student's experiences.

4. What is the family structure? What is the family's socioeconomic status? What are the ethnic background and religious affiliation of family members? Who cares for children if both parents work? What health practices are common (e.g., types of foods eaten, meal times, immunizations, bedtime, exercise)? What habits are common (e.g., do any family members smoke, drink to excess, or use drugs)? How does the family cope with stress? Do close friends or family members live nearby, and can they help if necessary?

REFLECTIVE PRACTICE USING CRITICAL THINKING SKILLS

Sample Answers

1. What basic human needs should be addressed by the nurse to provide individualized, holistic care for Mr. Kaplan?

When providing holistic nursing care, the nurse should consider all the dimensions that affect how the patient's basic human needs are met in health and in illness. For Mr. Kaplan, these needs include physiologic needs related to his and his wife's health condition; safety and security needs for a safe environment for a patient with Alzheimer's disease; love and belonging needs related to his desire to remain with, and care for, his wife; self-esteem needs based on his pride in taking care of

himself and his wife; and self-actualization needs or acceptance of himself and his current situation.

2. What would a successful outcome be for this patient? Mr. Kaplan verbalizes the reasons he is unable to care for his wife in his home and acknowledges a plan to provide a safe environment for himself and his wife.

3. What intellectual, technical, interpersonal, and/or ethical/legal competencies are most likely to bring about the desired outcome?

Intellectual: knowledge of Alzheimer's disease and its effect on the family

Interpersonal: using strong interpersonal skills to establish a trusting relationship with Mr. Kaplan that demonstrates respect for his human dignity and autonomy

Ethical/Legal: skill in working collaboratively with colleagues and community members to advocate for the healthcare needs of Mr. Kaplan and his wife

4. What resources might be helpful for Mr. Kaplan? Teaching aids for patients with Alzheimer's disease, counseling services, community services, skilled nursing care

CHAPTER 5

PRACTICING FOR NCLEX
MULTIPLE CHOICE QUESTIONS

1. d	**2.** a	**3.** c	**4.** b	**5.** a
6. d	**7.** c	**8.** b	**9.** a	

ALTERNATE-FORMAT QUESTIONS
Multiple Response Questions

1. b, e, f

2. a, b, e, f

3. c, d, f

4. b, c, e

5. a, e, f

6. b, c, e

DEVELOPING YOUR KNOWLEDGE BASE

FILL-IN-THE-BLANKS

1. Quantitative

2. Concepts

3. Adaptation

4. Informed consent

5. Evidence-based practice

MATCHING EXERCISES

1. f	**2.** c	**3.** i	**4.** h	**5.** d
6. e	**7.** b	**8.** a	**9.** g	

SHORT ANSWER

1. a. General systems theory: This theory explains breaking whole things into parts and then learning how these parts work together in systems. It includes the relationship between the whole and the parts and defines concepts about how the parts will function and behave.

b. Adaptation theory: This theory defines adaptation as the adjustment of living matter to other living things and to environmental conditions. Adaptation is a dynamic or continuously changing process that effects change and involves interaction and response. Human adaptation occurs on three levels—internal, social, and physical.

c. Developmental theory: Outlines the process of growth and development of humans as orderly and predictable, beginning with conception and ending with death. The growth and development of an individual are influenced by heredity, temperament, emotional and physical environment, life experiences, and health status.

2. a. Nursing theories identify and define interrelated concepts specific to nursing and clearly state the relation between these concepts.

b. Nursing theories must be logical and use orderly reasoning and identify relations that are developed using a logical sequence.

c. Nursing theories must be consistent with the basic assumptions used in their development. They should be simple and general.

d. Nursing theories should increase the nursing profession's body of knowledge by generating research and should guide and improve practice.

3. a. Cultural influences on nursing: Until the past 2 decades, nursing essentially had been considered "women's work," and women were considered inferior to men. After Nightingale established an acceptable occupation for educated women and facilitated improved attitudes toward nursing, the role of the woman as nurse became more favorably accepted.

b. Educational influences on nursing: The service orientation of nursing was the strongest influence on nursing practice until the 1950s. After World War II, women increasingly entered the workforce, became more independent, and sought higher education. Nursing education began to focus more on education instead of just training. In the 1960s, college- and university-based baccalaureate programs in nursing increased in number and enrollment, and master's and doctoral programs in nursing were established.

c. Research and publishing in nursing: Beginning in the 1950s, great advances were made in technology and medical research; nursing leaders realized that research about the practice of nursing was necessary to meet the health needs of modern society.

d. Improved communication in nursing: Nursing is based on communication with others—patients, other healthcare team members, community members, as well as with nurses practicing in a variety of specialty settings. Nurses need a knowledge base and common terminology to use in communicating with other professionals.

e. Improved autonomy of nursing: Nursing is in the process of defining its own independent functions and contributions to healthcare. The development and use of nursing theory provide autonomy in the practice of nursing.

4. Answers will vary with student's experiences.

REFLECTIVE PRACTICE USING CRITICAL THINKING SKILLS

Sample Answers

1. How might the nurse respond to Ms. Horn's concerns regarding the care of her mother?
The nurse should provide Ms. Horn with information and practical tips for inserting a nasogastric tube and checking its patency. After demonstrating the procedure, the nurse could ask for a return demonstration from Ms. Horn. The nurse should also reassure Ms. Horn that assistance will be available if any problems occur and provide her with the appropriate resources.

2. What would be a successful outcome for this patient?
Ms. Horn accurately demonstrates the procedure for nasogastric tube feedings and states confidence in her ability to take care of her mother.

3. What intellectual, technical, interpersonal, and/or ethical/legal competencies are most likely to bring about the desired outcome?
Intellectual: Knowledge of nasogastric tube feedings and associated care
Technical: ability to provide technical nursing assistance based on sound scientific rationales to meet the learning needs of Ms. Horn
Interpersonal: ability to demonstrate empathy and respect for Ms. Horn and her situation
Ethical/Legal: ability to provide patient education consistent with the nursing code of ethics and within the scope of legal practice

4. What resources might be helpful for Ms. Horn?
Reference materials for teaching the procedure for nasogastric tube feedings, home healthcare services if applicable.

CHAPTER 6

PRACTICING FOR NCLEX
MULTIPLE CHOICE QUESTIONS

1. c	2. b	3. a	4. b	5. c
6. a	7. b			

ALTERNATE-FORMAT QUESTIONS
Multiple Response Questions

1. c, f
2. d, e
3. a, b, e
4. c, e, f
5. b, d, e
6. a, b, d, f

DEVELOPING YOUR KNOWLEDGE BASE

FILL-IN-THE-BLANKS

1. Laissez-faire
2. Responsible choice
3. Values clarification
4. Prizing
5. Value system
6. Advocacy

MATCHING EXERCISES

1. g	**2.** d	**3.** a	**4.** f	**5.** i
6. b	**7.** e	**8.** c	**9.** d	**10.** e
11. a	**12.** c	**13.** b	**14.** e	**15.** d
16. a	**17.** c			

SHORT ANSWER

1. Sample answers:
   a. Values clarification: Have the mother state the three most important things in her life. Explore her answers with her and find out why she chose them and how her choices may affect her situation.
   b. Choosing: After exploring the mother's values, have her choose her key values freely. She may choose her child or profession.
   c. Prizing: Reinforce the mother's choices and, if possible, involve the husband and child in decision making.
   d. Acting: Assist the mother to plan new behaviors consistent with the values she has chosen and incorporate them into her life. For example, if she values her child, she may reduce the number of classes she takes at night and spend more time with her.
2. Sample answers:
   a. Cost-containment issues
   b. End-of-life decisions
   c. Incompetent, unethical, or illegal practices of colleagues
   d. Pain management
3. a. Autonomy: Respect the decision-making capacity of autonomous persons (e.g., patients have the right to refuse treatment they do not feel would be helpful to their condition).
   b. Nonmaleficence: Avoid causing harm (e.g., be sure you are fully knowledgeable about a procedure before performing it).
   c. Beneficence: Provide benefits and balance these benefits against risks and harms (e.g., securing a patient with restraints who is at high risk for falls).
   d. Justice: Distribute benefits, risks, and costs fairly (e.g., give service to all patients regardless of their life circumstances).
   e. Fidelity: Be faithful to promises you made to the public to be competent, and be willing to use your competence to benefit patients entrusted to your care (e.g., not abandoning a patient entrusted to your care without first seeing to his/her needs).

4. a. Ethical sensibility: The nurse would recognize that a patient's right to confidentiality has been breached.
   b. Ethical responsiveness: The nurse can decide to ignore his/her superior's breach of confidence, or he/she can confront his/her superior or report the superior to a higher authority.
   c. Ethical reasoning: The nurse confides in his/her mentor and discusses the options available.
   d. Ethical accountability: The nurse is willing to accept the repercussions of any actions he/she takes to rectify the situation.
   e. Ethical character: Because the nurse valued patient confidentiality, his/her course of action was obvious.
   f. Ethical valuing: The nurse could not ignore the situation because of good ethical character and personal integrity.
   g. Transformative ethical leadership: As a result of confronting his/her superior, the nurse was able to make a positive impact on the hospital environment.
5. Answers will vary with student's experiences.
6. Answers will vary with student's experiences.
7. Sample answers:
   a. Gather as much data as possible to support your diagnosis.
   b. Identify the ethical problem and explore solutions to the problem.
   c. Plan a course of action you can justify (e.g., seeking assistance for the patient at a higher level).
   d. Implement your decision by speaking to your superiors and presenting your case in a competent manner.
   e. Evaluate your decision: What was the outcome? How does this make me feel? Did I make the right decision?
8. Sample answers:
   a. Breach of confidentiality, incompetent practice
   b. Covering for another nurse who is not performing her job competently, short-staffing
   c. Physician incompetence, conflicts concerning the role of the nurse in certain situations
   d. Cost-containment vs. hospitalization, healthcare rationing

REFLECTIVE PRACTICE USING CRITICAL THINKING SKILLS

Sample Answers

1. How might the nurse react to Mr. Raines' response to filling his prescriptions?
   The nurse should protect and support Mr. Raines' rights by being a strong patient advocate. This could be accomplished by investigating available social services and community services for Mr. Raines. The nurse could also check with the drug manufacturer to see if the company has a discount for needy patients.
2. What would be a successful outcome for this patient? Mr. Raines vocalizes the health benefits of taking his blood pressure medication and lists three reasons for seeking social services and other available assistance.

3. What intellectual, technical, interpersonal, and/or ethical/legal competencies are most likely to bring about the desired outcome?
Intellectual: ability to integrate ethical principles and use an ethical framework and decision-making process to resolve ethical problems
Technical: ability to integrate ethical agency to provide the technical nursing assistance necessary to meet the needs of Mr. Raines
Interpersonal: ability to advocate for patients whose values may be different from personal ones
Ethical/Legal: ability to identify and develop the essential elements of ethical agency, cultivate the virtues of nursing, and understand ethical theories that dictate and justify professional conduct
4. What resources might be helpful for Mr. Raines?
Social services, counseling services, government assistance, community services, drug assistance programs

CHAPTER 7

PRACTICING FOR NCLEX
MULTIPLE CHOICE QUESTIONS

1. c	**2.** b	**3.** a	**4.** c	**5.** d
6. b	**7.** c	**8.** a	**9.** c	**10.** d

ALTERNATE-FORMAT QUESTIONS
Multiple Response Questions
1. a, d, e, f
2. b, e, f
3. c, d, e
4. a, c, e
5. c, d, e, f
6. a, c, d
7. b, d, f
8. a, c, e

Prioritization Question
1.

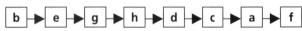

DEVELOPING YOUR KNOWLEDGE BASE

FILL-IN-THE-BLANKS
1. Public
2. Nurse Practice Act
3. Licensure
4. Expert witness
5. Collective bargaining
6. Incident
7. Sentinel event

MATCHING EXERCISES

1. g	**2.** e	**3.** a	**4.** c	**5.** h
6. f	**7.** b	**8.** i	**9.** i	**10.** h
11. a	**12.** l	**13.** c	**14.** d	**15.** k
16. b	**17.** f	**18.** g	**19.** j	**20.** c
21. g	**22.** a	**23.** b	**24.** d	**25.** e

SHORT ANSWER
1. Sample answers:
   a. Failure to ensure patient safety: Update knowledge on patient safety and new interventions to prevent and reduce injury.
   b. Improper treatment or performance of treatment: Use proper techniques when performing procedures and follow agency procedures.
   c. Failure to monitor and report: Follow physician orders regarding monitoring of patient unless changes in the patient's condition necessitate a change in the frequency of monitoring; report need for change to physician.
   d. Medication errors and reactions: Listen to patient's objections regarding medication and investigate patient concerns before administering the medication.
   e. Failure to follow agency procedure: Advise the appropriate person of procedures that need to be revised.
   f. Equipment misuse: Learn how to operate equipment in a safe and appropriate manner. Never operate equipment with which you are unfamiliar.
   g. Adverse incidents: Do not assume, voice, or record any blame for an incident.
   h. Improper use of infection control techniques: Know and follow agency policies and procedures for the care of patients with infectious disease.
2. a. Voluntary standards: Developed and implemented by the nursing profession itself; not mandatory; used for peer review. Example: professional nursing organizations.
   b. Legal standards: developed by legislative action; implemented by authority granted by the state (or province) to determine minimum standards for the education of nurses, set requirements for licensure or registration, and decide when to revoke or suspend nurse's licenses. Example: licensure.
3. a. For each specialized diagnostic procedure
   b. For experimentation involving patients
   c. On admission for routine treatment
   d. For medical or surgical treatment
4. Sample answers:
   a. Talking with patients in rooms that are not soundproof
   b. Pressing the patient for information not necessary for care planning
   c. Using tape recorders, dictating machines, computer banks, and so on without taking precautions to ensure patient confidentiality
5. a. Solid educational background
   b. Understanding of the legal aspects of nursing and malpractice liability
   c. Knowledge of the state (or province) Nurse Practice Act and standard of nursing care where the incident occurred
6. A contract must contain real consent of the parties, a valid consideration, a lawful purpose, competent parties, and the form required by law.

7. Sample answer:
Limit telephone orders to true emergency situations; repeat a telephone order back to the physician; document the order, its time and date, situation necessitating order, physician prescribing, reconfirming the order as it is read back, and signing name; and VO or TO. If possible, two nurses should listen to a questionable telephone order, with both nurses countersigning the order.

8. **a.** Contraindicated by normal practice
   b. Contraindicated by patient's present condition

9. Sample answers:
   a. The nurse is liable for her actions and should file an incident report.
   b. The incident report should contain the name of the patient; all witnesses; a complete factual account of the incident; the date, time, and place of the incident; pertinent characteristics of the person involved; and other relevant variables believed important to the incident.
   c. Answers will vary with student's experiences.

REFLECTIVE PRACTICE USING CRITICAL THINKING SKILLS

Sample Answers

1. How might the nurses involved in this scenario respond to Ms. Bedford's disclosure that she will be pressing charges against the hospital?
The nurse speaking to Ms. Bedford should not volunteer any information regarding the case and should refer her to the legal department of the hospital. It would also be appropriate for the nurse to seek advice from legal counsel. The nurses providing the care may be named as defendants and will need to work closely with an attorney while preparing the defense. Either the defense or the prosecuting attorney may call the first nurse to testify as a fact witness if he or she has knowledge of the actual incident prompting the legal case. This nurse must base testimony on only firsthand knowledge of the incident and not on assumptions. When in doubt about facts, the nurses should simply testify, "I do not remember that."

2. What intellectual, technical, interpersonal, and/or ethical/legal competencies are most likely to be used in this situation?
Intellectual: knowledge of law and sources of law and ability to identify potential areas of liability in nursing
Technical: ability to provide technical nursing assistance in a competent, legally appropriate manner
Interpersonal: ability to work collaboratively with other members of the healthcare team and legal department
Ethical/Legal: ability to identify errors in personal action

3. What resources might be helpful for the nurses in this case?
Hospital legal department, liability insurance, risk management programs, malpractice arbitration panel

CHAPTER 8

PRACTICING FOR NCLEX
MULTIPLE CHOICE QUESTIONS

1. a	**2.** b	**3.** a	**4.** d	**5.** c
6. c	**7.** d	**8.** b	**9.** a	**10.** a

ALTERNATE-FORMAT QUESTIONS
Multiple Response Questions

1. a, b, e
2. c, d, f
3. b, d, f
4. b, d, f

DEVELOPING YOUR KNOWLEDGE BASE

FILL-IN-THE-BLANKS

1. Inpatient
2. Ambulatory care
3. Respite
4. Hospice
5. Voluntary
6. Respiratory therapist

MATCHING EXERCISES

1. f	**2.** d	**3.** g	**4.** b	**5.** e
6. j	**7.** h	**8.** l	**9.** c	**10.** i
11. m	**12.** q	**13.** a	**14.** n	**15.** p
16. h	**17.** f	**18.** a	**19.** j	**20.** g
21. e	**22.** b	**23.** c	**24.** i	**25.** d

SHORT ANSWER

1. **a.** DRGs encourage early discharge from the hospital and have created a new acutely ill population who need skilled care at home.
   b. There are increasing numbers of older people living longer with multiple chronic illnesses who are not institutionalized.
   c. With more sophisticated technology, people can be kept alive and comfortable in their own homes.
   d. Healthcare consumers demand that services be humane and provisions be made for a dignified death at home.

2. **a.** Primary care offices: Make health assessments, assist physician, and provide health education
   b. Ambulatory care centers and clinics: A nurse practitioner may run these centers, which usually provide walk-in services and are open at times other than traditional office hours.
   c. Mental health centers: Nurses who work in crisis intervention centers must have strong communication and counseling skills and must be thoroughly familiar with community resources specific to the needs of patients being served.
   d. Rehabilitation centers: These centers use a healthcare team comprising physicians, nurses, physical therapists, occupational therapists, and counselors.
   e. Long-term care centers: Help patients maintain function and independence with concern for the

living environment as well as the healthcare provided. Provide direct care, supervise others, serve as an administrator, and teach.

3. With the trend toward discharging patients earlier, hospitals more often focus on the acute care needs of the patient. Along with this focus has come a proliferation of services offered by the hospital aimed at the outpatient.

4. **a.** Surgical procedures
   b. Diagnostic tests
   c. Medications
   d. Physical therapy
   e. Counseling
   f. Health education

5. DRGs: Diagnosis-related groups: This plan pays the hospital a predetermined, fixed amount defined by the medical diagnosis or specific procedure rather than by the actual cost of hospitalization and care. DRGs were implemented by the federal government in an effort to control rising healthcare costs. If the cost of hospitalization is greater than that assigned, the hospital must absorb the additional cost. However, if cost is less than that assigned, the hospital makes a profit.

6. When patients come in contact with many different healthcare providers (e.g., registered nurses, licensed practical nurses, nursing assistants, nurse specialists, physical therapists, dietitians, and students) and are frequently seen by other physician specialists called in on consultation or to do surgery, the patient may become confused about care and treatment. This fragmentation of care may result in the loss of continuity of care, resulting in conflicting plans of care, too much or too little medication, and higher healthcare costs.

REFLECTIVE PRACTICE USING CRITICAL THINKING SKILLS

Sample Answers

1. What nursing interventions might the nurse employ to assist Ms. Ritchie with her caregiver duties?
   The nurse can provide Ms. Ritchie with information about how to access respite care and make referrals for her. However, since Medicaid and most insurance providers do not cover the costs of respite care, the nurse should also check community services that may provide respite care for free. Ms. Ritchie's husband may qualify for hospice care, and the nurse can arrange for this service.

2. What would be a successful outcome for this patient?
   Ms. Ritchie vocalizes the benefits of respite care and hospice care programs and states that she will sign up for any services available to her.

3. What intellectual, technical, interpersonal, and/or ethical/legal competencies are most likely to bring about the desired outcome?
   Intellectual: knowledge of the various types of healthcare services and settings available to meet the needs of families caring for dying patients

Technical: ability to provide technical assistance to meet the needs of families of patients on hospice
Interpersonal: ability to work with different available resources to ensure everyone's access to safe, quality healthcare
Ethical/Legal: knowledge of ethical and legal principles related to patients with terminal illnesses

4. What resources might be helpful for Ms. Ritchie?
   Respite care, hospice services, community services

CHAPTER 9

PRACTICING FOR NCLEX
MULTIPLE CHOICE QUESTIONS

1. c	2. a	3. d	4. a	5. b
6. c				

ALTERNATE-FORMAT QUESTIONS
Multiple Response Questions

1. a, c, e
2. b, c, f
3. c, d, e, f
4. b, e, f
5. a, d, f

DEVELOPING YOUR KNOWLEDGE BASE

FILL-IN-THE-BLANKS

1. Community-based
2. Health Insurance Portability and Accountability Act (HIPAA)
3. Against medical advice (AMA)
4. Discharge planning

CORRECT THE FALSE STATEMENTS

1. False—nurse
2. False—Continuity of care
3. True
4. True
5. False—patient's name, ID number, and physician
6. False—decreasing
7. False—is indicated
8. True
9. False—remains at the hospital
10. False—physician's order

SHORT ANSWER

1. Sample answers:
   a. With patient's permission, check with relatives, neighbors, or fellow church or club members who could help; if necessary, check with social agencies.
   b. Describe the procedure to the patient in detail so he/she will know what to expect.
   c. Check the patient's insurance status, Medicare, or Medicaid; see if procedures are covered and what amount the patient will be responsible for. Refer to the appropriate agencies if necessary.
   d. With patient's permission, check with family; if necessary, check into home healthcare possibilities, hospice, or extended-care facilities.

2. **a.** Medications: Drug name, dosage, purpose, effect, and times taken, stated verbally and in writing
   b. Procedures and treatments: Demonstrate all steps, practice, and put in writing. Caregivers should demonstrate procedures.
   c. Diet: Explain diet and purpose; give examples of meals and provide written plans.
   d. Referrals: Instruct patient and family how to make follow-up visits and whom to call with problems.
   e. Health promotion: All aspects of the illness or effects of treatment should be described verbally, and written materials should be supplied.

3. **a.** Discharge planning: Exchanges information among the patient, caregivers, and those responsible for home care while the patient is in the institution and after the patient returns home.
   b. Collaboration with other members of the healthcare team: Meets the patient's and family's physical, psychological, sociocultural, and spiritual needs in all settings and at all levels of health.
   c. Involving patient and family in planning: Ensures that patient and family needs are consistently met as the patient moves from one level of care to another.

4. **a.** Assess the patient's need for nursing care related to admission.
   b. Include consideration of biophysical, psychosocial, environmental, self-care, educational, and discharge planning factors in each patient's assessment.
   c. Involve the patient and family in care as appropriate.
   d. Nursing staff members should collaborate, as appropriate, with physicians and members of other clinical disciplines to make decisions regarding the patient's need for nursing care.
   e. Assess need for continuing care in preparation for discharge, and document referrals for such care in the patient's medical record.

5. **a.** Establish the health database: age; sex; height; weight; medical history, including any prior miscarriages; and current medical treatment, follow-up treatment
   b. Assess for personal data: Personal feelings about her miscarriage, effectiveness of personal coping methods
   c. Explore husband's relationship with patient and ability to provide emotional support.
   d. Check if there are any support services (e.g., support groups, fertility clinics) that would be available to this couple.

6. **a.** Transfer within the hospital setting: Patient's belongings and/or furniture are moved; patient's chart, Kardex, care plan, and medications must be correctly labeled for the new room; and other departments must be notified as appropriate. If transfer is to a new floor, the nurse at the original area gives a verbal report about the patient to the nurse at the new area.
   b. Transfer to a long-term facility: All the patient's belongings are carefully packed and sent to the facility; prescriptions and appointment cards for return visits to the physician's office may be sent; patient is discharged from hospital setting, but a copy of the chart may be sent to long-term facility along with a detailed assessment and care plan.
   c. Discharge from a healthcare setting: Check patient discharge order, instructions, equipment and supplies, and financial arrangements. Assist patient to dress and pack belongings; check for written order for future services; transport patient to car and assist as necessary; make necessary recordings on records and complete discharge summary.

7. A form must be signed that releases the physician and healthcare institution from any legal responsibility for the patient's health status; the patient is informed of any possible risk before signing the form; the signature of the patient must be witnessed; and the form becomes part of the patient's record.

8. Position the bed in its highest position; arrange the furniture in the room to allow easy access to the bed. Open the bed by folding back the top bed linens. Assemble necessary equipment and supplies. Assemble special equipment and supplies (e.g., oxygen therapy equipment) and make sure it is working properly. Adjust the physical environment of the room.

REFLECTIVE PRACTICE USING CRITICAL THINKING SKILLS

Sample Answers

1. How might the admitting nurse respond to the grandmother's refusal to sign consent forms?
   The nurse should speak to the grandmother and ask her if there is another contact for Jeff, such as a parent. The nurse could also check if there is a durable power of attorney on file for Jeff, and if not, a legal consult may be in order.

2. What would be a successful outcome for this patient?
   Jeff's grandmother states the importance of getting medical attention for her grandson and cooperates with the staff to authorize the necessary care or assign this responsibility to another caretaker.

3. What intellectual, technical, interpersonal, and/or ethical/legal competencies are most likely to bring about the desired outcome?
   Intellectual: knowledge of mental retardation and the settings available to meet the needs of a patient with profound mental retardation
   Interpersonal: ability to establish trusting professional relationships with patients, family caregivers, and healthcare professionals in different practice settings to ensure continuity of care
   Ethical/Legal: knowledge of the nurse's legal and ethical obligations as patients are transferred between home and different practice settings

4. What resources might be helpful for the nurse working with this family?

Legal counsel, information on communicating with patients with mental retardation, other healthcare professionals who have worked with Jeff

CHAPTER 10

PRACTICING FOR NCLEX
MULTIPLE CHOICE QUESTIONS

1. d   **2.** c   **3.** a   **4.** b

ALTERNATE-FORMAT QUESTIONS
Multiple Response Questions

1. a, d, e, f
2. d, e, f
3. b, d, e
4. a, b, f
5. b, c, d, f

DEVELOPING YOUR KNOWLEDGE BASE

FILL-IN-THE-BLANKS

1. Home healthcare
2. 1965 Social Security Act

3. Advocacy
4. Home healthcare nurse
5. Older women

MATCHING EXERCISES

1. a   **2.** c   **3.** c   **4.** b   **5.** b
6. a

CORRECT THE FALSE STATEMENTS

1. False—hospital-based care to community-based care
2. True
3. False—chronic and acute
4. False—care must be adapted to patient's schedule
5. False—Mary Brewster
6. True
7. False—generalists
8. False—are responsible
9. True
10. True
11. False—short term
12. True
13. True

SHORT ANSWER

1. See table below.

Date	Home Healthcare Provider/Location	Type of Care
1893	Henry Street Settlement House, New York City	Visiting nurses cared for poor residents living in tenements.
Prior to WWII During and Post WWII	Physician Nurses	Often made home care visits to treat the sick. There was a shift in practice from the home to the hospital and office setting. Nurses provided most home care visits.
Mid 1960s	1965 Social Security Act	Home care services expanded to include the older population. The Social Security Act provided program coverage for older adults participating in Medicare.
Post 1980	Home care specialists	Many home care nurses have specialized in advanced practice skills to meet the growing demands of acutely ill patients cared for at home.
2000s	Nurses and families	More complex services provided at home. Increasing numbers of surgical procedures performed on outpatient basis; families have more responsibility providing care.

2. Sample answers:
   a. Knowledge and skills: Home care nurses must have knowledge of legal regulations, physical assessment, body mechanics, nursing diagnoses, and infection control.
   b. Independence: Home care nurses enjoy practicing in an autonomous setting where they can use their expertise in an expanded role.
   c. Accountability: Home care nurses are accountable to the patient, the family, and the primary healthcare provider.
3. a. Patient advocate: Protecting and supporting the patient's rights—the home care nurse helps a patient prepare a living will.
   b. Coordinator of services: The home care nurse is the coordinator of all other healthcare providers visiting the patient—the home care nurse helps arrange for rehabilitation services for a stroke patient.
   c. Educator: Home care nurses spend time teaching patients and families about the disease process, nutrition, medications, or treatment and care of wounds—the home care nurse teaches a patient with diabetes about diet.
4. a. Wash hands before removing supplies from the bag.
   b. Anything the nurse takes out of the bag must be cleaned before returning it to the bag.
   c. Anytime the nurse needs to access the bag, handwashing must take place first.
   d. The bag should be placed on a liner before setting it down in the patient's home.
5. Teaching is geared to the patient's readiness to learn and adapted to the patient's physical and emotional status. Information that is essential to keep patients safe until the next visit is the major focus. Teaching is adapted to what works best in the home. Incentives to learn include knowledge of serious consequences as well as positive benefits of carrying through with certain behaviors.
6. As healthcare continues to shift from the hospital setting to community-based care, families will bear the burden associated with this change. Patients are discharged sooner with a higher acuity level; chronically ill patients will need continued long-term personal care at home not covered by Medicare.
7. Sample answer:
   The nurse would work with an interdisciplinary team of other healthcare professionals such as social workers, pastoral counselors, home health aides, and volunteers to provide comprehensive palliative care. Emotional support would be provided for the husband and children as well as the patient, and pain and symptom management would be conducted. The focus is on improving the quality of life for the patient and preserving dignity for the patient in death. Bereavement care would continue for the family for 6 months after the patient's death.

REFLECTIVE PRACTICE USING CRITICAL THINKING SKILLS
Sample Answers
1. What is the role of the home healthcare nurse in providing continuity of care for Mr. Califano?
   The home healthcare nurse must identify the needs of the family and caregiver and assesses whether the patient and family understand and agree with the plan of care. The nurse can also help the patient and family identify and use community resources to meet various needs. If a caregiver is becoming overwhelmed, the nurse can provide resources to relieve the stress. In Mr. Califano's case, the nurse would need to coordinate care related to his diabetes, hypertension, and renal disease.
2. What would be a successful outcome for this patient?
   Mr. Califano and his caretakers verbalize the home treatment plan designed to care for his foot ulcers and other related diabetic conditions.
   Mr. Califano lists resources that may be contacted to assist with care in the home setting as necessary.
3. What intellectual, technical, interpersonal, and/or ethical/legal competencies are most likely to bring about the desired outcome?
   Intellectual: ability to incorporate knowledge of the healthcare delivery system to meet the needs of patients receiving care in the home
   Technical: ability to adapt technical nursing assistance as necessary for an older adult with numerous health concerns
   Interpersonal: ability to work with different resources to ensure safe quality home care
   Ethical/Legal: ability to practice in an ethically and legally defensible manner in home settings
4. What resources might be helpful for Mr. Califano?
   Community services, housekeeping services, home healthcare services

CHAPTER 11

PRACTICING FOR NCLEX
MULTIPLE CHOICE QUESTIONS
1. c   2. a   3. b   4. c   5. d
6. c   7. d

ALTERNATE-FORMAT QUESTIONS
Multiple Response Questions
1. a, b, c
2. c, e, f
3. a, c, d, e
4. b, e, f
5. b, d, e

Prioritization Questions
1.

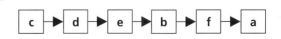

2.

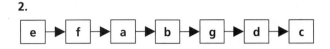

DEVELOPING YOUR KNOWLEDGE BASE

FILL-IN-THE-BLANKS

1. Standards of practice
2. Implementing
3. Concept mapping
4. Whistle-blower
5. Medical diagnosis, nursing diagnosis, all pertinent clinical data

MATCHING EXERCISES

1. a	**2.** d	**3.** e	**4.** b	**5.** c
6. a	**7.** e	**8.** b	**9.** c	**10.** e
11. d	**12.** a	**13.** c	**14.** b	**15.** d
16. a	**17.** d	**18.** b	**19.** a	**20.** c
21. b	**22.** d			

SHORT ANSWER

1. Patient:
   a. Scientifically based, holistic, individualized care
   b. The opportunity to work collaboratively with nurses
   c. Continuity of care
   Nursing:
   a. Achievement of a clear and efficient plan of action by which the entire nursing team can achieve results for patients
   b. Satisfaction that the nurse is making an important difference in the lives of patients
   c. Opportunity to grow professionally when evaluating the effectiveness of interventions and variables that contribute positively or negatively to the patient's goal achievement

2. a. Determining the need for nursing care: The nursing process provides a framework that enables the nurse to systematically collect patient data and clearly identify patient strengths and problems.
   b. Planning and implementing the care: The nursing process helps the nurse and patient develop a holistic plan of individualized care that specifies both the desired patient goals and the nursing actions most likely to assist the patient to meet those goals and execute the plan of care.
   c. Evaluating the results of the nursing care: The nursing process provides for evaluation of the plan of care in terms of patient goal achievement.

3. The nursing process is a systematic, patient-centered, goal-oriented method of caring that provides a framework for nursing practice.
   The goals of the nursing process are to help the nurse manage each patient's care scientifically, holistically, and creatively to promote wellness, prevent disease or illness, restore health, and facilitate coping with altered functioning.

The skills necessary to use the nursing process successfully include intellectual, technical, interpersonal, and ethical/legal skills, as well as the willingness to use these skills creatively when working with patients.

4. Sample answers:
   a. Systematic: Each nursing task is a part of an ordered sequence of activities, and each activity depends on the accuracy of the activity that precedes it and influences the actions that follow it.
   b. Dynamic: There is great interaction and overlapping among the five steps; no one step in the process is a one-time phenomenon; each step is fluid and flows into the next step.
   c. Interpersonal: The human being is always at the heart of nursing. The nursing process ensures that nurses are patient centered rather than task centered.
   d. Goal oriented: The nursing process offers a means for nurses and patients to work together to identify specific goals related to wellness promotion, disease and illness prevention, health restoration, and coping with altered functioning that are most important to the patient and match them with appropriate nursing actions.
   e. Universally applicable: Once nurses have a working knowledge of the nursing process, they can apply it to well or ill patients, young or old patients, in any type of practice setting.

5. a. Purpose of thinking: This helps to discipline thinking by keeping all thoughts directed to the goal.
   b. Adequacy of knowledge: It is important to judge whether the knowledge available to you is accurate, complete, and relevant. If you reason with false information or lack important data, it is impossible to draw a sound conclusion.
   c. Potential problems: As you become more skilled in critical thinking, you will learn to "flag" or remedy pitfalls to sound reasoning.
   d. Helpful resources: Wise professionals are quick to recognize their limits and seek help in remedying their deficiencies.
   e. Critique of judgment/decision: Ultimately, you must identify alternative judgments or decisions, weigh their merits, and reach a conclusion.

6. Sample answers:
   a. Practice a necessary skill until you feel confident in its execution before performing it on a patient.
   b. Take time to familiarize yourself with new equipment before using it in a clinical procedure.
   c. Identify nurses who are technical experts and ask them to share their secrets.
   d. Never be ashamed to seek assistance if you feel unsure of how to perform a procedure or manage equipment.

7. Answers will vary with student's experiences.
8. Answers will vary with student's experiences.
9. Sample answers:
   a. "I'm Nurse Brown and I'll be your nurse this week. What would you like to accomplish with this time, and how can I help you get through this period?"
   b. "What family members do you expect to see while you are here? Would you trust them to make decisions about your care if you were unable to do so yourself?"
   c. "What are your goals, hopes, and dreams in life? How do you hope to accomplish them? How will your hospitalization affect these goals?"
   d. "Tell me about your life at home/school/work. Is there anyone or anything in particular that you will miss during your recuperation?"
10. a. Do I know the legal boundaries of my practice?
    b. Do I own my personal strengths and weaknesses and seek assistance as needed?
    c. Am I knowledgeable about, and respectful of, patient rights?
    d. Does my documentation provide a legally defensible account of my practice?

REFLECTIVE PRACTICE USING CRITICAL THINKING SKILLS

Sample Answers

1. How might the nurse use blended nursing skills to respond to this patient situation?
   The nurse should investigate the reasons Ms. Horvath is not cooperating with the teaching session on wound care for her child. Possible reasons include fear, fatigue, lack of knowledge of possible consequences if the wound is not kept clean (i.e., infection), and being overwhelmed with family responsibilities. The nurse should use blended skills to advocate for this family and seek out possible resources (such as help from relatives or the community) to help remedy this situation.
2. What would be a successful outcome for this patient and her family?
   Ms. Horvath states the consequences of improper wound care and demonstrates changing the dressings on her daughter's wound.
3. What intellectual, technical, interpersonal, and/or ethical/legal competencies are most likely to bring about the desired outcome?
   Intellectual: knowledge of the science of nursing care related to wound care
   Technical: ability to competently change dressings on a wound and teach this skill to the caretaker
   Interpersonal: ability to counsel Ms. Horvath who is finding it difficult to respond to the challenge of caring for her daughter at home
   Ethical/Legal: commitment to patient safety and quality care, including the ability to report problem situations immediately

4. What resources might be helpful for Ms. Horvath?
   Counseling services, community services, help from relatives, printed materials on wound care

CHAPTER 12

PRACTICING FOR NCLEX
MULTIPLE CHOICE QUESTIONS

1. d	2. c	3. c	4. a	5. c
6. b	7. d	8. d		

ALTERNATE-FORMAT QUESTIONS
Multiple Response Questions

1. a, d, e
2. c, d, f
3. b, c, f
4. a, d, f

Prioritization Question

1.

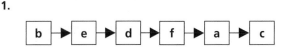

b → e → d → f → a → c

DEVELOPING YOUR KNOWLEDGE BASE

FILL-IN-THE-BLANKS

1. Patient support people, patient record
2. Database nursing assessment
3. Validation
4. Reflective
5. Focused
6. Time-lapsed
7. Minimum data set

MATCHING EXERCISES

1. f	2. j	3. e	4. c	5. g
6. i	7. k	8. a	9. b	10. d
11. a	12. b	13. a	14. a	15. b
16. b				

SHORT ANSWER

1. a. Make a judgment about a patient's health status.
   b. Make a judgment about a patient's ability to manage his/her own healthcare.
   c. Make a judgment about a patient's need for nursing.
   d. Refer the patient to a physician or other healthcare professional.
   e. Plan and deliver individualized, holistic nursing care that draws on the patient's strengths.
2. a. Patient: Most patients are willing to share information when they know it is helpful in planning their care.
   b. Support people: Family members, friends, and caregivers are helpful sources of data when a patient is a child or has a limited capacity to share information with the nurse.

c. Patient record: A review of the records prepared by different members of the healthcare team provides information essential to comprehensive nursing care.

d. Medical history, physical examination, and progress notes: Sources that record the findings of physicians as they assess and treat the patient.

e. Reports of laboratory and other diagnostic studies: These sources (e.g., x-rays and diagnostic tests) can either confirm or conflict with data collected during the nursing history or examination.

f. Reports of therapies by other healthcare professionals: Other healthcare professionals record their findings and note progress in specific areas (e.g., nutrition, physical therapy, or speech therapy).

g. Other healthcare professionals: Other nurses, physicians, social workers, and so on can provide information about a patient's normal health habits and patterns and response to illness.

h. Nursing and other healthcare literature: If a nurse is unfamiliar with a disease, it is important for him/her to read about the clinical manifestations of the disease and its usual progression to know what to look for when assessing the patient.

3. a. Purposeful: The nurse must identify the purpose of the nursing assessment (comprehensive, focused, emergency, time-lapsed) and then gather the appropriate data.

b. Complete: All patient data need to be identified to understand a patient's health problem and develop a plan of care to maximize health promotion.

c. Factual and accurate: Nurses concerned with accuracy and fact must continually verify what they hear with what they observe using other senses and validate all questionable data.

d. Relevant: Because recording data can become an endless task, nurses must determine what type of data and how much data to collect for each patient.

4. Sample answers:

a. What are the patient's current responses to his/her situation?

b. What is the patient's current ability to manage his/her care?

c. What is the immediate environment?

5. a. Patient should know the name of his/her primary nurse and what he/she can expect of nursing.

b. Patient should sense that the nurse is competent and cares about him/her.

c. Patient should know what is expected of him/her in terms of developing the plan of care and participating in its execution.

6. Sample answers:

a. Closed questions:
How long have you been experiencing these symptoms?
How many children do you have at home?

b. Open-ended questions:
How will you modify your diet now that you have been diagnosed with diabetes?
What do you know about insulin injections?

c. Reflective questions:
What effect will diabetes have on your life?
How do you feel about using insulin injections to control your diabetes?

7. a. Patient's health orientation: Patients must identify potential and actual health risks and explore habits, behaviors, beliefs, attitudes, and values that influence levels of health.

b. Patient's developmental stage: Nursing assessments are modified according to the patient's developmental stage.

c. Patient's need for nursing: Whether the nurse will interact with the patient for a short or long period and the nature of nursing care needs influence the type of data the nurse collects.

8. Sample answers:

a. When there are discrepancies (e.g., a patient claims he has no pain but grimaces when you touch his chest)

b. When the data lack objectivity (e.g., when a patient claims to have 20/20 vision but holds his reading material far away from his face)

9. Immediate communication of data is indicated whenever assessment findings reveal a critical change in the patient's health status that necessitates the involvement of other nurses or healthcare professionals.

REFLECTIVE PRACTICE USING CRITICAL THINKING SKILLS

Sample Answers

1. How might the nurse facilitate Ms. Morgan's ability to cope with disability?
The nurse should assess the patient's body image and self-esteem needs. Working collaboratively with other members of the healthcare team, the nurse could then prepare a nursing care plan that specifically addresses these needs.

2. What would be a successful outcome for this patient?
By discharge, Ms. Morgan will verbalize acceptance of her diagnosis of MS and state methods to keep herself as physically active as possible.

3. What intellectual, technical, interpersonal, and/or ethical/legal competencies are most likely to bring about the desired outcome?
Intellectual: knowledge of the signs and symptoms of MS and supportive services for patients with MS
Interpersonal: demonstration of strong people skills for dealing with individuals experiencing alterations in health
Ethical/Legal: strong advocacy skills and a willingness to use them for patients needing assistance

4. What resources might be helpful for Ms. Morgan?
Family counseling, printed materials on MS, support groups

CHAPTER 13

PRACTICING FOR NCLEX

MULTIPLE CHOICE QUESTIONS

1. c   **2.** a   **3.** d   **4.** c   **5.** d

ALTERNATE-FORMAT QUESTIONS

Multiple Response Questions

1. b, c, e, f
2. c, d, f
3. a, b, d
4. c, d, e
5. a, b, d

DEVELOPING YOUR KNOWLEDGE BASE

FILL-IN-THE-BLANKS

1. Collaborative
2. Cues
3. Standard or norm
4. Data cluster
5. Nursing diagnosis
6. Inability to accept the death of newborn child
7. Desire for a higher level of wellness, an effective present status or function
8. Syndrome

MATCHING EXERCISES

1. c   **2.** a   **3.** b   **4.** d   **5.** a
6. c   **7.** d

CORRECT THE FALSE STATEMENTS

1. False—nursing diagnoses
2. False—Nursing diagnoses
3. False—standard or norm
4. True
5. False—cluster of significant data
6. True
7. False—etiology
8. True
9. True
10. True
11. False—analyzes patient data
12. False—risk diagnosis

SHORT ANSWER

1. a. Using legally inadvisable language
   b. X
   c. Identifying responses not necessarily unhealthy
   d. X
   e. Both clauses say the same thing.
   f. X
   g. Including value judgment
   h. Identifying responses not necessarily unhealthy
   i. X
   j. Including medical diagnosis
   k. Identifying problems as signs and symptoms
   l. Reversing clauses
   m. X
   n. Both clauses say the same thing.
   o. Identifying problems/etiologies that cannot be altered
   p. Both clauses say the same thing.
   q. X
   r. Writing diagnosis in terms of needs
2. Sample answers:
   a. Were you able to pass urine this morning? Did you drink the fluids we brought you?
   b. Do you feel like talking to other patients who are undergoing the same treatment? Would you like to see your family today?
   c. Do you feel helpless to put your life back in order? Are you overwhelmed by the changes in your life?
   d. Were you able to get some sleep last night? Did the noise on the unit keep you awake?
3. a. No problem: Reinforce patient's health habits and patterns; initiate health promotion activities to prevent disease or illness or promote higher level of wellness.
   b. Possible problem: Collect more data to confirm or rule out suspected problem.
   c. Actual or potential nursing diagnosis: Unable to treat because patient denies problem or refuses treatment; begin planning, implementing, and evaluating care designed to prevent, reduce, or resolve problem.
   d. Clinical problem other than nursing diagnosis: Consult with appropriate healthcare professional and work collaboratively on problem; refer to medicine.
4. Sample answers:
   a. An infant who is below the normal growth standards for his age group may be experiencing "failure to thrive."
   b. A mother who has a history of mental illness shows little or no interest in her baby.
   c. A patient placed in a nursing home by her son becomes incontinent without a physical cause.
5. a. Are my data accurate and complete?
   b. Has the patient or the patient's surrogates (if able to do so) validated that these are important problems?
   c. Have I given the patient or the patient's surrogate an opportunity to identify problems that I have missed?
   d. Is each diagnosis supported by evidence? Might these cues signify a different problem or diagnosis?
   e. Have I tried to identify what is causing the actual or potential problem and what strengths/resources the patient might use to avoid or resolve the problem?
6. a. In the presence of known problems, nurses must predict the most common and most dangerous complications and take immediate action to prevent them or manage them in case they cannot be prevented.

b. Whether problems are present or not, nurses must look for evidence of risk factors, and if identified, aim to reduce or control them, thereby preventing the problems themselves.

c. In all situations, nurses must encourage behaviors that promote optimum function, independence, and a sense of well-being.

7. a. Mr. Klinetob, aged 86, has been seriously depressed since the death of his wife of 52 years, 6 months ago. Although he suffers from <u>degenerative joint disease</u> and has talked for years about having "just a touch of arthritis," this never kept him from being up and about. Recently, however, he spends all day sitting in a chair and seems to have no desire to engage in self-care activities. He tells the visiting nurse that <u>he doesn't get washed up anymore because he's "too stiff" in the morning to bathe and "I just don't seem to have the energy."</u> The visiting nurse notices that <u>his hair is matted and uncombed, his face has traces of previous meals, and he has a strong body odor</u>. His adult children have complained that their normally fastidious father seems not to care about personal hygiene any longer.

   Nursing Diagnosis: Bathing/Hygiene Self-Care Deficit, related to decreased strength and endurance, discomfort, and depression, as evidence by matted and uncombed hair, new beard, food particles on face, and strong body odor

b. Miss Adams sustained a right-sided cerebral infarct that resulted in <u>left hemiparesis</u> (paralysis on left side of body) and <u>left "neglect."</u> She <u>ignores the left side of her body</u> and actually denies its existence. <u>When asked about her left leg, she stated that it belonged to the woman in the next bed</u>—this while she was in a private room. <u>This patient was previously quite active: she walked for 45 to 60 minutes four or five times a week and was an avid swimmer</u>. At present, <u>she cannot move either her left arm or leg</u>.

   Nursing Diagnosis: Body Image Disturbance, related to left hemiparesis (paralysis), as evidenced by her ignoring the left side of her body following her inability to move it

c. After trying to conceive a child for 11 years, Ted and Rosemary Hines sought the assistance of a fertility specialist who was highly recommended by a friend. It was determined that Ted's sperm was inadequate, and Rosemary was inseminated with sperm from an anonymous donor. The couple was told that the donor was healthy and that he was selected because he resembled Ted. Rosemary became pregnant after the second in-vitro fertilization attempt and delivered a healthy baby girl named Sarah.

   Sarah is now 7 years old, and Ted and Rosemary have learned from blood tests that their fertility specialist is the biologic father of their child. It seems that he lied to some couples about using sperm from anonymous donors and deceived others into thinking the wives had become pregnant when he had simply injected them with hormones. Ted and Rosemary have joined other couples in pressing charges against this physician. Rosemary tells the nurse in her pediatrician's office that she is concerned about how all this is affecting her family. <u>"Ted and I both love Sarah and would do nothing to hurt her</u>, but I'm so angry about this whole situation that I'm afraid I may be taking it out on her," she says. Questioning reveals that Rosemary <u>has found herself yelling at Sarah for minor disobediences and spanking her, something she rarely did before</u>. Both Ted and Rosemary had commented before about Sarah's striking physical resemblance to the fertility specialist but attributed this to coincidence. Rosemary says, <u>"Whenever I see her now I can't help but see Dr. Clowser and everything inside me clenches up and I want to scream."</u> Both Ted and Rosemary express great remorse that Sarah, who is innocent, is bearing the brunt of something that is in no way her fault.

   Nursing Diagnosis: Parental Role Conflict related to unexpected discovery about their daughter's biologic father, as evidenced by parental concern about increased incidence of parental yelling and spanking and the anger the child evokes in her parents because of her physical resemblance to the fertility specialist who deceived them.

REFLECTIVE PRACTICE USING CRITICAL THINKING SKILLS

Sample Answers

1. What nursing diagnosis would be appropriate for Mr. Prescott? How might the nurse advocate for Mr. Prescott to ensure that he gets tested for colon cancer?
   Nursing Diagnosis: Anxiety related to constipation and possible bowel alterations
   Mr. Prescott would benefit from patient teaching/counseling regarding the need for stool testing. After checking with the primary care provider, the nurse could schedule a colonoscopy if ordered to check for colon cancer. The nurse should address the patient's constipation and check with the primary care provider about scheduling a consult with a gastroenterologist.

2. What would be a successful outcome for this patient?
   Mr. Prescott states the warning signs of colon cancer and agrees to schedule a colonoscopy

3. What intellectual, technical, interpersonal, and/or ethical/legal competencies are most likely to bring about the desired outcome?

Intellectual: knowledge of gastrointestinal elimination, including hemorrhoids and risk factors for possible colon cancer

Interpersonal: ability to work collaboratively with other members of the healthcare team to meet the needs of patients

Ethical/Legal: ability to serve as a trusted and effective patient advocate to counsel patients with bowel alterations

4. What resources might be helpful for Mr. Prescott? Consults with other healthcare professionals, educational materials on colon cancer, diet plans to prevent constipation

CHAPTER 14

PRACTICING FOR NCLEX
MULTIPLE CHOICE QUESTIONS

1. d   2. a   3. c   4. b   5. c
6. b   7. c

ALTERNATE-FORMAT QUESTIONS
Multiple Response Questions

1. a, c, d, f
2. a, c
3. c, d, e
4. b, d, e
5. a, d, f
6. c, d, e, f
7. c, d, f
8. b, d, f

DEVELOPING YOUR KNOWLEDGE BASE

FILL-IN-THE-BLANKS

1. Patient outcome
2. Informal planning
3. Initial, ongoing, discharge
4. Pain/the problem statement
5. Nursing Outcomes Classification (NOC)
6. Evaluative
7. Nursing intervention
8. Nurse-initiated
9. Physician-initiated
10. Algorithm
11. Plan of nursing care

MATCHING EXERCISES

1. a   2. e   3. f   4. b   5. d
6. c   7. g   8. b   9. i   10. b
11. a   12. b   13. c   14. a   15. c
16. b   17. a   18. b   19. c   20. c
21. a

SHORT ANSWER

1. a. Teach patient the proper technique and application for an inhaler.
   b. Walk with patient the length of the hallway every 5 hours, encouraging her to rely on the walker for support.
   c. Teach patient the importance of a well-balanced diet and daily exercise; have patient monitor daily caloric intake.
   d. Help patient sit up and dangle legs over side of bed; gradually help patient to stand and take several steps around the room.

2. a. Setting priorities: Before developing or modifying the plan of care, the prioritized list of nursing diagnoses should be reviewed to determine whether they are correctly ranked as high priority, medium priority, or low priority.
   b. Writing goals/outcomes that determine the evaluative strategy: For each nursing diagnosis in the plan of care, at least one goal must be written that, if achieved, demonstrates a direct resolution of the problem statement.
   c. Selecting appropriate evidence-based nursing interventions: Nursing interventions should be consistent with standards of care; realistic; compatible with patient's values, beliefs, and psychosocial background; valued by patient and family; and compatible with other planned therapies.
   d. Communicating the plan of nursing care: Nursing orders describe in writing, and thus communicate to the entire nursing staff and healthcare team the specific nursing care to be implemented for the patient.

3. Sample answers:
   Informal planning: A postpartum nurse learns that a patient is complaining of soreness related to unsuccessful attempts to breastfeed her infant and plans to spend more time with her. A home healthcare nurse quickly assesses safety in the home of a patient prone to accidents.

4. A formal plan of care allows the nurse to individualize care; set priorities; facilitate communication among nursing personnel; promote continuity of high-quality, cost-effective care; coordinate care; evaluate patient's response to nursing care; and promote the nurse's professional development.

5. a. Assess effectiveness of pain medication for patient every 4 hours.
   b. Speak to parents of patient to assess their ability to support patient.
   c. Assess patient's room for variety of colors, textures, visual stimulation.
   d. Teach patient to perform daily exercises and learn to ambulate with a walker.

6. **a.** Basic human needs: The nursing care plan should concisely communicate to caregivers data about the patient's usual health habits and patterns obtained during the nursing history that are needed to direct daily care (e.g., requires assistance setting up food tray).

   b. Nursing diagnoses: The plan should contain goals/outcomes and nursing interventions for every nursing diagnosis, as well as a place to note patient responses to the plan of care; for instance, if the nursing diagnosis is Impaired Skin Integrity related to mobility deficit, a goal should be written to turn patient frequently and assess for skin breakdown.

   c. Medical and interdisciplinary plan of care: The plan of care should record current medical orders for diagnostic studies and specified related nursing care; for instance, if a diagnostic test is scheduled for the morning, appropriate fasting measures should be included in the plan of care.

7. **a.** Have changes in the patient's health status influenced the priority of nursing diagnoses?

   b. Have changes in the way the patient is responding to health and illness or the plan of care affected those nursing diagnoses that can be realistically addressed?

   c. Are there relationships among diagnoses that require that one be worked on before another can be resolved?

   d. Can several patient problems be dealt with together?

8. **a.** Mrs. Myers learns one lesson on nutrition per day, beginning 2/16/12.

   b. After viewing film on smoking, Mrs. Gray identifies three dangers of smoking.

   c. X

   d. X

   e. By next visit, patient will list three benefits of psychotherapy.

   f. X

9. Sample answers:

   a. By 11/12/12, patient will reestablish fluid balance as evidenced by (1) an approximate balance between fluid intake and fluid output, to average approximately 2,500 mL; (2) urine specific gravity within the normal range (1.010–1.025).

   b. By next visit, patient will report a resumption of usual level of sexual activity following her acceptance of her new body image.

   c. By 6/4/12, patient will report a decrease in the number of stress incontinent episodes (less than one per day), following her use of Kegel exercises.

   d. By 8/10/12, patient reports he has sufficient energy to carry out the priority activities identified 8/2/12.

   e. By end of shift, patient reports better pain management (pain decreased to less than 3 on a scale of 10), related to new administration schedule.

10. **a.** Be familiar with standards and agency policies for setting priorities, identifying and recording expected patient outcomes, selecting evidence-based nursing interventions, and recording the plan of care.

    b. Remember that the goal of patient-centered care is to keep the patient and the patient's interests and preferences central in every aspect of planning.

    c. Keep the "big picture" in focus. What are the discharge goals for this patient, and how should this direct each shift's interventions?

    d. Trust clinical experience and judgment but be willing to ask for help when the situation demands more than your qualifications and experience can provide; value collaborative practice.

    e. Respect your clinical intuition, but before establishing priorities, identifying outcomes, and selecting nursing interventions, be sure that research supports your plan.

    f. Recognize personal biases and keep an open mind.

11. **a.** What problems need immediate attention, and which ones can wait?

    b. Which problems are your responsibility, and which do you need to refer to someone else?

    c. Which problems can be dealt with by using standard plans (e.g., critical paths, standards of care)?

    d. Which problems are not covered by protocols or standard plans but must be addressed to ensure a safe hospital stay and timely discharge?

REFLECTIVE PRACTICE USING CRITICAL THINKING SKILLS

Sample Answers

1. How might the nurse respond to Ms. Kronk's questions regarding fitness?

   The nurse can teach Ms. Kronk about low-salt, low-fat diets and encourage her to begin an exercise program, such as walking each day or joining a gym. The nurse could also refer Ms. Kronk to a dietitian to explain the types of diets and diet supplements that are available, including diets that are healthy and foods to avoid with high blood pressure.

2. What would be a successful outcome for this patient?

   Ms. Kronk lists 3 benefits of following a heart healthy diet and starting an exercise program to lose weight.

3. What intellectual, technical, interpersonal, and/or ethical/legal competencies are most likely to bring about the desired outcome?

   Intellectual: knowledge of what information is needed to develop a plan of care that meets the nursing needs of a woman who wants to improve her fitness level

Technical: ability to use the Internet to research literature to obtain knowledge to develop a plan of care for Ms. Kronk
Interpersonal: ability to empathize with patients, sharing their struggles and celebrating their achievement of valued goals
Ethical/Legal: ability to serve as a trusted and effective patient advocate
4. What resources might be helpful for Ms. Kronk? Printed materials on healthy diets, exercise plans, referrals to other healthcare professionals (such as fitness trainers)

CHAPTER 15

PRACTICING FOR NCLEX
MULTIPLE CHOICE QUESTIONS
1. b   2. c   3. d   4. c   5. b
ALTERNATE-FORMAT QUESTIONS
Multiple Response Questions
1. a, b
2. a, e, f
3. b, c, e, f
4. d, e, f

DEVELOPING YOUR KNOWLEDGE BASE
FILL-IN-THE-BLANKS
1. Physician-initiated intervention
2. Protocols
3. Community (or public health) interventions
4. Indirect care
5. Nursing Interventions Classification
6. Collaborative interventions
MATCHING EXERCISES
1. a   2. b   3. a   4. c   5. b
6. c
CORRECT THE FALSE STATEMENTS
1. False—nurse
2. True
3. False—Protocols
4. False—nurse
5. True
6. False—nothing about the plan of care is fixed
7. True
8. False—not sufficient
9. False—reassess the strategy
10. True
11. True
SHORT ANSWER
1. a. Interpret the specialists' findings for patients and family members.
   b. Prepare patients to participate maximally in the plan of care before and after discharge.

c. Serve as a liaison among the members of the healthcare team.
2. Sample answers:
   a. Nurse variable: A nurse with overwhelming outside concerns
   b. Patient variable: A patient who gives up
   c. Healthcare variable: Understaffing causes overworked nurses.
3. a. If patients and their families want to participate actively in seeking health, preventing disease and illness, recovering health, and learning to cope with altered functioning, they must possess effective self-care behavior.
   b. The nursing actions planned to promote patient goal/outcome achievement and the resolution of health problems should be carefully executed. It is important that the nurse use time wisely to maximize each patient encounter to help the patient achieve his/her goals/outcomes.
4. Sample answer:
   Mr. Franks may need a psychological evaluation to assess his adjustment to his new environment. Efforts should be made to get Mr. Franks involved in his new life so he shows interest in himself and others.
5. Sample answer:
   As well as care for pregnancy, this patient should receive counseling on planning economical, nutritious meals and should be alerted to any social services in her community that could provide some relief in this area.
6. Sample answers:
   a. Administering a prescribed medication to a patient
   b. A nurse lobbies for a new recreational facility in a nursing home
   c. A nurse participates in a free blood pressure screening at a local mall

REFLECTIVE PRACTICE USING CRITICAL THINKING SKILLS
Sample Answers
1. What might be the nurse's response when advocating for Antoinette and her family?
   The nurse's first responsibility is to her patient. In this case, the nurse must investigate the circumstances surrounding Antoinette's family life that are causing her failure to thrive. A referral to social services may be in order to help the family with childcare and the necessities of life. The nurse should also investigate any community services available to help this family.
2. What would be a successful outcome for this patient?
   By next visit, Antoinette is in the normal range of growth for her age and reaches the appropriate developmental milestones.
   Antoinette's grandmother states that she is less overwhelmed with her role as caregiver and is receiving help from community services

3. What intellectual, technical, interpersonal, and/or ethical/legal competencies are most likely to bring about the desired outcome?
Intellectual: knowledge of appropriate information necessary to implement the nursing interventions that effectively meet the nursing needs of a toddler with physical and developmental delays
Technical: ability to competently adapt procedures and equipment to meet the needs of patients across the life span
Interpersonal: ability to work collaboratively with members of the healthcare team to implement the interdisciplinary plan of care
Ethical/Legal: ability to participate as a trusted and effective patient advocate
4. What resources might be helpful for this family?
Social services, community services, counseling services

CHAPTER 16

PRACTICING FOR NCLEX
MULTIPLE CHOICE QUESTIONS
1. a   2. c   3. b   4. d   5. b
6. d   7. d   8. d

ALTERNATE-FORMAT QUESTIONS
Multiple Response Questions
1. a, d, e
2. a, b, c
3. c, e, f
4. a, b, d
5. b, c, f
6. a, d, f

DEVELOPING YOUR KNOWLEDGE BASE

FILL-IN-THE-BLANKS
1. Terminate, modify, continue
2. Patient
3. Outcome achievement
4. Criteria
5. Standards
6. Clinical practice guidelines (CPGs)
7. Quality assurance programs
8. Structure
9. Nursing audit

MATCHING EXERCISES
1. e   2. c   3. a   4. d   5. b
6. a   7. b   8. b   9. a   10. a

SHORT ANSWER
1. Sample answers:
  a. Cognitive goals: Ask the patient to repeat the information or ask the patient to apply the new knowledge to his/her everyday situations.

  b. Psychomotor goals: Ask the patient to demonstrate the new skill.
  c. Affective goals: Observe the patient's behavior and conversation for signs that the goals are achieved.
2. a. Identifying evaluative criteria: Evaluative criteria are the patient goals/outcomes developed during the planning step and must be identified to determine whether they can be met by the patient.
  b. Determining whether goals and criteria are met: Because evaluative criteria reflect desired changes or outcomes in patient behavior, and because nursing actions are directed toward these outcomes, they become the core of evaluation to determine whether the plan has been effective.
  c. Terminating, continuing, or modifying the plan: Reviewing each step of the nursing process helps to determine whether goals have been met and whether the plan should be terminated, continued, or modified.
3. Sample answers:
  a. Patient: Is the patient motivated to learn new health behaviors?
  b. Nurse: Do the nurses come to work well rested and ready to help their patients?
  c. Healthcare system: Is a healthy nurse-to-patient ratio important to the institution?
4. The nurse should reevaluate each preceding step of the nursing process for accuracy. After this is done, it may become necessary to collect new assessment data, add or revise diagnoses, modify or rewrite patient goals/outcomes, and change the nursing orders. In addition, patient evaluations may have to be targeted more frequently.
5. a. Structure: An audit focused on the environment in which care is provided. Evaluation is based on physical facilities and equipment, organizational characteristics, policies and procedures, fiscal resources, and personnel resources.
  b. Process: An audit that focuses on the nature and sequence of activities carried out by the nurse implementing the nursing process. Evaluation is based on acceptable levels of performance of nursing actions related to patient assessment, diagnosis, planning, implementation, and evaluation.
  c. Outcome: Outcome evaluations focus on measurable and demonstrable changes in the health status of the patient or the results of nursing care.
6. a. Delete or modify the nursing diagnosis: After evaluating the data, the nurse may decide the nursing diagnosis is inadequate and delete or change the diagnosis.
  b. Make the goal statement more realistic: The nurse should determine the effectiveness of the goal and adjust the goal to meet the patient's needs.

c. Adjust time criteria in the goal statement: If the time period was too short to accomplish the goal, it may need to be extended.

d. Change nursing interventions: Reevaluate the nursing interventions and change the ones that were ineffective; tailor the interventions to the patient's needs.

7. Answers will vary with student's experiences.

8. a. Nurses measure patient outcome achievement.

b. Nurses measure how effectively nurses help targeted groups of patients to achieve their specific goals.

c. Nurses measure the competence of individual nurses.

d. Nurses measure the degree to which external factors, such as different types of healthcare services, specialized equipment or procedures, or socioeconomic factors, influence health and wellness.

REFLECTIVE PRACTICE USING CRITICAL THINKING SKILLS

Sample Answers

1. What should be the focus of an evaluation of Ms. Otsuki's nursing care plan conducted by the home healthcare nurse?

The nurse should evaluate Ms. Otsuki's understanding of, and compliance with, the medication regime, since she admits to taking a double dose of diuretics related to confusion with brand/generic prescriptions. A secondary concern would be if Ms. Otsuki is capable of living by herself with only a daily visit from her daughter.

2. What would be a successful outcome for this patient? By next visit, Ms. Otsuki states the dosages and frequency of administration of the drugs she is taking. By next visit, Ms. Otsuki verbalizes that she feels comfortable with the medication administration and is receiving help with home management from her daughter/social services.

3. What intellectual, technical, interpersonal, and/or ethical/legal competencies are most likely to bring about the desired outcome?

Intellectual: ability to incorporate knowledge of assessment, diagnosing, planning, and implementing nursing care when evaluating care for an elderly patient taking too much prescribed medication

Technical: ability to use a documentation system competently to record the patient's progress toward outcome achievement

Interpersonal: ability to identify and respond to the changing needs of patient experiencing different alterations in health status

Ethical/Legal: commitment to evaluating patient achievement of outcomes in a timely fashion and to addressing whatever is interfering with outcome achievement within the scope of nursing practice

4. What resources might be helpful for Ms. Otsuki? Social services, community services, printed materials on the drugs she is taking, compartmentalized pill boxes

CHAPTER 17

PRACTICING FOR NCLEX
MULTIPLE CHOICE QUESTIONS

1. d	**2.** d	**3.** c	**4.** a	**5.** b
6. b	**7.** c	**8.** a	**9.** c	

ALTERNATE-FORMAT QUESTIONS
Multiple Response Questions

1. a, d, f
2. a, b, e
3. c, d, f
4. b, d, e
5. a, b, e, f
6. c, d, e

Hot Spot Question
See figures below.

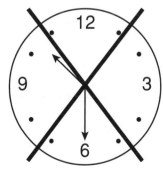 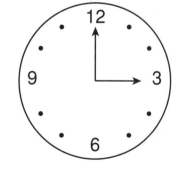 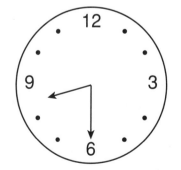

DEVELOPING YOUR KNOWLEDGE BASE

FILL-IN-THE-BLANKS

1. Patient record
2. Variance
3. Minimum data sets
4. Outcome and assessment information set
5. Resident assessment instrument (RAI)
6. Change-of-shift report
7. Incident report
8. Nursing care conference

MATCHING EXERCISES

1. c	**2.** f	**3.** i	**4.** e	**5.** h
6. a	**7.** g	**8.** b	**9.** j	**10.** k

SHORT ANSWER

1. a. Nursing care data related to patient assessments
   b. Nursing diagnoses or patient needs
   c. Nursing interventions
   d. Patient outcomes
2. a. Change-of-shift reports: Given by a primary nurse to the nurse replacing him/her or by the charge nurse to the nurse who assumes responsibility for continuing care of the patient. Can be written, oral, or audiotaped.
   b. Telephone reports: Telephones can link healthcare professionals immediately and enable nurses to receive and give critical information about patients in a timely fashion.
   c. Telephone orders: Policy must be followed regarding telephone orders; they must be transcribed on an order sheet and co-signed by the physician within a set time.
   d. Transfer and discharge reports: Nurses report a summary of a patient's condition and care when transferring or discharging patients.
   e. Reports to family members and significant others: Nurses must keep the patient's family and significant others updated about the patient's condition and progress toward goal achievement.
   f. Incident reports: A tool used by healthcare agencies to document the occurrence of anything out of the ordinary that results in or has the potential to result in harm to a patient, employee, or visitor.
   g. Conferring about care: To consult with someone to exchange ideas or to seek information, advice, or instructions.
   h. Consultations and referrals: When nurses detect problems they cannot resolve because they lie outside the scope of independent nursing practice, they make referrals to other professionals.
   i. Nursing care conference: Nurses and other healthcare professionals frequently confer in groups to plan and coordinate patient care.
   j. Nursing care rounds: Procedures in which a group of nurses visit selected patients individually at each patient's bedside to gather information, evaluate nursing care, and provide the patient with an opportunity to discuss his/her care.
3. a. Communication: The patient record helps healthcare professionals from different disciplines who interact with the same patient at different times to communicate with one another.
   b. Care planning: Each professional working with the patient has access to the patient's baseline and updated data and can see how he/she is responding to the treatment plan from day to day. Modifications of the plan are based on these data.
   c. Quality review: Charts may be reviewed to evaluate the quality of nursing care and the competence of the nurses providing that care.
   d. Research: The record may be studied by researchers to determine the most effective way to recognize or treat specific health problems.
   e. Decision analysis: Information from records review often provides the data needed by strategic planners to identify needs and the means and strategies most likely to address these needs.
   f. Education: Healthcare professionals and students reading a patient's chart can learn a great deal about the clinical manifestations of health problems, effective treatment modalities, and factors that affect patient goal achievement.
   g. Legal documentation: Patient records are legal documents that may be entered into court proceedings as evidence and play an important role in implicating or absolving health practitioners charged with improper care.
   h. Reimbursement: Patient records are used to demonstrate to payers that patients received the care for which reimbursement is being sought.
   i. Historical document: Because the notations in patient records are dated, they provide a chronologic account of services provided.
4. a. Nurses should identify themselves and the patient and state their relationship to the patient.
   b. Nurses should report concisely and accurately the change in the patient's condition and what has already been done in response to this change.
   c. Nurses should report the patient's current vital signs and clinical manifestations.
   d. Nurses should have the patient record at hand so that knowledgeable responses can be made to the physician's inquiries.
   e. Nurses should record concisely the time and date of the call, what was said to the physician, and the physician's response.
5. a. Residents respond to individualized care.
   b. Staff communication becomes more effective.
   c. Resident and family involvement increases.
   d. Documentation becomes clear.

6. See table below.

Documentation Method	Description/Advantages/Disadvantages
SOURCE-ORIENTED RECORD	Each healthcare group keeps data on its own separate form. Notations are entered chronologically, with most recent entry being nearest the front of the record. **Advantages:** Each discipline can easily find and chart pertinent data. **Disadvantages:** Data are fragmented, making it difficult to track problems chronologically with input from different groups of professionals.
PROBLEM-ORIENTED MEDICAL RECORDS	Organized around a patient's problems; contributes collaboratively to plan of care. SOAP is used to organize data entries in the progress notes. **Advantages:** Entire healthcare team works together in identifying a master list of patient problems and contributes collaboratively to plan of care. **Disadvantages:** Some nurses believe that SOAP method focuses too narrowly on problems and advocates a return to the traditional narrative format.
PIE—PROBLEM, INTERVENTION, EVALUATION	Unique in that it does not develop a plan of care; the plan of care is incorporated into the progress notes in which problems are identified by a number. A complete assessment is performed and documented at the beginning of each shift. **Advantages:** It promotes continuity of care and saves time since there is no separate plan of care. **Disadvantages:** Nurses need to read all the nursing notes to determine problems and planned interventions before initiating care.
FOCUS CHARTING	Its purpose is to bring the focus of care back to the patient and the patient's concerns. A focus column is used that incorporates many aspects of a patient and patient care. The focus may be a patient strength, problem, or need. **Advantages:** Holistic emphasis on the patient and patient's priorities; ease of charting. **Disadvantages:** Some nurses report that DAR categories (Data, Action, Response), are artificial and not helpful when documenting care.
CHARTING BY EXCEPTION	Shorthand documentation method that makes use of well-defined standards of practice; only significant findings or "exceptions" to these standards are documented in the narrative notes. **Advantages:** Decreased charting time, greater emphasis on significant data, easy retrieval of significant data, timely bedside charting, standardized assessment, greater communication, better tracking of important responses and lower costs. **Disadvantages:** None noted.
CASE MANAGEMENT MODEL	Interdisciplinary documentation tools clearly identify those outcomes that select groups of patients are expected to achieve on each day of care. Collaborative pathway is part of a computerized system that integrates the collaborative pathway and documentation flowsheets designed to match each day's expected outcomes. **Advantages:** Reduced charting time by 40% and increased staff satisfaction with the amount of paperwork from 0–85%. **Disadvantages:** Works best for "typical" patients with few individualized needs.
VARIANCE CHARTING	Variances from the plan are documented; for example, when a patient fails to meet an expected outcome or a planned intervention is not implemented in the case management model. **Advantages:** Decreased charting time; only variances are charted. **Disadvantages:** Loss of individualized care.
COMPUTERIZED RECORDS	Comprehensive computer systems have revolutionized nursing documentation in the patient record. **Advantages:** The nurse can call up the admission assessment tool and key in the patient data, develop the plan of care using computerized care plans, add new data to the patient data base, receive a work list showing treatments, procedures and medications, and document care immediately. **Disadvantages:** Policies should specify what type of patient information can be retrieved, by whom, and for what purpose (privacy).

REFLECTIVE PRACTICE USING CRITICAL THINKING SKILLS

Sample Answers

1. What should be the focus of discharge teaching for Mr. Baron and his wife?

   The nurse should provide a report of Mr. Baron's condition and care that concisely summarizes all the patient data that his wife will need to provide immediate care. In this case, Mr. Baron's medication administration and any follow-up appointments should be discussed and written in the discharge summary.

2. What would be a successful outcome for this patient?

   Mr. Baron and his wife describe the medication dosage and frequency and state the date and time of a follow-up appointment

3. What intellectual, technical, interpersonal, and/or ethical/legal competencies are most likely to bring about the desired outcome?

   Intellectual: knowledge of colonoscopy as a diagnostic measure and need for follow-up
   Interpersonal: ability to demonstrate that what matters is communicating the plan of care so that coordination of care is achieved
   Ethical/Legal: ability to incorporate ethical and legal principles that guide decision making related to a patient needing discharge teaching

4. What resources might be helpful for Mr. Baron?

   Discharge teaching including medication administration and follow-up appointments

CHAPTER 18

PRACTICING FOR NCLEX

MULTIPLE CHOICE QUESTIONS

1. a   2. d   3. a   4. a   5. b
6. c   7. c   8. d   9. d

ALTERNATE-FORMAT QUESTIONS

Multiple Response Questions

1. c, e, f
2. b, d, e
3. a, b, e
4. c, d, e
5. a, c, f

Prioritization Questions

1.

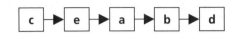

2.

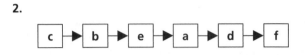

DEVELOPING YOUR KNOWLEDGE BASE

FILL-IN-THE-BLANKS

1. Proximodistal development
2. Genital
3. James Fowler
4. Middle adult years
5. Libido
6. Assimilation
7. Formal operational
8. Individual life structure

MATCHING EXERCISES

1. d	2. a	3. f	4. e	5. h
6. e	7. g	8. c	9. b	10. g
11. e	12. c	13. f	14. a	15. d
16. b				

CORRECT THE FALSE STATEMENTS

1. True
2. False—regular and predictable
3. False—different
4. False—sexuality
5. False—id
6. True
7. True
8. False—preconventional level, stage 1, punishment and obedience orientation
9. False—29 to 34

SHORT ANSWER

1. See table below.

Theorist and Theory	Basic Concepts of Theory	Stages of Development
EXAMPLE **Sigmund Freud** Psychoanalytic theory	Stressed the impact of instinctual drives on determining behavior: Unconscious mind, the id, the ego, the superego, stages of development based on sexual motivation.	Oral stage Anal stage Phallic stage Latent stage Genital stage
Eric Erikson Psychosocial theory	Based on Freud, expanded to include cultural and social influences in addition to biologic processes: (1) stages of development, (2) developmental goals or tasks, (3) psychosocial crises, (4) process of coping	Trust vs. mistrust Autonomy vs. shame/doubt Initiative vs. guilt Industry vs. inferiority Identity vs. role confusion Intimacy vs. isolation Generativity vs. stagnation Ego integrity vs. despair
Robert J. Havighurst Developmental tasks	Living and growing are based on learning; person must continually learn to adjust to changing social conditions, developmental tasks	Infancy and early childhood Middle childhood Adolescence Young adulthood Middle adulthood Later maturity
Jean Piaget Cognitive development	Learning occurs as result of internal organization of an event, which forms a mental schemata and serves as a base for further schemata as one grows and develops.	Sensorimotor stage Preoperational stage Concrete operational stage Formal operational stage
Lawrence Kohlberg Moral development	Levels closely follow Piaget's; preconventional level, conventional level, postconventional level; moral development influenced by cultural effects on perceptions of justice or interpersonal relationships	Preconventional level Stage 1: punishment and obedience orientation Stage 2: instrumental relativist orientation conventional level Stage 3: "good boy–good girl" orientation Stage 4: "law and order" orientation Postconventional level Stage 5: social contract, utilitarian orientation Stage 6: universal ethical principle orientation
Carol Gilligan Moral development	Conception of morality from female point of view (ethic of care); selfishness, goodness, nonviolence; female: morality of response and care; male: morality of justice.	Level 1—selfishness Level 2—goodness Level 3—nonviolence
James Fowler Faith development	Theory of spiritual identity of humans; faith is reason one finds life worth living; six stages of faith.	Intuitive–projective faith Mythical–literal faith Synthetic–conventional faith Individuative–reflective faith Conjunctive faith Universalizing faith

2. a. Preconventional level: Follows intuitive thought and is based on external control as child learns to conform to rules imposed by authority figures. Example: Child learns that he will be sent to his room if he writes on the walls.

   b. Conventional level: This level is obtained when person becomes concerned with identifying with significant others and shows conformity to their expectations. Example: A college student gets all A's in college so his parents will think he is a good son.

   c. Postconventional level: This level is associated with moral judgment that is rational and internalized into one's standards or values. Example: A bank teller resists the urge to steal money from a patient's account because it is against the law.

3. Sample answers:

   a. Freud: The 6-year-old is between the phallic and latency stage and will be experiencing increased interest in gender differences and conflict and resolution of that conflict with parent of same sex.

   b. Erikson: The 6-year-old is becoming achievement oriented, and the acceptance of parents and peers is paramount.

   c. Havighurst: The 6-year-old is ready to learn the developmental tasks of developing physical skills, wholesome attitudes toward self, getting along with peers, sexual roles, conscience, morality, personal independence, and so on. An illness could stall these processes.

   d. Piaget: The 6-year-old is in the preoperational stage, including increased language skills and play activities allowing child to better understand life events and relationships.

   e. Kohlberg: Moral development is influenced by cultural effects on perceptions of justice in interpersonal relationships. Moral development begins in early childhood and could be affected by a traumatic illness.

   f. Gilligan: Females develop a morality of response and care, level one being selfishness: a woman may tend to isolate herself to avoid getting hurt.

   g. Fowler: The 6-year-old is in stage 1—intuitive–projective faith. Children imitate the religious gestures and behaviors of others, primarily their parents, without a thorough understanding of them.

4. a. Superego

   b. Identity vs. role confusion

   c. Formal operations stage

   d. Synthetic–conventional faith

5. Sample answer:
The family plays a vital role in wellness promotion and illness prevention. Family values and cultural heritage influence interpretation of illness. A health problem of any family member can affect the remainder of the unit. Many health practices are shared by the family. Sometimes the family may be the cause of illness.

REFLECTIVE PRACTICE USING CRITICAL THINKING SKILLS

Sample Answers

1. What developmental considerations may affect care planning for Mr. Logan?
According to Havighurst, the developmental tasks of later adulthood include adjusting to decreasing physical strength and health, adjusting to retirement and reduced income, and establishing physical living arrangements. The nurse should assess Mr. Logan's self-esteem needs related to his feelings of dependency on healthcare providers and his family. The nurse could then base the nursing plan of care on interventions to foster feelings of personal dignity and worth.

2. What would be a successful outcome for this patient?
Mr. Logan states that he is willing to participate in his care plan and do everything in his power to adjust to his situation by accepting the assistance of others when necessary

3. What intellectual, technical, interpersonal, and/or ethical/legal competencies are most likely to bring about the desired outcome?
Intellectual: ability to apply knowledge of developmental theories to nurse care planning
Technical: ability to provide technical nursing assistance to Mr. Logan as needed
Interpersonal: ability to use therapeutic communication to meet the emotional and spiritual needs of Mr. Logan
Ethical/Legal: ability to advocate for the unmet developmental needs of Mr. Logan

4. What resources might be helpful for Mr. Logan and his family?
Home healthcare services, community services, support groups

CHAPTER 19

PRACTICING FOR NCLEX

MULTIPLE CHOICE QUESTIONS

1. c	**2.** a	**3.** b	**4.** b	**5.** c
6. b	**7.** b	**8.** b	**9.** a	**10.** c
11. c	**12.** b	**13.** d		

ALTERNATE-FORMAT QUESTIONS

Multiple Response Questions

1. a, d, e, f
2. b, c, e
3. b, d, e
4. a, b, e
5. a, c, e, f
6. a, b, f

Chart/Exhibit Questions

1. 7
2. 3
3. 10

DEVELOPING YOUR KNOWLEDGE BASE

FILL-IN-THE-BLANKS

1. Endoderm, mesoderm, ectoderm
2. Embryonic
3. Apgar rating scale
4. Bonding
5. Failure to thrive (FTT)
6. Sudden infant death syndrome (SIDS)
7. Denver Developmental Screening Test (DDST)

MATCHING EXERCISES

1. f	**2.** d	**3.** d	**4.** f	**5.** a
6. c	**7.** b	**8.** e		

SHORT ANSWER

1. Age group—Physiologic characteristics and behaviors
   P—Motor abilities include skipping, throwing and catching, copying figures, and printing letters and numbers.
   A—Puberty begins.
   I—Brain grows to about half the adult size
   N—Reflexes include sucking, swallowing, blinking, sneezing, and yawning
   N—Temperature control responds quickly to environmental temperatures
   T—Walks forward and backward, runs, kicks, climbs, and rides tricycle
   T—Drinks from a cup and uses a spoon
   A—Sebaceous and axillary sweat glands become active
   S—Height increases 2 to 3 inches, weight increases 3 to 6 lbs a year
   A—The feet, hands, and long bones grow rapidly; muscle mass increases.
   N—Alert to environment, sees color and form, hears and turns to sound
   I—Birth weight usually triples.
   P—Full set of 20 deciduous teeth; baby teeth fall out and are replaced.
   P—Body is less chubby and becomes leaner and more coordinated.
   A—Primary and secondary development occurs with maturation of genitals.
   T—Typically four times the birth weight and 23 to 37 inches in height
   I—Body temperature stabilizes.
   P—Average weight is 45 lbs.
   S—Brain reaches 90% to 95% of adult size; nervous system almost mature.
   P—Head is close to adult size.
   I—Motor abilities develop, allowing feeding self, crawling, and walking.
   N—Can smell and taste and is sensitive to touch and pain
   N—Begins to eliminate stool and urine
   I—Deciduous teeth begin to erupt.
   S—All permanent teeth present except for second and third molars
   T—Attains bladder control during the day and sometimes during the night
   S—Holds a pencil and eventually writes in script and sentences
   A—Full adult size is reached.
   N—Drinks breast milk, glucose water, and plain water
   I—Eyes begin to focus and fixate.
   T—Turns pages in a book and by age 3 draws stick people
   I—Heart doubles in weight, heart rate slows, blood pressure rises.
   T—Rapid brain growth; increase in length of long bones of the arms and legs.
   T—Uses fingers to pick up small objects
   S—Sexual organs grow but are dormant until late in this period.

2. Age group—Psychosocial characteristics and behaviors
   I—Is in oral stage (Freud); strives for immediate gratification of needs; strong sucking need.
   S—Developmental task of learning appropriate sex's social role
   A—In Freud's genital stage, libido reemerges in mature form.
   T—Is in anal stage (Freud); focus on pleasure of sphincter control
   A—Self-concept is being stabilized, with peer group as greatest influence.
   I—Develops trust (Erikson) if caregiver is dependable to meet needs
   S—Achieves personal independence; develops conscience, morality, and scale of values
   A—Tries out different roles, personal choices, and beliefs (identity versus role confusion)
   I—Meets developmental tasks (Havighurst) by learning to eat, walk, and talk
   S—Develops skill in reading, writing, and calculating, as well as concepts for everyday living
   A—More mature relationships with both males and females of same age
   T—Enters Erikson's stage of autonomy versus shame and doubt
   P—Is in Erikson's stage of initiative versus guilt
   A—Inner turmoil/examination of propriety of actions by rigid conscience
   P—Getting ready to read and learning to distinguish right from wrong
   A—One's personal appearance accepted; set of values internalized
   S—Freud's latency stage—strong identification with own sex
   T—Developmental tasks of learning to control elimination; begins to learn sex differences, concepts, learn language, learn right from wrong
   P—Focus on learning useful skills with an emphasis on doing, succeeding, and accomplishing
   P—Developmental tasks of describing social and physical reality through concept formation and language development
   P—Is in phallic stage (Freud) with biologic focus on genitals
   A—Superego and conscience begin to develop

P—Developmental tasks of learning sex differences and modesty

S—Developmental task of learning physical game skills

S—Is in Erikson's industry versus inferiority stage

3. **a.** Preembryonic stage: Lasts about 3 weeks; zygote implants in the uterine wall and has three distinct cell layers: ectoderm, endoderm, and mesoderm.

b. Embryonic stage: fourth through eighth week; rapid growth and differentiation of the germ cell layers, all basic organs established, bones ossify, and human features are recognizable.

c. Fetal stage: 9 weeks to birth; continued growth and development of all body organs and systems take place.

4. **a.** Gross motor behavior and skills

b. Fine motor behavior and skills

c. Language acquisition

d. Personal and social interaction

5. Sample answers:

a. Infant sleeps, eats, and eliminates easily; smiles spontaneously; cries in response to significant needs.

b. Infant is more passive and distant than the "easy" infant.

c. Infant has volatile and labile responses, often is restless sleeper, is highly sensitive to noises and eats poorly.

6. **a.** Colic is acute abdominal pain caused by spasmodic contractions of the intestine during the first 3 months of life. The nurse should educate the parents about colic and teach them measures to help relieve the symptoms.

b. Failure to thrive is a condition thought to be related to a disturbed interaction between the infant and the primary caregiver that results in severely inadequate physiologic development. Underlying physical causes should be ruled out first; if the cause is psychosocial, specialized health interventions are warranted.

c. Sudden infant death syndrome is the sudden, unexpected death of an infant or young child in which a postmortem examination fails to reveal a cause of death. Parents should be aware that the highest incidence occurs in families who are poor or live in crowded housing in cold months of the year during sleep periods. Maternal health, smoking, and nutrition are being investigated; infants should sleep on their side or back.

d. Child abuse is the intentional, nonaccidental, physical, or sexual abuse of a child by a parent or other caregiver. Healthcare professionals must recognize and report abuse of children and provide interventions for high-risk families.

7. Sample answers:

a. Toddler: A toddler begins to understand object permanence, following simple commands, and anticipating events. The perception of body image begins, and the toddler uses short sentences. The nurse should be aware that the toddler may experience separation anxiety; parents should be included in the preparation; language should be clear and simple.

b. Preschooler: A preschooler may have fear of pain and body mutilation as well as separation anxiety that must be recognized by the nurse. The child needs much reassurance and parental support. A preprocedure visit should be scheduled if possible; allowing the child to practice on a doll may be helpful.

c. School-aged child: Body image, self-concept, and sexuality are interrelated. The school-aged child has well-developed language skills and ability to store information in long-term memory. The procedure should be explained clearly and thoroughly to child and caregivers.

d. Adolescent and young adult: The adolescent tries out different roles, personal choices, and beliefs in the stage called identity versus role confusion. Self-concept is being stabilized, with the peer group acting as the influential body. The nurse should be aware of the adolescent's need to understand the procedure and its benefits/risks.

8. Sample answers:

a. Infant: The most important role of the nurse is the prevention of illness and promotion of wellness through teaching family members. Teaching may range from scheduling immunizations to counseling parents who have a baby born with AIDS.

b. Toddler: The role of the nurse is in wellness promotion, helping caregivers find the means of helping toddlers through encouraging independence while setting firm limits. Safety measures for parents of active toddlers should be taught.

c. Preschooler: Promoting wellness continues for the preschooler, with emphasis on teaching accident prevention and safety, infection control, dental hygiene, and play habits and encouraging self-esteem.

d. School-aged child: Areas of concern for school-aged children are traffic, bicycle, and water safety. Substance abuse teaching should be included, and communicable conditions should be discussed. Nurses should work with parents and teachers to recognize mental health disorders and to encourage physical fitness and positive self-identity.

e. Adolescent and young adult: Nurses should educate adolescents and family members about substance abuse, motor vehicle accidents, nutrition, and sex. Nurses and parents should be aware of the adolescent's need to belong to a peer group, be like everyone else, and try on different roles.

9. **a.** Prepubescence: Secondary sex characteristics begin to develop, but the reproductive organs do not yet function.

b. Pubescence: Secondary sex characteristics continue to develop, and ova and sperm begin to be produced by the reproductive organs.

c. Postpubescence: Reproductive functioning and secondary sex characteristics reach adult maturity.

REFLECTIVE PRACTICE USING CRITICAL THINKING SKILLS
Sample Answers

1. What should be the focus of the nursing care plan developed for Ms. Leming?

The immediate focus should be the health habits of the mother and their effect on the fetus. Ms. Leming's nursing care plan should include patient teaching regarding the detrimental effects of smoking and drinking alcohol on the fetus, and the necessity to control nausea and eat a proper diet. Ms. Leming could benefit from a referral to counseling and/or social services.

2. What would be a successful outcome for this patient?

By end of visit, Ms. Leming states that she values her health and the health of her fetus enough to stop smoking and drinking alcohol.

By next visit, Ms. Leming reports that her nausea is under control and she is able to eat three healthy meals a day.

3. What intellectual, technical, interpersonal, and/or ethical/legal competencies are most likely to bring about the desired outcome?

Intellectual: knowledge of the developmental needs of fetuses and the effects of maternal behaviors, such as smoking and alcohol consumption on the fetus

Technical: ability to provide the technical nursing assistance necessary to assess and meet the needs of a pregnant woman and her fetus

Interpersonal: ability to demonstrate nonjudgmental attitude when interacting in potentially emotionally charged situations, such as a high-risk pregnancy

Ethical/Legal: knowledge of the nurse's legal and ethical obligations in cases of maternal–fetal conflict

4. What resources might be helpful for Ms. Leming?

Counseling services, social services, community services, support groups, printed materials on healthy pregnancy behaviors

CHAPTER 20

PRACTICING FOR NCLEX
MULTIPLE CHOICE QUESTIONS

1. c	**2.** a	**3.** d	**4.** b	**5.** c
6. a	**7.** d	**8.** b	**9.** b	

ALTERNATE-FORMAT QUESTIONS
Multiple Response Questions

1. c, e, f
2. a, c, d, e
3. a, b, e, f
4. c, d, e
5. a, c, f

DEVELOPING YOUR KNOWLEDGE BASE
FILL-IN-THE-BLANKS

1. Cross-linkage
2. 40 to 65 years
3. Sandwich generation
4. 60 to 74, 75 to 84, 85 and older
5. Ageism
6. Identity-continuity
7. Life review, reminiscence
8. Alzheimer's disease
9. Reality orientation
10. Gerontology

SHORT ANSWER

1. a. Middle adulthood:

Physiologic development: The early years are marked by maximum physical development and functioning. As time passes, gradual internal and external changes occur.

Psychosocial development: Usually a time of increased personal freedom, economic stability, social relationships, increased responsibility, and awareness of one's own mortality

Cognitive, moral, and spiritual development: Intellectual abilities change from those of the young adult. There is increased motivation to learn. Problem-solving abilities remain, although response time may be slightly longer.

b. Older adulthood:

Physiologic development: The process of aging becomes more rapid. All organ systems undergo some degree of decline, and the body becomes less efficient.

Psychosocial development: Most continue their activities from middle adulthood and adapt intuitively to gradual limitations of aging.

Cognitive, moral, and spiritual development: Cognition does not change appreciably with aging; an older adult continues to learn and solve problems, and intelligence and personality remain consistent.

2. Sample answers:

a. Complete physical examination every 2 years
b. Annual dental examination
c. Eye examination every 1 to 2 years
d. Maintenance of current immunizations
e. Cancer screening for women

3. a. Genetic theory: Explains that life span depends to a great extent on genetic factors

b. Immunity theory: Focuses on the functions of the immune system, which declines steadily after young adulthood

c. Cross-linkage theory: As one ages, cross-links accumulate, leading to essential molecules in the cell binding together and interfering with normal cell function.

d. Free radical theory: Free radicals formed during cellular metabolism are molecules with separated high-energy electrons that can have adverse effects on and attack adjacent molecules.

e. Disengagement theory: Maintains that an older adult withdraws from societal interactions because it is mutually desired and satisfying for both the individual and society

f. Activity theory: Successful aging involves the ability to maintain high levels of activity and functioning.

g. Identity-continuity theory: Assumes that healthy aging is related to the ability of the older adult to continue similar patterns of behavior that existed in young to middle adulthood

4. Alzheimer's disease affects brain cells and is characterized by patchy areas of the brain that degenerate, or break down. At first, forgetfulness and impaired judgment may be evident; over a period of several years, the person becomes progressively more confused, forgetting family and becoming disoriented in familiar surroundings.

5. a. Integumentary: Wrinkling and sagging of skin occur with decreased skin elasticity; dryness and scaling are common.

   b. Musculoskeletal: Muscle mass and strength decrease.

   c. Neurologic: Temperature regulation and pain perception become less efficient.

   d. Cardiopulmonary: The body is less able to increase heart rate and cardiac output with activity.

   e. Gastrointestinal: Malnutrition and anemia become more common.

   f. Genitourinary: Blood flow to the kidneys decreases with diminished cardiac output.

REFLECTIVE PRACTICE USING CRITICAL THINKING SKILLS

Sample Answers

1. How might the nurse use blended nursing skills to provide holistic, developmentally sensitive care for Mr. and Mrs. Jenkins?
   The nurse should aim to facilitate the Jenkins' achievement of the developmental tasks of older adulthood, such as, adjusting to the changes of older adulthood and retirement, relating to one's age group, maintaining social roles, and continuing moral and spiritual development. The Jenkins would benefit from a referral to community services, such as physical fitness programs and social clubs designed for older adults.

2. What would be a successful outcome for this patient?
   By next visit, Mr. Jenkins will report being involved in social and physical activities and drinking less.

3. What intellectual, technical, interpersonal, and/or ethical/legal competencies are most likely to bring about the desired outcome?
   Intellectual: knowledge of the theories of aging as they relate to the changes faced by the aging adult
   Technical: ability to adapt necessary skills and techniques to address the changes associated with the aging adult

Interpersonal: ability to establish trusting professional relationships with adult patients of different ages, respecting their developmental needs
Ethical/Legal: ability to practice in an ethically and legally defensible manner, maintaining the rights of the aging adult

4. What resources might be helpful for Mr. and Mrs. Jenkins?
   Community services, social networks, physical fitness programs, nutrition classes

CHAPTER 21

PRACTICING FOR NCLEX
MULTIPLE CHOICE QUESTIONS

1. d	**2.** a	**3.** b	**4.** a	**5.** c
6. c	**7.** d	**8.** d	**9.** c	**10.** c

ALTERNATE-FORMAT QUESTIONS
Multiple Response Questions

1. a, b, d
2. b, c, f
3. b, d, f
4. c, e, f
5. a, c, f
6. c, e, f
7. a, c, f
8. c, d, e

DEVELOPING YOUR KNOWLEDGE BASE
FILL-IN-THE-BLANKS

1. Stimulus
2. Channel
3. Feedback
4. Nonverbal
5. Helping
6. Orientation
7. Validating
8. Horizontal violence

MATCHING EXERCISES

1. b	**2.** d	**3.** g	**4.** a	**5.** c
6. e	**7.** b	**8.** c	**9.** a	**10.** a
11. c	**12.** b	**13.** c	**14.** a	**15.** b
16. b	**17.** c	**18.** a	**19.** e	**20.** d
21. c				

SHORT ANSWER

1. Sample answers:
   a. Touch: The nurse gently squeezes a patient's hand before surgery. The patient's response to this touch may express fear, gratitude, acceptance, and so on.
   b. Eye contact: A patient avoids eye contact. The patient may be expressing defenselessness or avoidance of communication.
   c. Facial expressions: A patient grimaces when looking at his surgical incision. The patient

may be experiencing anxiety over the alteration in his/her physical appearance.

d. Posture: A patient stands erect with good body alignment. The patient may be experiencing good health.

e. Gait: A patient walks slightly bent over. The patient may be accommodating an illness.

f. Gestures: A patient gives you a thumbs-up sign after receiving test results. The patient is most likely happy with the results.

g. General physical appearance: A patient is sweating and having difficulty breathing. The patient may be experiencing a life-threatening condition.

h. Mode of dress and grooming: A patient who has been bedridden for a week asks to take a shower and get dressed. The patient is probably feeling better.

i. Sounds: A patient sighs whenever you mention her significant other. The patient may be experiencing difficulty with this relationship.

j. Silence: A patient who has undergone a mastectomy remains silent when asked how she is feeling. The patient may be overwhelmed with emotion and unable to express her feelings.

2. Sample answers:

a. An 8-year-old boy: An 8-year-old has limited understanding of surgical procedures. Therefore, the nurse must explain the procedure in simple terms so that the child will cooperate without being frightened.

b. A 16-year-old girl: Adolescents are developing their ability to think abstractly and can understand fairly detailed descriptions of clinical procedures.

c. A 65-year-old man with a hearing impairment: The nurse should talk directly to the patient while facing him. When necessary, nonverbal communication should be used (e.g., sign language or finger spelling, or by writing any ideas that cannot be conveyed in another manner).

3. Occupation may reveal a person's abilities, talents, interests, and economic status.

4. a. Assessing: Verbal and nonverbal communication are essential nursing tools because the major focus of patient assessment is information gathering. Written words, patient records, spoken words, and observational skills are employed.

b. Diagnosing: Once a nurse formulates a diagnosis, it must be communicated through the spoken and written word to other nurses as well as to the patient.

c. Planning: The patient, nurse, and other healthcare team members must communicate with each other as patient goals and outcomes are developed and interventions selected.

d. Implementing: Verbal and nonverbal communication allows nurses to enhance basic caregiving measures and to teach, counsel, and support patients and their families.

e. Evaluating: Nurses often rely on the verbal and nonverbal clues they receive from their patients to determine whether patient objectives or goals have been achieved.

f. Documenting: The documentation of data promotes the continuity of care given by nurses and other healthcare providers.

5. a. Having specific objectives: Having a purpose for an interaction guides the nurse toward achieving a meaningful encounter with the patient.

b. Providing a comfortable environment: A comfortable environment in which the patient and nurse are at ease helps to promote meaningful interactions. Relationships are enhanced when the atmosphere is relaxed and unhurried.

c. Providing privacy: Every effort should be made to provide privacy during nurse–patient conversations.

d. Maintaining confidentiality: The patient should know his/her right to specify who may have access to clinical or personal information.

e. Maintaining patient focus: Communication in the nurse–patient relationship should focus on the patient and the patient's needs, not on the nurse or an activity in which the nurse is engaged.

f. Using nursing observations: Observation is especially valuable in validating information and helping the nurse become aware of the patient's nonverbal communication. It also demonstrates the nurse's caring and interest in the patient.

g. Using optimal pacing: The nurse must consider the pace of any conversation or encounter with a patient and let the patient set the pace.

h. Providing personal space: Nurses must try to determine each patient's perception of personal space; invasion of this zone can evoke uncomfortable feelings.

i. Developing therapeutic communication skills: Nurses must train and practice using therapeutic skills by controlling the tone of their voices, being knowledgeable about the topic, being flexible, being clear and concise, avoiding words that may be interpreted differently, being truthful and open minded, and taking advantage of opportunities for communicating.

j. Developing listening skills: Nurses should sit when communicating with a patient, be alert and relaxed, keep the conversation natural, maintain eye contact if culturally correct, indicate they are paying attention, think before responding to the patient, and listen for themes in the patient's comments.

k. Using silence as a tool: The nurse can use silence appropriately by taking the time to wait for the patient to initiate or continue speaking. Nurses should be aware of the different possible meanings of silence (the patient is comfortable with the nurse, the patient is demonstrating stoicism or exploring inner thoughts, the patient may be fearful, etc.).

6. Sample answers:
   a. "Tell me about the night you had."
   b. "Let's try walking on that foot now."
   c. "What things prompted you to stop taking your insulin?"
   d. "Tell me what makes you afraid of taking the test."
   e. "Your procedure has been performed successfully every time here."
   f. Should not be said at all

7. Mrs. Clarke, age 42, underwent a mastectomy. She has a husband and two children, ages 10 and 5. When the nurse enters Mrs. Clarke's room, she finds her patient's eyes are teary and there is a worried expression on her face. When asked how she is feeling, Mrs. Clarke replies "fine," although her face is rigid and her mouth is drawn in a firm line. She is moving her foot back and forth under the covers. On further investigation, the nurse finds out Mrs. Clarke is worried about her children and her own ability to be a healthy, functioning wife and mother again. After prompting, Mrs. Clarke says, "I don't know if my husband will still love me like this." She sighs and falls silent, reflecting upon her recovery. The nurse tries to make Mrs. Clarke comfortable and puts her hand over Mrs. Clarke's hand. She establishes eye contact with Mrs. Clarke and reassures her that things have a way of working out and suggests that she give her situation some time.

8. Sample answers:
   a. Orientation phase:
      1. By 8/6/12, Mr. Uhl will call Nurse Parish by her name.
      2. By 8/6/12, Mr. Uhl will describe his freedoms/responsibilities within the institute.
   b. Working phase:
      1. By 8/10/12, Mr. Uhl will list various classes/activities available to patients.
      2. By 8/10/12, Mr. Uhl will express any anxieties he may have in his new environment to the nurse.
   c. Termination phase:
      1. By 8/25/12, Mr. Uhl will be introduced to the new nurse in charge of his case by Nurse Parish, who will continue to oversee the new relationship until her departure.
      2. By 8/27/12, Mr. Uhl will report feeling good about his past care and look forward to his new relationship.

9. Sample answers:
   a. Warmth and friendliness: A nurse who greets a patient with a pleasant smile
   b. Openness: A nurse who provides an honest explanation of a procedure
   c. Empathy: A nurse who listens to a woman's lament over her miscarriage while helping her bathe

d. Competence: A nurse who competently and smoothly inserts a Hep-Lock into a patient's vein
e. Consideration of patient variables: A nurse who finds another nurse who speaks Spanish for her Hispanic patient

10. Sample answers:
    a. Empathic component: "Mr. Johnson, you've always been so independent, it must be difficult for you to accept the fact that you need medical care."
    b. Description: "Mr. Johnson, you've been diagnosed with prostate cancer. There are several options for treatment."
    c. Expectation: "Mr. Johnson, your prognosis for leading a normal life is good, but we need your cooperation to make this treatment work."
    d. Consequence: "When you are discharged on Tuesday, we'll set you up with a schedule for your radiation treatments and let you know what you can expect. I'd like to work with you to help you understand your illness and its treatments better."

11. Sample answers:
    a. Failure to perceive the patient as a human being: The nurse should focus on the whole person, not simply the illness or dysfunction.
    b. Failure to listen: Nurses should be open to opportunities for communication by keeping an open mind and focusing on the patient's needs instead of their own needs.
    c. Use of inappropriate comments or questions: The nurse should avoid certain types of comments and questions (clichés, questions that probe for information, leading questions, comments that give advice, judgmental comments) that tend to impede communication.
    d. Changing the subject: The nurse should avoid changing the subject; the patient may be ready to discuss something and may be frustrated if put off by a change in topic.
    e. Giving false assurance: The nurse should not try to convince the patient that things are going to turn out well when knowing the chances are not good. False assurance may give patients the impression the nurse is not interested in their problems.

REFLECTIVE PRACTICE USING CRITICAL THINKING SKILLS

Sample Answers

1. What communication skills might the nurse use to complete an assessment of Mrs. Russellinski?
   The nurse should orient Mrs. Russellinski to his or her presence before initiating conversation and talk directly to her while facing her. Important information should be communicated in a quiet environment where there is little to distract Mrs. Russellinski's attention and conversation should be kept simple and concrete. The nurse must be patient and give Mrs. Russellinski time to respond.

An interpreter should be called if the language barrier is too great, and attempts should be made to contact Mrs. Russellinski's daughter for information since she is listed as the contact person.

2. What would be a successful outcome for this patient? Mrs. Russellinski provides information to the nurse for the assessment and agrees to her daughter's participation in the interview.

3. What intellectual, technical, interpersonal, and/or ethical/legal competencies are most likely to bring about the desired outcome?
Intellectual: ability to incorporate knowledge of the goals and phases of helping relationships as a component of the patient's plan of care
Interpersonal: strong people skills including the ability to communicate and interact effectively with patients who have hearing or cognitive deficits
Ethical/Legal: ability to advocate for patients like Mrs. Russellinski who are unable to do so themselves due to language and hearing problems

4. What resources might be helpful for Mrs. Russellinski?
An interpreter, other family members, consultation with an audiologist

CHAPTER 22

PRACTICING FOR NCLEX
MULTIPLE CHOICE QUESTIONS
1. a **2.** c **3.** b **4.** d **5.** a
6. c **7.** b **8.** d **9.** c **10.** c

ALTERNATE-FORMAT QUESTIONS
Multiple Response Questions
1. a, c, d
2. a, b, f
3. b, e, f
4. c, d, f
5. a, e, f
6. a, c, f
7. b, c, d

DEVELOPING YOUR KNOWLEDGE BASE

FILL-IN-THE-BLANKS
1. Promoting health
2. Helping
3. Cognitive
4. Affective
5. Patients
6. Motivation
7. Evidence-based
8. Counselor

MATCHING EXERCISES
1. b **2.** a **3.** d **4.** h **5.** f
6. g **7.** e **8.** g **9.** d **10.** c
11. c **12.** b **13.** a **14.** d **15.** b
16. a **17.** d **18.** c **19.** b **20.** d
21. b **22.** a **23.** b **24.** c **25.** c
26. a

SHORT ANSWER
1. Sample answers:
   a. Promoting health: Nurses can teach/counsel patients concerning health practices that lead to a higher level of wellness.
   b. Preventing illness: Nurses can teach patients health practices that help prevent specific illnesses or dangerous situations.
   c. Restoring health: Nurses can teach patients self-care practices that will facilitate recovery.
   d. Facilitating coping: Nurses can teach patients and their families to come to terms with the patient's illness and necessary lifestyle modifications.
2. Sample answers:
   a. The sensitivity and concern of the nurse in the helping relationship are the foundation for a nonthreatening learning environment for the adult patient.
   b. Honest and open communication can provide the adult learner with a realistic preview of what will be involved and allow him/her to retain some control over what is taught.
   c. New information must be presented clearly and in amounts that patients can comprehend to prevent them from becoming discouraged or overwhelmed.
3. Sample answers:
   a. Demonstration: Take Mr. Lang through the exercises and have him demonstrate them in return.
   b. Print material: Give Mr. Lang a brochure that explicitly describes and diagrams the exercises you wish him to learn.
   c. Discussion: Have a conversation with Mr. Lang about the exercises and his desire and ability to perform them.
4. a. Content must be prioritized such that essential information is taught thoroughly and promptly and less important content is saved for last or for another time.
   b. Teamwork and cooperation allow nurses to meet deadlines for teaching. If teaching continues beyond hospitalization, the nurse can schedule additional learning opportunities through outpatient programs or referrals to community-based programs.
5. a. Formal: Planned teaching that is provided to fulfill learner objectives (e.g., viewing a film on diabetes)
   b. Informal: Unplanned teaching that represents the majority of nurse–patient interactions (e.g., a nurse showing a mother the proper way to hold an infant)
6. a. Cognitive domain: Oral questioning
   b. Affective domain: Patient's response
   c. Psychomotor domain: Return demonstration
7. A summary of the learning need, plan, implementation of the plan, and evaluated results should be documented in the patient chart. The evaluative

statement should indicate whether the patient has displayed concrete evidence of learning how to bathe her infant.

8. **a.** Short-term counseling: Situational crisis (e.g., a nurse counsels a housebound patient after a fire destroys her bedroom)
   b. Long-term counseling: Developmental crisis (e.g., a nurse counsels an adolescent about the dangers of drugs and alcohol)
   c. Motivational counseling: Discussion of feelings and incentives with the patient (e.g., a nurse counsels a woman in a shelter about leaving her abusive spouse)

9. **a.** Identifying the new knowledge, attitudes, or skills that are necessary for patients and family members to manage their healthcare
   b. Assessing learning readiness
   c. Assessing the patient's ability to learn
   d. Identifying patient strengths and personal resources the nurse can tap

10. Answers will vary with student's experiences.

11. **a.** Be certain that healthcare instructions are understandable and designed to support patient goals.
    b. Include patient and family as partners in the teaching–learning process.
    c. Use interactive teaching strategies.
    d. Remember that teaching and learning are processes that rely on strong interpersonal relationships with patients and their families.

12. **a.** Ignoring the restrictions of the patient's environment
    b. Failing to accept that patients have the right to change their mind
    c. Using medical jargon
    d. Failing to negotiate goals
    e. Duplicating teaching that other team members have done

REFLECTIVE PRACTICE USING CRITICAL THINKING SKILLS

Sample Answers

1. What should be the focus of patient teaching for this couple?
   Patient teaching should focus on health maintenance and promotion for the mother and fetus. Teaching topics might include proper nutrition including the benefits of folic acid supplements and prenatal vitamins, substances to avoid when pregnant (tobacco, alcohol, cat litter, x-rays, etc.), methods of childbirth, and parenting skills. The nurse should encourage the couple's choice of childbirth planning and provide as much information as possible on home births.

2. What would be a successful outcome for Mr. and Mrs. Ramirez?
   By next visit, Mrs. Ramirez lists the benefits of home childbirth and signs up for a parenting class

3. What intellectual, technical, interpersonal, and/or ethical/legal competencies are most likely to bring about the desired outcome?

Intellectual: knowledge of how to design an appropriate teaching program for childbirth and parenting
Interpersonal: ability to establish trusting relationships with patients to foster teaching and learning
Ethical/Legal: strong sense of accountability for the health and well-being of patients that translates into a commitment to getting patients the information they need

4. What resources might be helpful for this couple?
   Parenting classes, prenatal classes, printed and AV materials on pregnancy, childbirth, and parenting

CHAPTER 23

PRACTICING FOR NCLEX
MULTIPLE CHOICE QUESTIONS

1. a	2. c	3. b	4. c	5. b
6. a				

ALTERNATE-FORMAT QUESTIONS
Multiple Response Questions

1. c, e, f
2. a, c, f
3. b, c, d
4. a, b, f
5. b, d, f
6. c, d, f

DEVELOPING YOUR KNOWLEDGE BASE

FILL-IN-THE-BLANKS

1. Explicit
2. Autocratic
3. Democratic
4. Quantum
5. Power
6. Mentorship

MATCHING EXERCISES

1. d	2. b	3. a	4. d	5. e
6. c	7. b	8. c	9. a	10. a
11. f				

SHORT ANSWER

1. Answers will vary with student's experiences.
2. Sample answers:
   a. Communication skills: The nurse explains to Mr. Eng that she realizes he is in a lot of pain, and she will be available to administer medication if he feels he needs more pain relief.
   b. Problem-solving skills: When the nurse learns that Mr. Eng's pain is not being relieved by the medication prescribed by his doctor, she calls the doctor to have it adjusted. She also teaches Mr. Eng some visualization exercises to help take his mind off the pain.
   c. Management skills: The nurse meets with Mr. Eng's family to involve them in his care. She also instructs the staff to monitor Mr. Eng for signs of stress due to pain.

d. Self-evaluation skills: The nurse realizes she is being effective in relieving Mr. Eng's suffering and vows to research techniques for pain management.

3. Sample answer:
Step 1. Identify problems with the old system and specific processes that need to be changed.
Step 2. Analyze several potential solutions to the problems, including a computerized system, and discuss the advantages and disadvantages of each.
Step 3. Select a course of action to initiate change.
Step 4. Plan for changes by developing specific objectives and a timetable to meet them and identifying the people who will be involved in the change process.
Step 5. Implement the change, evaluate its effects, and revise accordingly to stabilize the new system.
Resistance to change: Determine why resistance exists and what technique will be most effective in helping employees overcome it.

4. a. Threat to self: Loss of self-esteem: belief that more work will be required and that social relationships will be disrupted. Explain the proposed change to everyone affected in simple, concise language so they know how they will be affected by it.
b. Lack of understanding: The people who will be affected by the change should be involved in the change process. When they understand the reason for and benefits of the change, they are more likely to accept it.
c. Limited tolerance for change: Some people do not like to function in a state of flux or disequilibrium. Expedite the change so there is only a short period of confusion, and explain this tactic to the employees involved.
d. Disagreements about the benefits of the change: Resistance may occur when the information available to the change agent is different from that received by individuals resisting the change. If the information available to the resisters is more accurate and relevant than the information available to the change agent, then resistance may be beneficial.
e. Fear of increased responsibility: People often worry about having more complex responsibilities placed on them, particularly if they are unprepared for them. Since communication is the key to understanding, opportunities should be provided for open communication and feedback. Incentives may be helpful in obtaining a commitment to change.

5. Nurses can change negative portrayals of nursing in the media by organizing, monitoring the media, reacting to the media, and fostering an improved image.

6. Sample answers:
a. Planning: Identify the problem and establish goals and a timeline for effecting change.

b. Organizing: Mobilize all available people and resources to educate the students about the dangers of binge drinking.
c. Motivating: Lead organized groups dedicated to stop binge drinking on campus.
d. Controlling: Evaluate the plan of action and degree of effectiveness.

7. Answers will vary with students' experiences.

8. a. Identifying strengths: A nurse manager might accomplish this through feedback analysis that supports a focus on continually improving those things that he/she does best; discovering intellectual arrogance—being bright is no substitute for knowledge; initiating work on acquiring the skills and knowledge he/she needs to fully realize strengths; remedying bad habits.
b. Evaluating work accomplishment: The manager should ask: Am I a visual or auditory learner? Do I learn best by reading or writing? Do I work more productively in teams or alone? Am I more productive as a decision maker or as an advisor?
c. Clarifying values: Working in an organization or on a particular unit whose value system is unacceptable or incompatible condemns a person to frustration and poor performance. The nurse manager should identify his/her own values and seek a work environment that is complementary, not adversarial.
d. Determining where he/she belongs and what he/she can contribute: In small or large organizations, the nurse manager should prepare for opportunities that emerge in response to these queries; in this dynamic industry, he/she should set reasonable short- to medium-range goals.
e. Assuming responsibility for relationships: The nurse manager should cultivate them, nurture them, and respect the differences they might have.

9. a. What is amenable to change?
b. How does the group function as a unit?
c. Is the person or group ready for change and, if so, at what rate can that change be expected to be accepted?
d. Are the changes major or minor?

10. a. The patient's condition
b. The complexity of the activity
c. The potential for harm
d. The degree of problem solving and innovation necessary
e. The level of interaction required with the patient
f. The capabilities of the NAP
g. The availability of professional staff to accomplish the unit workload

11. a. The right task: The task should be one that can be delegated.
b. The right circumstance: The patient setting should be appropriate and resources and other relevant factors considered.
c. The right person: The person should be qualified to do the job.

d. The right direction/communication: The communication should be a clear, concise description of the objective and expectations.

e. The right supervision: There should be appropriate monitoring, evaluation as needed, and feedback.

REFLECTIVE PRACTICE USING CRITICAL THINKING SKILLS

Sample Answers

1. How might the nurse empower Ms. Kohls with the knowledge and ability to be a leader of her peers? The nurse could help Ms. Kohls identify her strengths, evaluate how she acomplishes work, clarify her values, and determine how she can contribute to the community by being a leader in her school. The nurse can also empower Ms. Kohls by teaching her how to find the resources necessary to be knowledgeable about STIs and feel confident in her role as a leader.

2. What would be a successful outcome for Ms. Kohls? By next visit, Ms. Kohls describes the incidence of STIs and lists interventions to prevent spreading these diseases.
   By next visit, Ms. Kohls states that she feels confident in her ability to lead fellow students in a group discussion on STIs

3. What intellectual, technical, interpersonal, and/or ethical/legal competencies are most likely to bring about the desired outcome?
   Intellectual: ability to identify leadership skills appropriately and apply personal leadership skills to a variety of patient situations; knowledge of the incidence and prevention of STIs
   Interpersonal: strong people skills; ability to communicate with and instill confidence in patients
   Ethical/Legal: ability to advocate for patients and provide them with legally sound counsel

4. What resources might be helpful for Ms. Kohls? Information on STIs, information on leadership styles and how to propose and overcome resistance to change

CHAPTER 24

PRACTICING FOR NCLEX

MULTIPLE CHOICE QUESTIONS

1. a	2. c	3. c	4. d	5. b
6. a	7. d	8. b	9. b	

ALTERNATE-FORMAT QUESTIONS

Multiple Response Questions

1. a, b, e
2. a, e, f
3. b, c, e
4. c, d, f
5. a, d, e
6. b, c, d, f
7. a, c, e

Fill-in-the-Blank Questions

1. 5.2 L/minute
2. Width 8 cm, length 21 cm
3. 2+
4. 100°F
5. 102.2°F
6. 37.5°C

DEVELOPING YOUR KNOWLEDGE BASE

IDENTIFICATION

1. a. Temporal
   b. Carotid
   c. Brachial
   d. Radial
   e. Femoral
   f. Popliteal
   g. Posterior tibial
   h. Dorsalis pedis

MATCHING EXERCISES

1. b	2. i	3. d	4. g	5. a
6. h	7. e	8. j	9. c	10. f
11. l	12. i	13. g	14. d	15. a
16. f	17. j	18. h	19. e	20. c
21. k	22. e	23. g	24. f	25. a
26. c	27. d			

SHORT ANSWER

1. a. Circadian rhythms: Predictable fluctuations in measurements of body temperature and blood pressure exhibit a circadian rhythm (e.g., body temperature is usually approximately 0.6°C lower in the early morning than in later afternoon and early evening)

   b. Age: Body temperatures of infants and children respond more rapidly to heat and cold air temperatures than in adults. The older adult loses some thermoregulatory control and is at risk for harm from extremes in temperature.

   c. Gender: Body temperature tends to fluctuate more in women than in men, probably as a result of normal, cyclic fluctuations in the release of their sex hormones.

   d. Stress: The body responds to both physical and emotional stress by increasing the production of epinephrine. As a result, the metabolic rate increases, raising the body temperature.

   e. Environmental temperature: Exposure to extreme cold without adequate protective clothing can result in heat loss severe enough to cause hypothermia. Exposure to extreme heat may result in hyperthermia.

2. See table below.

Type of Thermometer	Brief Description	Contraindication	Normal Reading
A. GLASS oral	Calibrated in degrees Centigrade or Fahrenheit	Unconscious, irrational, seizure-prone, infants, oral disease	98.6°F 37.0°C
rectal	Calibrated in degrees Centigrade or Fahrenheit	Newborns, diseases of rectum, certain heart diseases	99.5°F 37.5°C
B. ELECTRONIC	Two nonbreakable probes, disposable probe covers		Site dependent
C. TYMPANIC MEMBRANE	Infrared sensors off membrane	Infants to 3 months Tympanic membrane damage	99.5°F 37.5°C
D. TEMPERATURE SENSITIVE PATCH	Forehead or abdomen; changes color at different temperatures	Newborns	94.0°F 34.4°C
E. AUTOMATED MONITORING DEVICE	Measure body temperature, pulse, and blood pressure automatically		Site dependent

3. a. The middle three fingers may be used to palpate all peripheral pulse sites.
  b. A stethoscope may be used to auscultate the apical pulse.
  c. Doppler ultrasound may be used to assess pulses that are difficult to palpate or auscultate.
4. a. Pumping action of the heart: When the amount of blood pumped into the arteries increases, the pressure of blood against arterial walls also increases.
  b. Blood volume: When blood volume is low, blood pressure is also low because there is less fluid within the arteries.
  c. Viscosity of blood: The more viscous the blood, the higher the blood pressure.
  d. Elasticity of vessel walls: The elasticity of the walls, in addition to the resistance of the arterioles, helps to maintain normal blood pressure.
5. a. Impaired Gas Exchange: Excess or deficit in oxygenation and/or carbon dioxide elimination at the alveolar–capillary membrane
  b. Ineffective Airway Clearance: Inability to clear secretions or obstructions from the respiratory tract to maintain a clear airway
  c. Ineffective Breathing Pattern: Inspiration and/or expiration that does not provide adequate ventilation

  d. Inability to Sustain Spontaneous Ventilation: A state in which the response pattern of decreased energy reserves results in an individual's inability to maintain breathing adequate to support life
6. a. Altered Tissue Perfusion: A decrease in oxygen, resulting in the failure to nourish the tissues at the capillary level
  b. Risk for Fluid Volume Imbalance: A risk for a decrease, increase, or rapid shift from one to the other of intravascular, interstitial, or intracellular fluid
  c. Fluid Volume Excess: The state in which an individual experiences increased isotonic fluid retention
  d. Fluid Volume Deficit: The state in which an individual experiences decreased intravascular, interstitial, or intracellular fluid
  e. Decreased Cardiac Output: A state in which the blood pumped by the heart is inadequate to meet the metabolic demands of the body
7. a. Stethoscope: Used to auscultate and assess body sounds, including the apical pulse and blood pressure. The acoustical stethoscope has an amplifying mechanism connected to earpieces by tubing.

b. Sphygmomanometer: Consists of a cuff and the manometer. The cuff contains an airtight, flat, rubber bladder covered with cloth, which is closed around the limb with contact closures. Two tubes are attached to the bladder within the cuff; one is connected to a manometer, the other to a bulb used to inflate the bladder.

REFLECTIVE PRACTICE USING CRITICAL THINKING SKILLS

Sample Answers

1. What might be causing Noah's reaction to the nurse's attempt to assess a tympanic temperature? Noah may be reacting out of fear of strange people and situations. Noah may also have an earache and in that case, a tympanic temperature is contraindicated because the movement of the tragus may cause severe discomfort.

2. What would be a successful outcome for Noah? Noah exhibits calmness upon examination and allows the nurse to perform necessary assessments

3. What intellectual, technical, interpersonal, and/or ethical/legal competencies are most likely to bring about the desired outcome?
Intellectual: knowledge of how to tailor vital signs technology to meet the needs of a 2-year-old
Technical: ability to correctly use the equipment necessary to assess and document vital signs
Interpersonal: ability to establish a trusting relationship with children and their families.

4. What resources might be helpful for the nurse caring for Noah?
Stuffed animal to demonstrate the procedures for taking vital signs, knowledge of distraction techniques to use when performing procedures on children

CHAPTER 25

PRACTICING FOR NCLEX
MULTIPLE CHOICE QUESTIONS

1. b	**2.** c	**3.** a	**4.** c	**5.** d
6. b	**7.** a	**8.** d	**9.** c	**10.** a
11. c	**12.** b	**13.** d	**14.** a	**15.** c
16. a	**17.** d	**18.** b		

ALTERNATE-FORMAT QUESTIONS
Multiple Response Questions

1. c, d, e
2. a, b, e
3. b, c, f
4. b, d, e
5. a, d, f
6. c, e, f
7. c, d, e
8. a, b, e

Hot Spot Question
1. See figure below.

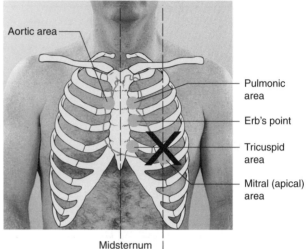

Aortic area
Pulmonic area
Erb's point
Tricuspid area
Mitral (apical) area
Midsternum
Midclavicular line

DEVELOPING YOUR KNOWLEDGE BASE

IDENTIFICATION QUESTIONS

1. a. Liver
 b. Stomach
 c. Spleen
 d. Transverse colon
 e. Descending colon
 f. Small intestine
 g. Sigmoid colon
 h. Bladder
 i. Appendix
 j. Cecum
 k. Ascending colon
2. a. Malleus
 b. Incus
 c. Semicircular canals
 d. Facial nerve
 e. Cochlear and vestibular branch
 f. Cochlea
 g. Oval window
 h. Round window
 i. Eustachian tube
 j. Stapes and footplate
 k. Tympanic membrane

MATCHING EXERCISES

1. a	**2.** b	**3.** a	**4.** d	**5.** c
6. b	**7.** e	**8.** d	**9.** c	**10.** a
11. b	**12.** d	**13.** c	**14.** a	**15.** b
16. e	**17.** g	**18.** d	**19.** h	**20.** f
21. f	**22.** b	**23.** d	**24.** j	**25.** a
26. c	**27.** e	**28.** h	**29.** i	**30.** g
31. d	**32.** f	**33.** a	**34.** c	**35.** b
36. e				

SHORT ANSWER

1. **a.** Establish a nurse–patient relationship
   b. Gather data about the patient's general health status, integrating physiologic, psychological, cognitive, sociocultural, developmental, and spiritual dimensions.
   c. Identify patient strengths.
   d. Identify existing and potential health problems.
   e. Establish a base for the nursing process.
2. **a.** Ophthalmoscope: Lighted instrument used for visualization of interior structures of the eye
   b. Otoscope: Lighted instrument used for examining external ear canal and tympanic membrane
   c. Snellen chart: Screening test for vision
   d. Nasal speculum: Instrument that allows visualization of lower and middle turbinates of the nose
   e. Vaginal speculum: Two-bladed instrument used to examine vaginal canal and cervix
   f. Tuning fork: Two-pronged metal instrument used for testing auditory function and vibratory perception

   g. Percussion hammer: Instrument with a rubber head, used to test reflexes and determine tissue density
3. **a.** patient's age
   b. patient's physical condition
   c. patient's energy level
   d. need for privacy
4. **a.** Patient: Consider physiologic and psychological needs of the patient. Explain that a physical assessment will be done by the nurse, that body structures will be examined, and that such assessments are painless. Have patient put on a gown and empty bladder.
   b. Environment: The time of the assessment should be mutually agreed on and should not interfere with meals or daily routines. The patient should be as free of pain as possible, and the room should be quiet and private.
5. See table below.

Technique	Definition	Assessment/Observation
a. Inspection:	Process of deliberate, purposeful observations performed in a systematic manner.	Body size, color, shape, position, symmetry, norms, and deviations from norm.
b. Palpation:	Technique that uses sense of touch.	Temperature, turgor, texture, moisture, vibrations, shape.
c. Percussion:	The act of striking an object against another object to produce a sound.	Location, shape, size, and density of tissues.
d. Auscultation:	The act of listening to sound produced in the body, using stethoscope.	Lung and bowel sounds; heart and vascular sounds.

6. **a.** Pitch—ranging from high to low
   b. Loudness—ranging from soft to loud
   c. Quality—for example, swishing or gurgling
   d. Duration—short, medium, or long
7. **a.** Edema: Palpate edematous area with the fingers; an indentation may remain after the pressure is released.
   b. Dehydration: Pick up the skin in a fold; when dehydration exists, normal elasticity and fullness are decreased, and skin fold returns to normal slowly.
8. **a.** Reaction to light: Ask patient to look straight ahead, bring the penlight from side of patient's face, and shine the light on one of the pupils. Observe pupil's reaction; normally it will constrict. Repeat procedure in the same eye, and observe the other eye—normally it too will

   constrict. Repeat the entire procedure with the other eye.
   b. Accommodation: Hold the forefinger about 10 to 15 cm in front of the bridge of the patient's nose. Ask the patient to first look at the forefinger, then at a distant object, then the forefinger again. Normally, the pupil constricts when the patient looks at the finger and dilates when he/she looks at a distant object.
   c. Convergence: Move a finger toward the patient's nose. Normally, the patient's eyes converge.
9. **a.** Weber: Hold the tuning fork at its base and strike it against the palm of the opposite hand so that the fork vibrates. Place the base of the fork on the center of the top of the patient's head; ask patient where the sound is heard. Normal findings: sound is heard in both ears or in midline.

b. Rinne: Activate tuning fork. Hold base of fork against patient's mastoid process and ask him/her to tell you when the sound can no longer be heard. Immediately place the still-vibrating fork close to the external ear canal and ask the patient if he/she can hear the sound. A normal ear will hear the sound. Repeat procedure with other ear.

10. Equipment: Vials of aromatic substances, visual acuity chart, penlight, sharp object, cotton balls, vials of solution to test taste, tuning fork, tongue depressor, reflex hammer, and familiar objects. Position: sitting.

11. Sample answers:
    a. Orientation: What is today's date?
    b. Immediate memory: What did you eat for lunch today?
    c. Past memory: When is your wedding anniversary?
    d. Abstract reasoning: Explain the proverb "a stitch in time, saves nine."
    e. Language: Would you read this passage from this book?

12. a. lub; b. mitral; c. tricuspid; d. ventricular; e. S1; f. apical; g. S2; h. systole; i. aortic; j. pulmonic; k. dub; l. one

REFLECTIVE PRACTICE USING CRITICAL THINKING SKILLS

Sample Answers

1. What type of health assessments would the nurse caring for Billy conduct?
   In the emergency room, the nurse should perform an emergency assessment to determine the effects of the bee sting and the allergic reaction that occurred. Once Billy is stabilized, the nurse should perform a focused assessment of Billy's allergies and answer the parent's questions at this time.

2. What would be a successful outcome for Billy and his family?
   Billy demonstrates the proper method for self-injecting epinephrine
   Billy and his family state methods to avoid bee stings in the future and emergency interventions in the event a bee sting occurs

3. What intellectual, technical, interpersonal, and/or ethical/legal competencies are most likely to bring about the desired outcome?
   Intellectual: knowledge of the typical assessment findings associated with an allergic reaction
   Interpersonal: ability to communicate and interact effectively with patients and their families during times of stress
   Ethical/Legal: knowledge of special regulations and legislation detailing nursing responsibilities when providing first aid in camp situations

4. What resources might be helpful for this family?
   Printed or AV materials on allergic reactions to insect bites and how to treat them.

CHAPTER 26

PRACTICING FOR NCLEX
MULTIPLE CHOICE QUESTIONS

1. a   2. c   3. d   4. b   5. a
6. b   7. a

ALTERNATE-FORMAT QUESTIONS
Multiple Response Questions

1. b, d, e
2. a, b, e
3. a, c, d
4. b, c, d
5. a, b, c, e
6. c, d, f
7. a, c, f

Prioritization Questions
1.

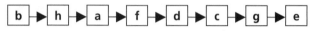

DEVELOPING YOUR KNOWLEDGE BASE

MATCHING EXERCISES

1. d. Contact poison control center. In ED, stomach lavage (may remove unabsorbed pills); possible use of cathartic. If dose is toxic, use of chelating agent
2. b. Never induce vomiting; dilute poison with milk or water, take to ED immediately.
3. a. In ED, activated charcoal or acetylcysteine either orally or via NG tube.
4. e. Chelating therapy and monitor lead levels
5. c. Never induce vomiting; contact physician or poison control center.
6. d   7. g   8. e   9. a   10. f
11. c   12. b

CORRECT THE FALSE STATEMENTS

1. True
2. True
3. True
4. False—home
5. False—children
6. True
7. True
8. False—preschooler
9. False—falls
10. False—unjustified
11. False—children under 5
12. True

SHORT ANSWER

1. a. Neonates and infants: mother who smokes; mother who drinks alcohol
   b. Toddler and preschooler: child abuse; expanded environment
   c. School-aged child: accidents, fire

d. Adolescent: drug and alcohol consumption; motor vehicle crashes
e. Adult: spousal abuse; using alcohol to relieve stress
f. Older adult: motor impairment; elder abuse

2. Sample answers:
   a. Developmental considerations: A teenager who drinks and drives is at risk for accidents; an adult who is under stress at work is at risk for drug or alcohol abuse.
   b. Lifestyle: A person who lives in a high-crime neighborhood is at risk for violence; a person who has a dangerous job is at risk for accidents.
   c. Limitation in mobility: An older patient with an unsteady gait is at risk for falls; recent surgery or prolonged illness can temporarily affect mobility.
   d. Limitation in sensory perception: Visual changes may cause a person to stumble, lose balance, and fall; a hearing deficit interferes with normal communication and may result in a patient who is insensitive to alarms, horns, sirens, and so on.
   e. Limitation in knowledge: A mother who does not know how to childproof her home puts her toddler at risk for accidents; an elderly person who does not know how to use her walker is at risk for falls.
   f. Limitation in ability to communicate: Fatigue or stress, certain medications, aphasia, and language barriers are factors that can affect personal interchange and compromise the patient's ability to express urgent safety concerns.
   g. Limitation in health status: A patient recovering from a stroke may have muscle impairment; many patients who fall also have a primary or secondary diagnosis of cardiovascular disease.
   h. Limitation in psychosocial state: Depression may result in confusion and disorientation, accompanied by reduced awareness of environmental hazards; social isolation may be responsible for a reduced level of concentration.

3. a. Nursing history: The nurse must be alert for any history of falls because a person with a history of falling is likely to fall again. Assistive devices should be noted. A history of drug or alcohol abuse should also be noted.
   b. Physical assessment: Nurses need to assess the patient's mobility status, ability to communicate, level of awareness or orientation, and sensory perception.
   c. Accident-prone behavior: Some people seem to be more likely than others to have accidents.
   d. The environment: The nurse must assess every setting in which the patient is at risk for injury, including the home, community, and healthcare agency.

4. Sample answers:
   a. Age older than 65 years
   b. Documented history of falls
   c. Slowed reaction time
   d. Disorientation or confusion

5. Sample answers:
   The mother should be informed about safety for toddlers, and a plan should be devised to help her childproof her home. The plan should include the installation of cabinet locks; electrical outlet covers; moving medications, cleaners, poisonous plants, and so on to higher levels; and keeping small or sharp objects out of reach.

6. Sample answers:
   a. Do your children's toys have small or loose parts?
   b. Have you ever left your infant in the bathtub to answer the phone?
   c. Do you have soft pillows or thick blankets in your infant's crib?

7. a. Risk for Injury related to refusal to use child safety seat
   b. Risk for Poisoning related to reduced vision
   c. Risk for Aspiration or Trauma (burns) related to child left unattended in bathtub
   d. Risk for Trauma related to history of previous falls
   e. Impaired Home Maintenance related to insufficient finances

8. a. Screening programs for vision and hearing
   b. Fire prevention programs
   c. Drug and alcohol prevention programs

9. Sample answers:
   a. Impaired circulation
   b. Pressure ulcers and diminished bone mass
   c. Fractures
   d. Altered nutrition and hydration
   e. Incontinence

10. Documentation should include alternative strategies that were ineffective, the reason for restraining the patient, the type of restraint and time it was applied, pertinent nursing assessments, and regular intervals when restraints were removed.

11. The nurse completes the safety event report immediately after an accident and is responsible for recording the occurrence of the accident and its effect on the patient in the medical record. The report should objectively describe the circumstances of the accident and provide details concerning the patient's response and the examination and treatment of the patient after the event.

12. Have the patient sit in a straight-backed chair. Observe his posture while seated. Instruct the patient to stand. Assess if he can stand in one fluid motion or needs the use of his hands to push up to a standing position. Does he need multiple attempts to stand? Once standing, ask the patient to keep his eyes open and stand as still as possible. Then ask him to close his eyes and observe his stability with eyes closed. Ask him to open his eyes

and walk 10 feet (3 meters), and then turn around and walk back to the chair. Using a timed Get Up and Go test: 9 seconds or less indicates full mobility and 10 to 19 seconds means person is almost completely independent. Higher times can indicate impaired mobility.

REFLECTIVE PRACTICE USING CRITICAL THINKING SKILLS

Sample Answers

1. What safety interventions might the nurse implement for this patient?
   Ms. Washington should be advised to have clutter removed from the home, remove throw rugs and fire hazards, and have smoke detectors installed. She should be advised to wear shoes with rubber soles when walking in her home. Ms. Washington might also benefit from a home alert system in case she falls and needs help.
2. What would be a successful outcome for Ms. Washington?
   By end of visit, Ms. Washington points out three safety issues in her home and formulates a plan to correct them.
   By next visit, Ms. Washington demonstrates walking freely through a clutter-free home with fire alarms installed
3. What intellectual, technical, interpersonal, and/or ethical/legal competencies are most likely to bring about the desired outcome?
   Intellectual: knowledge of the safety and security needs of older adults and related nursing responsibilities and care
   Interpersonal: ability to establish a therapeutic relationship with an older adult in order to communicate the need for safety interventions in the home
   Ethical/Legal: Commitment to patient safety and quality care, including ability to report problem situations immediately
4. What resources might be helpful for Ms. Washington?
   Home healthcare services, housekeeping services, smoke detectors, home alert system

CHAPTER 27

PRACTICING FOR NCLEX
MULTIPLE CHOICE QUESTIONS

1. b	2. d	3. c	4. b	5. a
6. c	7. a			

ALTERNATE-FORMAT QUESTIONS
Multiple Response Questions

1. c, d
2. a, c, d
3. b, f
4. a, b, c
5. b, c, e
6. b, d, e
7. a, d, f

Prioritization Questions

1.
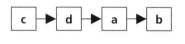

2.
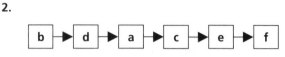

DEVELOPING YOUR KNOWLEDGE BASE

FILL-IN-THE-BLANKS

1. Infection
2. Bacteria
3. Aerobic
4. Fungi
5. Normal flora
6. Reservoirs
7. Portal of entry
8. Antibody
9. Healthcare-associated infection

MATCHING EXERCISES

1. k	2. f	3. a	4. b	5. j
6. i	7. m	8. c	9. e	10. g
11. d	12. n			

13. c. Blood, semen, vaginal secretions
14. e. Ticks
15. d. Sputum
16. a. Skin surface
17. b. Blood, feces, body fluids
18. a. Mouth
19. a. Throat

20. d	21. a	22. c	23. b

CORRECT THE FALSE STATEMENTS

1. True
2. True
3. False—Washing hands
4. False—Transient bacteria
5. True
6. True
7. True
8. False—surgical asepsis
9. True

SHORT ANSWER

1. a. Number of organisms
   b. Virulence of the organism
   c. Competence of a person's immune system
   d. Length and intimacy of the contact between a person and the microorganism
2. Sample answers:
   a. Other humans: Tuberculosis
   b. Animals: Rabies
   c. Soil: Gas gangrene
3. a. Gastrointestinal
   b. Genitourinary tracts
   c. Blood and tissue

4. Sample answers:
   a. Direct contact: Transmission of disease through touching, kissing, or sexual contact
   b. Indirect contact: Personal contact with contaminated blood, food, water, etc.
   c. Vectors: Mosquitoes, ticks, and lice transmit organisms from one host to another.
   d. Airborne: Spread of droplet nuclei through coughing, sneezing, or talking
5. a. Inflammatory response: A protective mechanism that eliminates the invading pathogen and allows tissue repair to occur
   b. Immune response: Involves specific reactions in the body as it responds to an invading foreign protein such as bacteria or, in some cases, the body's own proteins. The body responds to an antigen by producing an antibody.
6. a. Intact skin and mucous membranes protect the body against microbial invasion.
   b. The normal pH levels of gastric secretions and of the genitourinary tract help to ward off microbial invasion.
   c. The body's white blood cells influence resistance to certain pathogens.
   d. Age, sex, race, and hereditary factors influence susceptibility.
7. a. Assessing: Early detection and surveillance techniques are critical. The nurse should inquire about immunization status and previous or recurring infections, observe nonverbal cues, and obtain the history of the current disease.
   b. Diagnosing: The direction or focus of nursing care depends on a nursing diagnosis that accurately reflects the patient's condition.
   c. Planning: Effective nursing interventions can control or prevent infection. Nurses should review assessment data and consider the cycle of events that results in infection control as patient goals are formulated.
   d. Implementing: The nurse uses principles of aseptic technique to halt the spread of microorganisms and minimize the threat of infection.
   e. Evaluating: The nurse can intervene in, and improve, a patient's outcome by assessing the person at risk, selecting appropriate nursing diagnoses, planning and intervening to maintain a safe environment, and evaluating the plan of care to determine whether it is working.
8. Sample answers:
   a. Patient's home: Wash hands before preparing food and before eating; use individual personal care items such as washcloths, towels, and toothbrushes.
   b. Public facilities: Wash hands after using any public bathroom; use individually wrapped drinking straws.
   c. Community: Use sterilized combs and brushes in beauty and barber shops; examine food handlers for evidence of disease.

   d. Healthcare facility: Use standard aseptic techniques to prevent further spread of a present organism and prevent nosocomial infections.
9. a. Instituting constant surveillance by infection-control committees and nurse epidemiologists
   b. Having written infection-prevention practices for all agency personnel
   c. Using practices that help promote the best possible physical condition in patients
10. a. Nature of organisms present: Some organisms are easily destroyed, whereas others can withstand certain commonly used sterilization and disinfection methods.
   b. Number of organisms present: The more organisms present on an item, the longer it takes to destroy them.
   c. Type of equipment: Equipment with narrow lumens, crevices, or joints requires special care. Certain items may be damaged by sterilization methods.
   d. Intended use of equipment: The need for medical or surgical asepsis influences the methods used in the preparation and cleaning of equipment.
   e. Available means for sterilization and disinfection: The choice of chemical or physical means of sterilization and disinfection takes into consideration the availability and practicality of the means.
   f. Time: Time is a key factor. Failure to observe recommended time periods for disinfection and sterilization significantly increases the risk for infection and is grossly negligent.
11. a. Hospital: The infection-control nurse is responsible for educating patients and staff about effective infection-control techniques and for collecting statistics about infections.
   b. Home care setting: The infection-control nurse's duties include surveillance for agency-associated infections, as well as education, consultation, performance of epidemiologic investigations and quality improvement activities, and policy and procedure development.
12. a. Risk for Infection related to altered skin integrity/burns
   b. Effective nursing interventions can control or prevent infection. The nurse should review patient data, consider the cycle of events that result in the development of an infection, and incorporate infection control as a patient goal.
13. Use standard precautions for the care of all patients in the ER. The additional concern with TB necessitates using airborne precautions in addition to standard precautions.

REFLECTIVE PRACTICE USING CRITICAL THINKING SKILLS
Sample Answers
1. How might the nurse respond to Ms. Turheis in a holistic manner that respects her human dignity, while at the same time, maintaining a safe environment for her?

Patients in isolation may suffer from sensory deprivation and loss of self-esteem may occur. The nurse can reinforce Ms. Turheis's self-identity by using looks, speech, and judicious touch to communicate worth, speaking to her respectfully, spending time in conversations with her about her life experiences, and allowing her to express negative feelings. The nurse can then help Ms. Turheis to recognize her strengths and explore other options to fulfill her self-esteem needs.

2. What would be a successful outcome for Ms. Turheis? By next visit, Ms. Turheis will report feeling better about her situation and will state three positive experiences that occurred in the last week.

3. What intellectual, technical, interpersonal, and/or ethical/legal competencies are most likely to bring about the desired outcome?
Intellectual: knowledge of the effects of isolation on the self-esteem of patients and interventions to minimize these effects
Technical: ability to use appropriate infection-control precautions and barrier techniques for infection prevention
Interpersonal: ability to communicate care and compassion to patients requiring infection-control precautions
Ethical/Legal: demonstration of a commitment to safety and quality; strong advocacy abilities

4. What resources might be helpful for Ms. Turheis? Referral to counseling services, home healthcare visits

CHAPTER 28

PRACTICING FOR NCLEX
MULTIPLE CHOICE QUESTIONS

1. a   **2.** c   **3.** b   **4.** c   **5.** a
6. d

ALTERNATE-FORMAT QUESTIONS
Multiple Response Questions

1. a, b, f
2. b, c, e
3. a, b, c, f
4. c, d, e
5. b, d, f
6. a, c, d

DEVELOPING YOUR KNOWLEDGE BASE

FILL-IN-THE-BLANKS

1. Yin
2. Holism
3. Acupuncture
4. Imagery
5. Nutritional supplements
6. Aromatherapy

MATCHING EXERCISES

1. d   **2.** f   **3.** b   **4.** e   **5.** a
6. c

SHORT ANSWER

1. a. Allopathy: Generally used to describe "traditional medicine." Has spearheaded remarkable advances in biotechnology, surgical interventions, pharmaceutical approaches, and diagnostic tools.
  b. Holism: A theory and philosophy that focuses on connections and interactions between parts of the whole; focuses on reductionism.
  c. Integrative care: Uses some combination of allopathic and complementary/alternative therapies; coordinates best possible treatment plan for patient

2. a. Ayurveda: Central to this CAT is understanding the patient's basic constitution or "dosha."
    Nursing Considerations: May include dietary needs, time set aside for self-care such as meditation, and desire to continue an herbal/supplement regimen
  b. Yoga: A set of exercises that consist of various physical postures practiced to promote strength and flexibility, increase endurance, or promote relaxation
    Nursing Considerations: Encourage patients to find a type of yoga that is compatible with their physical condition and goals. Some positions are contraindicated in patients with certain physical conditions.
  c. Traditional Chinese Medicine: Believes that the interaction of people with their environment is most significant in creating health
    Nursing Considerations: Teaching about acupuncture, diet, herbs, massage, and energy exercises
  d. Qi gong: System of posture, exercise, breathing techniques, and visualization regulating qi
    Nursing considerations: Can be learned from videos/DVDs or in a class; encourage students to explore background of instructor.

3. a. Relaxation techniques: Ultimate goal is to increase the parasympathetic system influence in the body–mind and reduce the effect of stress and stress-related illness.
  b. Meditation: Seeks to change one's physiology to a more relaxed state and alter one's perception to an increased acceptance of reality
  c. Imagery: Involves using all five senses to imagine an event or body process unfolding according to a plan

4. a. All the life sciences agree that physically a human being is an open energy system.
  b. Anatomically, a human being is bilaterally symmetric.

c. Illness is an imbalance in an individual's energy field.
d. Human beings have natural abilities to transform and transcend their conditions of living.
5. Sample answers:
   a. Shamanism: Treatment would consist of first restoring the patient's power and then treating symptoms.
   b. Native American tradition: Healing techniques may include native plants and herbs, animals, ritual, ceremony, and purification techniques.
   c. Intercessory prayer: Treatment would involve praying for the patient to the Judeo-Christian god.
6. Sample answers:
   a. Nutritional therapy: It is believed that people have individual needs and preferences with respect to foods.
   b. Aromatherapy: It is believed that the fragrance of oils can evoke powerful memories in a split second and change people's perceptions and behaviors.
   c. Music: It is believed that music is effective in reducing pain, decreasing anxiety, and promoting relaxation, thereby distracting persons from unpleasant sensations.
   d. Humor: It is believed that a good "belly laugh" can help treat acute and debilitating illness.
7. a. Biology-based practices: using herbs and special diets
   b. Mind–body medicine: using meditation or yoga
   c. Energy medicine: using energy fields or magnetic fields
   d. Manipulative and body-based practices: manipulating body parts

REFLECTIVE PRACTICE USING CRITICAL THINKING SKILLS

Sample Answers

1. What type of Complementary and Alternative Therapies might the nurse suggest to promote relaxation for Ms. Puentes?
   The nurse could teach Ms. Puentes mind–body techniques, such as meditation, guided imagery, biofeedback, and relaxation, to reduce stressful emotions. Energy healing techniques would also be helpful for pain that lingers after an injury heals, as well as pain complicated by trauma, anxiety, or depression. These CATs include acupuncture, acupressure, Qi gong, and Reiki. Movement-based therapies are also appropriate for postoperative pain. These include physical therapy, yoga, pilates, and tai chi.
2. What would be a successful outcome for Ms. Puentes?
   Upon next visit, Ms. Puentes lists two CAT measures that promote relaxation and demonstrates the proper use of them.

3. What intellectual, technical, interpersonal, and/or ethical/legal competencies are most likely to bring about the desired outcome?
   Intellectual: knowledge of available and appropriate complementary and alternative modalities
   Technical: ability to properly perform CAT and integrate these measures into patient care
   Interpersonal: ability to work collaboratively with other members of the healthcare team to promote culturally competent care that includes the use of CAT
4. What resources might be helpful for Ms. Puentes?
   Other healthcare professionals using CAT, printed and AV materials on CAT, referral to special programs delivering CAT

CHAPTER 29

PRACTICING FOR NCLEX
MULTIPLE CHOICE QUESTIONS

1. d	2. a	3. c	4. d	5. b
6. a	7. b	8. d	9. b	10. a
11. c	12. d	13. b	14. c	15. b
16. a	17. d			

ALTERNATE-FORMAT QUESTIONS
Multiple Response Questions

1. a, c, d
2. b, e, f
3. a, b, c
4. d, e
5. a, c, d
6. b, e, f
7. c, d, f
8. a, b, d

Fill-in-the-Blank Questions

1. 1.5 mL
2. 0.5 tab (½ tab)
3. 3 tabs
4. 0.5 tab (½ tab)
5. 3 tabs
6. 0.5 tab (½ tab)
7. 0.5 tab (½ tab)
8. 2 tabs
9. 4 mL

DEVELOPING YOUR KNOWLEDGE BASE
MATCHING EXERCISES

1. f	2. a	3. c	4. k	5. b
6. j	7. d	8. g	9. i	10. h
11. l	12. m	13. c	14. i	15. b
16. e	17. f	18. d	19. g	20. a

SHORT ANSWER

1. Drugs may be classified by:
   a. body systems
   b. the symptom relieved by the drug
   c. the clinical indication for the drug
2. a. Drug–receptor interactions: The drug interacts with one or more cellular structures to alter cell function.
   b. Drug–enzyme interactions: The drug combines with enzymes to achieve the desired effect.
3. Sample answers:
   a. Developmental stage of patient: A child's dose of medication is smaller than an adult's dose.
   b. Weight: Drug doses for children should be calculated on weight or body surface area. Doses for adults are based on a reference adult (i.e., a healthy adult of 18 to 65 years weighing 150 lb).
   c. Sex: Hormonal fluctuations can affect drug action.
   d. Genetic factors: Asian patients may require smaller doses of a drug because they metabolize it at a slower rate. Cultural: Herbal remedies may interfere with or counteract the action of the prescribed medication.
   e. Psychological factors: Patients may attain the same effect with a placebo as with an active drug.
   f. Pathology: Liver disease may affect drug action by slowing the metabolism of drugs.
   g. Environment: The lower oxygen concentration of air at high altitudes may increase sensitivity to some drugs.
   h. Time of administration: The presence of food in the stomach generally delays the absorption of oral medications.
4. Sample answers:
   a. The nurse knows that the patient is allergic to the drug.
   b. The nurse has difficulty reading the order.
   c. The nurse knows the drug will be harmful to the patient.
5. a. Stock supply system: Large quantities of medications are kept on the nursing unit.
   b. Individual supply system: Each patient is supplied with the medication needed for a period of time.
   c. Unit-dose system: The pharmacist simplifies medication preparation by packaging and labeling each dosage for a 24-hour period.
6. a. Three checks: The medication label should be checked (1) when the nurse reaches for the container; (2) after retrieval from the drawer and compared with the CMAR, or compared with the CMAR immediately before pouring from a multidose container; and (3) when replacing the container to the drawer or shelf or before giving the unit dose medication to the patient.
   b. Five rights: (1) Give the right medication (2) to the right patient (3) in the right dosage (4) through the right route (5) at the right time.
7. Sample answers:
   a. Crush the medication or add it to food.
   b. Allow the patient to suck on a piece of ice to numb the taste buds.
   c. Give the medication with generous amounts of water.
8. Sample answers:
   a. Route of administration: A longer needle is needed for an intramuscular injection than for an intradermal or subcutaneous injection.
   b. Viscosity of the solution: Some medications are more viscous than others and require a large-lumen needle to be injected.
   c. Quantity to be administered: The larger the amount of medication to be injected, the greater the capacity of the syringe.
   d. Body size: An obese person requires a longer needle to reach muscle tissue than a thin person.
   e. Type of medication: There are special syringes for certain uses.
9. a. Check the patient's condition immediately when the error is noted. Observe for adverse effects.
   b. Notify the nurse manager and the physician to discuss possible courses of action based on the patient's condition.
   c. Write a description of the error on the patient's medical record, including remedial steps that were taken.
   d. Complete a special form for reporting errors, as dictated by agency policy.
10. a. Ampules: An ampule is a glass flask that contains a single dose of medication for parenteral administration. Medication is removed from an ampule after its thin neck is broken.
    b. Vials: A vial is a glass bottle with a self-sealing stopper through which medication is removed. The nurse can remove several doses from the same container.
    c. Prefilled cartridges: These provide a single dose of medication. The nurse inserts the cartridge into a reusable holder and clears the cartridge of excess air.

11. See Medical Administration Record below.

Medical Administration Record

Ord date	PRN MEDS.		
2/24/11	Dalmane 30 mg	Date	
	PO hs prn	Time	
		Init / Site	
2/24/11	Tylenol with codeine #2	Date	2/24/11
	PO q4h prn	Time	10 AM
		Init / Site	CL/PO

SINGLE ORDERS–PREOPERATIVES

Ord date	Medication–Dosage–Route of Admin	Date/Time	Site/Initials
2/24/11	Regular Insulin U-100	2/24/11 ® thigh/CL	
	10U SQ STAT		

INJECTION SITES MUST BE CHARTED

Ord date	Medication–Dosage–Route of Admin	Hr	2/25	2/26	2/27	2/28	3/1	3/2	3/3
2/24/11	Tenormin 50 mg PO od	10AM	CL						
2/24/11	Hydrodiuril 50 mg PO od	10AM	CL						
			130/90						
2/24/11	NPH Insulin U-100 45U	7:30AM	CL						
	SQ daily in AM		Ⓛ arm						
2/24/11	Cipro 500 mg PO q12h	10AM	CL						
		10PM							
2/24/11	Timoptic 0.25% †gtt	10AM	CL						
	OD bid	6PM							
2/24/11	Nitropaste 1/2" q8h	8AM	CL 130/90						
	to chest wall	4PM							
		12PM							
2/24/11	Colace 100 mg PO od	10AM	CL						

CL: Claire Long, RN

12. See medication chart below.

Method	Xanax	Zantac	Cipro
Dosage	0.25–0.5 mg	150–300 mg	250–750 mg
Route of administration	PO	PO	PO
Frequency/schedule	tid	bid	bid
Desired effects	Relief of anxiety	Cure/relief of peptic ulcer	Cure/treat infection
Possible adverse effects	Drowsiness, lightheadedness, dry mouth, constipation	Malaise, rash, GI upset	GI upset, nausea, diarrhea
Signs and symptoms of toxic drug effects	Diminished reflexes, somnolence, confusion	Tachycardia, GI upset	CNS stimulation
Special instructions	No alcohol	None	No antacids
Recommended course of action with problems	Gastric lavage	None	None

REFLECTIVE PRACTICE USING CRITICAL THINKING SKILLS
Sample Answers
1. How might the nurse use blended nursing skills to respond to this medication error?

The nurse would use the five rights of medication administration ([1] Give the right medication [2] to the right patient [3] in the right dosage [4] through the right route [5] at the right time) to determine that the medication was labeled incorrectly. The nurse could then call the pharmacy and have new medication delivered with the right patient name.

2. What would be a successful outcome for this patient? Mr Baptiste receives the prescribed medication with his name on the label.

3. What intellectual, technical, interpersonal, and/or ethical/legal competencies are most likely to bring about the desired outcome?

Intellectual: knowledge of intravenous antibiotic therapy including correct dosages for IV medications
Technical: ability to safely administer IV antibiotics to a patient
Legal/Ethical: ability to provide patient safety via accurate patient identification to ensure medications are delivered in the right dosage to the right patient.

CHAPTER 30

PRACTICING FOR NCLEX
MULTIPLE CHOICE QUESTIONS

1. a	**2.** c	**3.** b	**4.** d	**5.** b
6. a	**7.** c	**8.** c	**9.** a	**10.** c
11. b	**12.** d	**13.** b	**14.** a	**15.** c
16. a				

ALTERNATE-FORMAT QUESTIONS
Multiple Response Questions

1. a, d, f
2. b, c, d, f
3. b, e, f
4. a, c, d
5. a, b, d, e
6. b, c, e
7. c, d, f
8. a, b, e
9. c, e, f

Prioritization Questions

1.

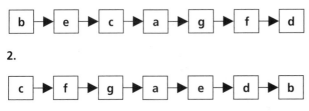

b → e → c → a → g → f → d

2.

c → f → g → a → e → d → b

DEVELOPING YOUR KNOWLEDGE BASE

FILL-IN-THE-BLANKS

1. Perioperative nursing
2. Urgency, risk, purpose
3. Elective surgery
4. Degree of risk
5. Regional
6. Induction, maintenance, emergence
7. Conscious
8. Informed consent
9. Living wills, durable power of attorney

MATCHING EXERCISES

1. a   **2.** c   **3.** d   **4.** b   **5.** d
6. b

SHORT ANSWER

1. **a.** Preoperative phase: Begins with the decision that surgical intervention is necessary and lasts until the patient is transferred to the operating room table
   b. Intraoperative phase: Extends from admission to the surgical department to transfer to the recovery area
   c. Postoperative phase: Lasts from admission to the recovery area to the complete recovery from surgery
2. **a.** Based on urgency: May be classified as elective surgery (preplanned; patient choice), urgent surgery (necessary for patient's health; not emergency), or emergency surgery (preserves patient's life, body part, or body function)
   b. Based on degree of risk: May be classified as minor (performed in physician's office, same-day surgery setting, or outpatient clinic) or major (requires hospitalization, is prolonged and has higher degree of risk, involves major body organs)

   c. Based on purpose: Descriptors include diagnostic, ablative, palliative, reconstructive, transplant, and constructive.
3. **a.** Induction: Begins with administration of the anesthetic agent and continues until patient is ready for incision
   b. Maintenance: Continues from point of incision until near completion of procedure
   c. Emergence: Starts as patient begins to emerge from the anesthesia and usually ends when patient is ready to leave the operating room
4. **a.** Description of the procedure or treatment
   b. Name and qualifications of the person performing the procedure or treatment
   c. Explanation of the risks involved, including potential for damage, disfigurement, or death
   d. Patient's right to refuse treatment and withdraw consent
5. **a.** Cardiovascular disease: Increased potential for hemorrhage and hypovolemic shock, hypotension, venous stasis, thrombophlebitis, and overhydration with IV fluids
   b. Pulmonary disorders: Increased possibility of respiratory depression from anesthesia, postoperative pneumonia, atelectasis, and alterations in acid–base balance
   c. Kidney and liver function disorders: Influence the patient's response to anesthesia, affect fluid and electrolyte as well as acid–base balance, alter metabolism and excretion of drugs, and impair wound healing
   d. Metabolic disorders: Increased potential for hypoglycemia or acidosis and slow wound healing
6. **a.** Fear of the unknown: Encourage the patient to identify and verbalize fears; identify and correct incorrect knowledge; identify patient strengths.
   b. Fear of pain and death: Support the patient's spiritual needs through acceptance, participation in prayer, or referral to clergy or chaplain.
   c. Fear of changes in body image and self-concept: Identify the need for support systems during initial interview; arrange a preoperative visit from a person who has had the same operation and adapted successfully.
7. The nurse is responsible for ensuring that the tests are ordered and performed, that the results are recorded in the patient's record before surgery, and that abnormal findings are reported.
8. **a.** Surgical events and sensations: Tell the patient and family when surgery is scheduled; how long it will last; what will be done before, during, and after surgery; and what sensations the patient will be experiencing during the perioperative period.
   b. Pain management: The patient should be informed that pain reported by the patient is the determining factor of pain control, pain will be assessed as often as every 2 hours after major surgery, there is little danger of addiction

to pain medications, and nonpharmacologic methods of pain control (relaxation techniques, TENS, and PCA) are available.

9. a. Hygiene and skin preparation: Clean the skin with antibacterial soap to remove bacteria (the patient can do this in a bath or shower), shampoo the hair, and clean the fingernails. Remove hair from incisional area with depilatory cream or hair clipper if indicated.
    b. Elimination: Emptying the bowel of feces is no longer a routine procedure, but the nurse should use preoperative assessments to determine the need for an order for bowel elimination. If indwelling catheter is not in place, the patient should void immediately before receiving preoperative medications.
    c. Nutrition and fluids: Diet depends on the type of surgery; patients need to be well nourished and hydrated before surgery to counterbalance fluid, blood, and electrolyte loss during surgery.
    d. Rest and sleep: The nurse can facilitate rest and sleep in the immediate preoperative period by meeting psychological needs, carrying out teaching, providing a quiet environment, and administering prescribed bedtime sedative medication.

10. a. Maintain intact skin surfaces
    b. Remain free of neuromuscular damage
    c. Have symmetric breathing patterns

11. a. Unconsciousness
    b. Response to touch and sounds
    c. Drowsiness
    d. Awake but not oriented
    e. Awake and oriented

12. Sample answer:
    The person who will be changing the patient's dressing at home should demonstrate proper techniques in wound care and dressing change. Teaching should include the following information: (1) where to buy dressing materials and medical supplies, (2) signs and symptoms of infection, (3) need to eat well-balanced meals and drink fluids, (4) how to modify activities of daily living (as needed), (5) need to wear disposable gloves when changing the dressing and wash hands before and after donning gloves, and (6) how to dispose of old dressings.

13. Sample answers:
    a. Developmental considerations: Infants and older adults are at a greater risk from surgery than are children and young or middle-aged adults.
    b. Medical history: Pathologic changes associated with past and current illnesses increase surgical risk.
    c. Medications: Use of anticoagulants before surgery may precipitate hemorrhage.
    d. Previous surgery: Previous heart or lung surgery may necessitate adaptations in the anesthesia used and in positioning during surgery.
    e. Perceptions and knowledge of surgery: The patient's questions or statements are important for meeting his/her psychological needs and

those of the family when preparing the patient for surgery.
    f. Lifestyle: Cultural and ethnic background of the patient may affect surgical risk.
    g. Nutrition: Malnutrition and obesity increase surgical risk.
    h. Use of alcohol, illicit drugs, nicotine: Patients with a large habitual intake of alcohol require larger doses of anesthetic agents and postoperative analgesics, increasing the risk for drug-related complications.
    i. Activities of daily living: Exercise, rest, and sleep habits are important for preventing postoperative complications and facilitating recovery.
    j. Occupation: Surgical procedures may require a delay in returning to work.
    k. Coping patterns: The patient needs information and emotional support to recover from surgery.
    l. Support systems: Family members should be encouraged to provide support before and after surgery.
    m. Sociocultural needs: The patient's cultural background may require that nursing interventions be individualized to meet needs in such areas as language, food preferences, family interaction and participation, personal space, and health beliefs and practices.

14. a. Vital signs: Assess temperature, blood pressure, and pulse and respiratory rates; note deviations from preoperative and PACU data as well as symptoms of complications.
    b. Color and temperature of skin: Assess for warmth, pallor, cyanosis, and diaphoresis.
    c. Level of consciousness: Assess for orientation to time, place, and person as well as reaction to stimuli and ability to move extremities.
    d. Intravenous fluids: Assess type and amount of solution, flow rate, securement and patency of tubing, and infusion site.
    e. Surgical site: Assess dressing and dependent areas for drainage. Assess drains and tubes and be sure they are intact, patent, and properly connected to drainage systems.
    f. Other tubes: Assess indwelling urinary catheter, gastrointestinal suction, and so forth for drainage, patency, and amount of output.
    g. Pain management: Assess for pain and determine whether analgesics were given in the PACU. Assess for nausea and vomiting.
    h. Position and safety: Place patient in the ordered position; if the patient is not fully conscious, place him/her in the side-lying position. Elevate side rails and place bed in low position.
    i. Comfort: Cover the patient with a blanket, reorient him/her to the room as necessary, and allow family members to remain with the patient after the initial assessment is completed.

15. Sample answers:
    a. Nausea and vomiting: Provide oral hygiene as needed; avoid strong-smelling foods.

b. Thirst: Offer ice chips; maintain oral hygiene.

c. Hiccups: Rebreathe into paper bag; eat a teaspoon of granulated sugar.

d. Surgical pain: Assess pain frequently; offer nonpharmacologic measures to supplement medications.

APPLYING YOUR KNOWLEDGE

REFLECTIVE PRACTICE USING CRITICAL THINKING SKILLS

Sample Answers

1. How might the nurse use blended nursing skills to implement the perioperative plan of care in a manner that respects Ms. Greenbaum's human dignity and addresses her fears and concerns about the surgical experience?

   The nurse should assess the patient's psychological, sociocultural, and spiritual dimension since surgery is a major psychological stressor that causes anxiety and fear. The nurse can use cues obtained in a health history to plan nursing interventions to provide information and emotional support for a successful recovery.

2. What would be a successful outcome for this patient? Following the nursing history, Ms. Greenbaum verbalizes her fears regarding the surgery and lists three coping methods to reduce stress.

3. What intellectual, technical, interpersonal, and/or ethical/legal competencies are most likely to bring about the desired outcome?

   Intellectual: ability to identify the common psychological patient responses before and after surgery.
   Interpersonal: ability to communicate to the patient concerns about the patient and his or her well-being.
   Ethical/Legal skills: ability to participate in care as a trusted and effective advocate, including advocating for a patient who is fearful.

4. What resources might be helpful for Ms. Greenbaum? Printed or AV materials of hysterectomies, counseling, support groups

CHAPTER 31

PRACTICING FOR NCLEX

MULTIPLE CHOICE QUESTIONS

1. c   2. a   3. c   4. b   5. b
6. d

ALTERNATE-FORMAT QUESTIONS

Multiple Response Questions

1. a, b, d, e
2. d, e, f
3. a, c, e
4. b, d, f
5. a, c, e

Prioritization Question

1.
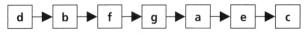

DEVELOPING YOUR KNOWLEDGE BASE

FILL-IN-THE-BLANKS

1. Gingivitis
2. Alopecia
3. Pediculosis
4. Hour of sleep
5. Bag bath

MATCHING EXERCISES

1. d	2. c	3. h	4. j	5. a
6. i	7. f	8. b	9. e	10. g
11. k				

CORRECT THE FALSE STATEMENTS

1. False—ceruminal glands
2. True
3. False—yellowish
4. True
5. False—lowest
6. True
7. False—Oily
8. False—lack of blood circulation
9. True
10. True
11. False—Pediculus humanis corpus
12. False—podiatrist
13. False—morning care

SHORT ANSWER

1. a. Culture: Many people in North America place a high value on personal cleanliness, shower frequently, and use many products to mask odors. Culture may also dictate whether bathing is private or communal.

   b. Socioeconomic class: Financial resources often define the hygiene options available to individuals. The availability of running water and finances for soap, shampoo, and so on affects hygiene.

   c. Spiritual practices: Religion may dictate ceremonial washing and purification, which may be a prelude to prayer or eating.

   d. Developmental level: Children learn different hygiene practices while growing up. Family practices may dictate morning or evening baths, frequency of shampooing, feelings about nudity, frequency of clothing changes, and so on.

   e. Health state: Disease or injury may hinder an individual's ability to perform hygiene measures or motivation to follow usual hygiene habits.

   f. Personal preference: People have personal preferences with regard to shower versus tub baths, bar soap versus liquid soap, and so on.

2. **a.** Feeding
   b. Bathing and hygiene
   c. Dressing and grooming
   d. Toileting
3. Bathing/Hygiene Deficit related to mother's lack of knowledge about bathing infants. The mother must be educated on the proper method of bathing her infant. She should be made aware of the need for good hygiene for her baby, and a bath should be demonstrated with a return demonstration. Investigate whether the mother has the financial means to buy the materials necessary for her baby's hygiene (shampoo, oil, powder, diaper rash ointment, etc.).
4. **a.** Early morning care: The patient should be assisted with toileting and provided comfort measures designed to refresh the patient and prepare him/her for breakfast. The face and hands should be washed and mouth care provided.
   b. Morning care: After breakfast, the nurse offers assistance with toileting, oral care, bathing, back massage, special skin care measures, hair care, cosmetics, dressing, and positioning. Bed linens are refreshed or changed.
   c. Afternoon care: The nurse should ensure the patient's comfort after lunch and offer assistance with toileting, handwashing, and oral care to nonambulatory patients.
   d. Hour of sleep care: The nurse again offers assistance with toileting, washing of face and hands, and oral care. A back massage helps the patient relax and fall asleep. Soiled bed linens or clothing should be changed and the patient positioned comfortably.
   e. As-needed care: The nurse offers individual hygiene measures as needed. Some patients require oral care every 2 hours. Patients who are diaphoretic may need their clothing or linens changed several times a shift.
5. Answers may include: Bathing cleanses the skin, acts as a conditioner, relaxes a restless person, promotes circulation, serves as musculoskeletal exercise, stimulates the rate and depth of respirations, promotes comfort, provides sensory input, improves self-esteem, and strengthens the nurse–patient relationship.
6. Provide the patient with articles for bathing and a basin of water that is at a comfortable temperature; place these items conveniently for the patient. Provide privacy for the patient; remove top linens on patient's bed and replace with a bath blanket. Place cosmetics in a convenient place with a mirror and light, and supply hot water and a razor for a patient who wishes to shave. Assist patients who cannot bathe themselves completely.
7. **a.** A towel bath can be accomplished with little fatigue to the patient.
   b. The towel remains warm during the short procedure.
   c. Patients state that they feel clean and refreshed.
   d. The oil in the bathing solution eliminates dry, itchy skin.
8. **a.** A back rub acts as a body conditioner.
   b. Giving a back rub provides an opportunity for the nurse to observe the skin for signs of breakdown.
   c. A back rub improves circulation and provides a means of communication with the patient through the use of touch.
9. **a.** Ventilation: It is wise to air the room when the patient is away for a diagnostic or therapeutic procedure to remove pathogens and unpleasant odors associated with body secretions and excretions.
   b. Odors: Odors can be controlled by promptly emptying bedpans, urinals, and emesis basins and by being careful not to dispose of soiled dressings or anything with a strong odor in the waste receptacle in the patient's room. Deodorizers may be needed.
   c. Room temperature: Whenever possible, patient preference should be followed regarding room temperature. In general, the temperature should be 20° to 23°C.
   d. Lighting and noise: The nurse should reduce harsh lighting and noises whenever possible. Conversations should not be carried on immediately outside the patient's room.
10. Sample answers:
    a. Rinse off soaps or detergents well when they are used for cleaning the skin.
    b. Add moisture to the air through a humidifier.
    c. Increase fluid intake.
    d. Use an emollient after cleansing the skin.
11. **a.** Lips: Color, moisture, lumps, ulcers, lesions, and edema
    b. Buccal mucosa: Color, moisture, lesions, nodules, and bleeding
    c. Gums: Lesions, bleeding, edema, and exudate; loose or missing teeth
    d. Tongue: Color, symmetry, movement, texture, and lesions
    e. Hard and soft palates: Intactness, color, patches, lesions, and petechiae
    f. Eye: Position, alignment, and general appearance; presence of lesions, nodules, redness, swelling, crusting, flaking, excessive tearing, or discharge; color of conjunctivae; blink reflex; and visual acuity
    g. Ear: Position, alignment, and general appearance; buildup of wax; dryness, crusting, discharge, or foreign body; and hearing acuity
    h. Nose: Position and general appearance; patency of nostrils; presence of tenderness, dryness, edema, bleeding, and discharge or secretions
12. **a.** Eye: Clean the eye from the inner canthus to the outer canthus using a wet, warm washcloth; cotton ball; or compress to soften crusted secretions. Avoid cross-contamination.

b. Ear: Clean the ear with a washcloth-covered finger, instructing patient never to insert objects into the ear for cleaning purposes.

c. Nose: Clean the nose by instructing patient to blow nose while both nares are patent (nasal suctioning may be indicated), remove crusted secretions around the nose, and apply petroleum jelly to tissue.

13. a. Contact lenses: Wash hands before touching eye surfaces or lenses; remove the lenses by gently grasping the lens near the lower edge and lifting it from eye. Soft lenses are cleaned, rinsed, and placed in a container of solution for storage. Identify as right or left lens.

b. Artificial eye: Assemble a small basin, soap and water, and solution for rinsing the prosthesis. Ask the patient how he/she cleans the eye area (usually flushed with normal saline before replacing the eye).

c. Hearing aids: Batteries should be checked routinely and earpieces cleaned daily with mild soap and water.

d. Dentures: Dentures should not be wrapped in tissue or disposable wipes. Dentures should be stored in water to prevent drying and warping of plastic materials. A few drops of essence of peppermint may be added to the water. Don gloves and hold dentures over a basin of water or a soft towel. Cleanse with cool or lukewarm water with a brush and nonabrasive powder or paste. Dentures can be soaked with special preparations to remove stains and hardened particles. Rinse well after cleaning; rinse mouth before replacing dentures.

14. Answers may include: Deficient self-care abilities, vascular disease, arthritis, diabetes mellitus, history of biting nails or trimming them improperly, frequent or prolonged exposure to chemicals or water, trauma, ill-fitting shoes, or obesity

APPLYING YOUR KNOWLEDGE

REFLECTIVE PRACTICE USING CRITICAL THINKING SKILLS

Sample Answers

1. What patient teaching should be implemented to help meet the hygienic needs of Ms. Delamordo? The nurse should investigate Ms. Delamordo's feelings about being cared for by her daughter since hygiene is such a personal matter. The nurse should encourage her to take care of as many hygienic practices as possible using her left side. Teaching should include how to adapt a bathroom to the needs of a disabled person, for example, placing a chair in the shower and using hand-held shower heads, checking water temperature, ensuring privacy, helping the patient get in and out of the shower, keeping the bathroom door unlocked, and helping to wash and dry areas that Ms. Delamordo can't reach

(such as the back). Ms. Delamordo's daughter should be taught the proper techniques for caring for her mother's hair, dentures, and hearing aids.

2. What would be a successful outcome for this patient? By next visit, Ms. Delamordo demonstrates washing areas of her body that she can reach. By next visit, Ms. Delamordo's daughter states that she is comfortable with the plan of care for hygienic measures instituted for her mother.

3. What intellectual, technical, interpersonal, and/or ethical/legal competencies are most likely to bring about the desired outcome?
Intellectual: having basic knowledge about hygiene, hygiene measures, and the products and equipment that facilitate care.
Technical: ability to adapt hygiene care measures to meet the needs of an older adult with right-sided paralysis.
Interpersonal: ability to encourage patients and their caregivers, as appropriate, in learning new self-care measures related to hygiene.

4. What resources might be helpful for Ms. Delamordo and her daughter?
Home healthcare services, information on adaptive devices for people with paralysis

PATIENT CARE STUDY

1. Objective data are underlined; subjective data are in boldface.
Dominic Gianmarco, a 78-year-old retired man with a history of Parkinson's disease, lives alone in a small home. He was recently hospitalized for problems with cardiac rhythm, and a pacemaker was installed. The home healthcare nurse visits 1 week after he was discharged to monitor his recovery and compliance with his medication regimen. The nurse observes that his appearance is disheveled and there are multiple stains on his clothing. Several food items are in various stages of preparation on the kitchen counter, and some appear to have spoiled. Mr. Gianmarco has several days' growth of beard and a body odor is apparent. He is pleasant and oriented to place and person but cannot identify the time or day of the week. **"I lose track of what day it is. Time is not important when you are my age. The most important thing to me right now is to be able to take care of myself and stay in this house near my friends."** There is a walker visible in a corner of the living room, but Mr. Gianmarco ambulates slowly around the house with a minimum of difficulty and does not use the walker. He comments that he keeps busy **"reading, watching old movies, and going to senior citizen activities with friends who stop by for me."** His daughter, who lives several hours away, visits him every weekend and prepares his medications for the week in a plastic container that is easy for him to open. The nurse observes that all medications appeared to have been taken to date: **"I don't mess**

around with my medicines. One helps my ticker and the others keep me from shaking so much."

2. Nursing Process Worksheet
   Health Problem: Self-care deficit: bathing/hygiene, dressing/grooming
   Etiology: Neuromuscular impairment secondary to Parkinson's disease, effects of aging
   Signs and Symptoms: Inability to bathe and groom self independently (disheveled appearance, stains on clothing, unshaven, presence of body odor)
   Expected Outcome: Within 2 weeks, patient will be able to perform self-care grooming activities with assistance of home healthcare aide.
   Nursing Interventions:
   a. Assess patient's ability to care for self in home setting.
   b. Explore availability of home healthcare aide to visit patient and assist with personal hygiene activities on a regular basis.
   c. Maintain safe environment.
   d. Encourage patient's independent activities.
   e. Investigate need for any adaptive equipment.
   Evaluative Statement: 3/28/11: Expected outcome partially met. Home healthcare aide assisting patient for several hours, 3 mornings/week. Continue to evaluate patient's ability to manage treatment regimen and need for any adaptive equipment.—*M. Gomez, RN*

3. Patient strengths: Has previously been able to care for self, motivated to maintain independence, caring family member able to visit on a regular basis
   Personal strengths: Commitment to caring, experienced home healthcare nurse, strong interpersonal skills, good knowledge of gerontologic nursing

4. 3/28/11: Revisited patient 2 weeks after initial visit. Patient alert and oriented. Neat personal appearance—clean shaven, absence of body odor, hair shampooed and combed, wearing clean clothes. Stated, "my girlfriends love me now." Conforming to medication schedule and participating in social activities. Continue periodic observations.—*M. Gomez, RN*

CHAPTER 32

PRACTICING FOR NCLEX
MULTIPLE CHOICE QUESTIONS

1. b	2. d	3. a	4. c	5. d
6. c	7. b	8. d	9. d	10. a
11. b	12. c			

ALTERNATE-FORMAT QUESTIONS
Multiple Response Questions

1. a, b, e
2. b, c, f
3. a, d, e
4. c, d, e
5. a, b, c
6. b, c, d
7. a, e, f
8. b, c, e
9. c, d, e
10. a, d, e
11. b, c, f

Prioritization Question

1.

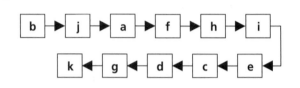

DEVELOPING YOUR KNOWLEDGE BASE
FILL-IN-THE-BLANKS

1. Intentional wounds
2. Exudate
3. Neutrophils, polymorphonuclear
4. Granulation
5. Fistula
6. Sterile 0.9% sodium chloride solution
7. Circular turn
8. Pressure ulcer

MATCHING EXERCISES

1. a	2. f	3. q	4. j	5. e
6. n	7. k	8. p	9. i	10. m
11. o	12. c	13. d	14. h	15. l
16. f	17. a	18. g	19. a	20. b
21. d	22. c	23. e	24. g	25. e

SHORT ANSWER

1. a. Protect the body
   b. Regulate body temperature
   c. Sense stimuli from the environment and transmit these sensations
   d. Excrete waste products
   e. Help maintain water and electrolyte balance
   f. Produce and absorb vitamin D
2. a. External pressure: Compresses blood vessels and causes friction
   b. Friction and shearing forces: Tear and injure blood vessels
3. a. Nutrition: Poorly nourished cells are easily damaged (e.g., vitamin C deficiency causes capillaries to become fragile, and poor circulation to the area results when they break).
   b. Hydration: Dehydration can interfere with circulation and subsequent cell nourishment.
   c. Moisture on the skin: Moisture associated with urinary incontinence increases the risk for skin damage more than chemical irritation from the ammonia in urine.
   d. Mental status: The more alert a patient is, the more likely it is that he/she will relieve pressure periodically and manage adequate skin hygiene.

e. Age: Older people are good candidates for pressure ulcers because their skin is susceptible to injury.

f. Immobility: Causes prolonged pressure on body areas

4. Sample answer:
Provide the caregivers with a simple, easy-to-understand list of instructions about caring for the pressure ulcer; address the causative factor for the pressure ulcer before proceeding with the plan of care; consult frequently with the physician about the progress of wound healing and products being used; use clean dressings; teach caregivers good handwashing technique; review signs of infection with caregivers and encourage them to contact a physician or home health nurse about any problems.

5. a. Hemostasis: Hemostasis occurs immediately after the initial injury. Involved blood vessels constrict and blood clotting begins through platelet activation and clustering. After only a brief period of constriction, these same blood vessels dilate and capillary permeability increases, allowing plasma and blood components to leak out into the area that is injured, forming a liquid called exudate.

b. Inflammatory phase: The inflammatory phase follows hemostasis and lasts about 4 to 6 days. White blood cells, predominantly leukocytes and macrophages, move to the wound. About 24 hours after the injury, macrophages enter the wound area and remain for an extended period. Macrophages are essential to the healing process. They not only ingest debris, but also release growth factors that are necessary for the growth of epithelial cells and new blood vessels. These growth factors also attract fibroblasts that help to fill in the wound, which is necessary for the next stage of healing. Acute inflammation is characterized by pain, heat, redness, and swelling at the site of the injury.

c. Proliferative phase: Begins about day 2 or 3 up to 2 to 3 weeks. New tissue is built to fill the wound space (action of fibroblasts). Capillaries grow across the wound, fibroblasts form fibrin that stretches through the clot, a thin layer of epithelial cells forms across the wound, and blood flow is reinstituted. Granulation tissue forms the foundation for scar tissue.

d. Maturation phase: Begins about 3 weeks after injury, up to 6 months if wound is large. Collagen is remodeled, new collagen is deposited, and avascular collagen tissue becomes a flat, thin white line.

6. Sample answers:
a. The patient will participate in the prescribed treatment regimen to promote wound healing.

b. The patient will remain free of infection at the site of the pressure ulcer.

c. The patient will demonstrate self-care measures necessary to prevent the development of a pressure ulcer.

7. Sample answers:
a. Overall appearance of skin: Are there any areas on your body where your skin feels paper thin? How does your skin feel in relation to moisture—dry, clammy, oily?

b. Recent changes in skin condition: Have you noticed any sores anywhere on your body? Do you ever notice any redness over a bony area when you stay in one position for a while?

c. Activity/mobility: Do you need assistance to walk to the bathroom? Can you change your position freely and painlessly?

d. Nutrition: Have you lost weight lately? Do you eat well-balanced meals?

e. Pain: Do you have any painful sores on your body? Do you take any medications for pain?

f. Elimination: Do you have any problems with incontinence? Have you ever used any briefs or pads for incontinence problems?

8. a. Appearance: Assess for the approximation of wound edges, color of the wound and surrounding areas, drains or tubes, sutures, and signs of dehiscence or evisceration.

b. Wound drainage: Assess the amount, color, odor, and consistency of wound drainage. Drainage can be assessed on the wound, the dressings, in drainage bottles or reservoirs, or under the patient.

c. Pain: Assess whether the pain has increased or is constant; pain may indicate delayed healing or an infection.

d. Sutures and staples: Assess the type of suture and whether enough tensile strength has developed to hold the wound edges together during healing.

9. Provide physical, psychological, and aesthetic comfort; remove necrotic tissue; prevent, eliminate, or control infection; absorb drainage; maintain a moist wound environment; protect the wound from further injury; and protect the skin surrounding the wound.

10. a. R = red = protect: Red wounds are in the proliferative stage of healing and are the color of normal granulation. They need protection by gentle cleansing, using moist dressings, applying a transparent or hydrocolloid dressing, and changing the dressing only when necessary.

b. Y = yellow = cleanse: Yellow wounds are characterized by oozing from the tissue covering the wound, often accompanied by purulent drainage. They need to be cleansed using irrigation; wet-to-moist dressings; using nonadherent, hydrogel, or other absorptive dressings; and topical antimicrobial medication.

c. B = black = débride: Black wounds are covered with thick eschar, which is usually black but may also be brown, gray, or tan. The eschar must be débrided before the wound can heal by using sharp, mechanical, chemical, or autolytic débridement.

11. a. Hot water bags or bottles: Relatively inexpensive and easy to use; may leak, burn, or make the patient uncomfortable from their weight

b. Electric heating pad: Can be used to apply dry heat locally; it is easy to apply and relatively safe and provides constant and even heat. Improper use can result in injury.

c. Aquathermia pad: Commonly used in healthcare agencies for various problems including back pain, muscle spasms, thrombophlebitis, and mild inflammation. Safer than a heating pad but still must be checked carefully.

d. Heat lamps: Provide dry heat to increase circulation to a small area, such as a pressure ulcer. Assess skin exposed to the heat every 5 minutes.

e. Heat cradles: A heat cradle is a metal half-circle frame that encloses the body part to be treated with heat. Precautions should be taken to prevent burning.

f. Hot packs: Commercial hot packs provide a specified amount of dry heat for a specific period.

g. Warm moist compresses: Used to promote circulation and reduce edema. Must be changed frequently and covered with a heating agent.

h. Sitz baths: Patient is placed in a tub filled with sufficient water to reach the umbilicus; the legs and feet remain out of the water.

i. Warm soaks: The immersion of a body area into warm water or a medicated solution to increase blood supply to a locally infected area; to aid in cleaning large sloughing wounds, such as burns; to improve circulation; and to apply medication to a locally infected area. Makes manipulation of a painful area much easier because of the buoyancy.

APPLYING YOUR KNOWLEDGE

REFLECTIVE PRACTICE USING CRITICAL THINKING SKILLS

Sample Answers

1. What nursing intervention would be appropriate to prevent skin irritation and the development of pressure ulcers for Mr. Bentz?

The nurse should review the patient chart to determine the cause and extent of previous wounds and institute measures to minimize these risks in the future. The nurse should be aware that larger than normal amounts of subcutaneous and tissue fat (which has fewer blood vessels) in people who are

obese may slow wound healing because fatty tissue is more difficult to suture, is more prone to infection, and takes longer to heal.

To protect Mr. Bentz, the nurse should implement turning and positioning schedules, as well as the use of appropriate support surfaces (tissue load management surfaces) and reposition him at least every 2 hours.

In the event of a reoccurrence of pressure ulcers, nursing interventions should focus on preventing infection, promoting wound healing, preventing further injury or alteration in skin integrity, promoting physical and emotional comfort, and facilitating coping.

2. What would be a successful outcome for this patient? Following discharge instructions, Mrs. Bentz will vocalize proper measures to assist her husband with hygiene, diet, positioning, and turning in bed. At follow-up appointment, Mr. Bentz will manifest intact skin free of skin irritations, infections, and wounds.

3. What intellectual, technical, interpersonal, and/or ethical/legal competencies are most likely to bring about the desired outcome?

Intellectual: knowledge of the phases of wound healing and factors that affect wound healing

Technical: ability to correctly use the products, protocols, and equipment necessary to prevent and treat pressure ulcers and other skin alterations

Interpersonal: ability to establish trusting professional relationships that enlist patients and their caregivers in a plan to prevent or treat pressure ulcers and other skin alterations

4. What resources might be helpful for Mr. Bentz and his wife?

Home healthcare visits, printed and/or AV materials on prevention of pressure ulcers

PATIENT CARE STUDY

1. Objective data are underlined; subjective data are in boldface.

Mrs. Chijioke, an 88-year-old woman who lived alone for years, was brought to the hospital after neighbors found her lying at the bottom of her cellar steps. She had broken her hip and underwent hip repair surgery 3 days ago. The nurse assigned to care for Mrs. Chijioke noticed during the patient's bath that the skin of her coccyx, heels, and elbows was reddened. The skin returned to a normal color when pressure was relieved in these areas. There was no edema, nor was there induration or blistering. Although Mrs. Chijioke can be lifted out of bed into a chair, she spends most of the day in bed, lying on her back with an abductor pillow between her legs. At 5 feet tall and 89 pounds, Mrs. Chijioke looks lost in the big hospital bed. Her eyes are bright, and she usually attempts a warm smile, but she has little physical strength and lies seemingly motionless for hours. Her skin is wrinkled and paper thin, and her arms are already bruised from unsuccessful attempts at intravenous therapy. She was dehydrated on admission since she had **spent almost 48 hours crumpled at the bottom of her steps before being found by her neighbors**, and she was clearly in need of nutritional, fluid, and electrolyte support. A long-time diabetic, Mrs. Chijioke is now spiking a <u>fever (39.0°C, or 102.2°F),</u> which concerns her nurse.

2. Nursing Process Worksheet

   Health Problem: Risk for impaired skin integrity

   Etiology: Immobility; effects of aging, dehydration, and illness

   Signs and Symptoms: Skin of her coccyx, heels, and elbows is reddened—returns to normal color when pressure is relieved; lies motionless on her back when unattended; skin is wrinkled and thin; elevated temperature (39°C).

   Expected Outcome: Whenever observed, the patient's skin will appear clean and intact (no redness, blistering, indurations).

   Nursing Interventions:

   a. Reposition patient in correct alignment at least every 1 to 2 hours and ensure protection of pressure points where possible; examine skin for signs of breakdown with each position change.

   b. Massage pressure points and keep skin clean and dry.

   c. Keep bed linens dry and free of wrinkles.

   d. Monitor high-risk factors: dehydration, effects of illness.

   Evaluative Statement: 10/6/11: Goal met—patient's skin is clean and intact and shows no signs of breakdown. Continue prevention program.
   —*M. Wong, RN*

3. Patient strengths: Concerned neighbors; until now has been able to care for herself and keep herself in good health

   Personal strengths: Ability to recognize patients at high risk for problems such as impaired skin integrity; strong commitment to meeting the needs of geriatric patients; experienced clinician

4. 10/6/11: Patient remains on an every-2-hour positioning regimen. The protective heel and elbow pads have resulted in intact skin in these areas—no redness. The skin on her coccyx appears reddened after she lies on her back, but the redness disappears when the pressure is relieved. No constant redness, edema, or induration. Skin remains dry; lotion applied with each position change.—*M. Wong, RN*

CHAPTER 33

PRACTICING FOR NCLEX
MULTIPLE CHOICE QUESTIONS

1. b	**2.** a	**3.** c	**4.** d	**5.** a
6. c	**7.** b	**8.** c	**9.** d	**10.** c
11. a	**12.** a	**13.** b	**14.** d	**15.** d

ALTERNATE-FORMAT QUESTIONS
Multiple Response Questions

1. c, d, f
2. a, c, e
3. b, c, d
4. a, e, f
5. b, d, e
6. c, e, f
7. a, b, c
8. b, c, e

DEVELOPING YOUR KNOWLEDGE BASE
IDENTIFICATION

1. a. Fowler's position
   b. Protective supine position
   c. Protective side-lying or lateral position
   d. Protective Sims' position
   e. Protective prone position

MATCHING EXERCISES

1. e	**2.** c	**3.** f	**4.** b	**5.** a
6. l	**7.** a	**8.** g	**9.** o	**10.** d
11. k	**12.** b	**13.** n	**14.** c	**15.** m
16. j	**17.** h	**18.** e	**19.** i	**20.** b
21. e	**22.** f	**23.** a	**24.** i	**25.** c
26. d	**27.** g			

CORRECT THE FALSE STATEMENTS

1. False—irregular bones
2. True
3. True
4. True
5. False—Body mechanics
6. True
7. False—wider
8. False—proprioceptor or kinesthetic
9. False—basal ganglia
10. True
11. True
12. True
13. False—facing
14. True
15. False—slide, roll, push, or pull

SHORT ANSWER

1. See table below.

Body System	Effects of Exercise	Effects of Immobility
Cardiovascular	↑ Efficiency of heart ↓ Resting heart rate and blood pressure ↑ Blood flow and oxygenation of all body parts	↑ Cardiac workload ↑ Risk for orthostatic hypotension ↑ Risk for venous thrombosis
Respiratory	↑ Depth of respiration ↑ Respiratory rate ↑ Gas exchange at alveolar level ↑ Rate of carbon dioxide excretion	↓ Depth of respiration ↓ Rate of respiration Pooling of secretions Impaired gas exchange
Gastrointestinal	↑ Appetite ↑ Intestinal tone	Disturbance in appetite Altered protein metabolism Altered digestion and utilization of nutrients
Urinary	↑ Blood flow to kidneys ↑ Efficiency in maintaining fluid and acid–base balance ↑ Efficiency in excreting body wastes	↑ Urinary stasis ↑ Risk for renal calculi ↓ Bladder muscle tone
Musculoskeletal	↑ Muscle efficiency ↑ Coordination ↑ Efficiency of nerve impulse transmission	↓ Muscle size, tone, and strength ↓ Joint mobility, flexibility Bone demineralization ↓ Endurance, stability ↑ Risk for contracture formation
Metabolic	↑ Efficiency of metabolic system ↑ Efficiency of body temperature regulation	↑ Risk for electrolyte imbalance Altered exchange of nutrients and gases
Integumentary	Improved tone, color, and turgor, resulting from improved circulation	↑ Risk for skin breakdown and formation of decubitus ulcers
Psychological Well-Being	Energy, vitality, general well-being Improved sleep Improved appearance Improved self-concept Positive health behaviors	↑ Sense of powerlessness ↓ Self-concept ↓ Social interaction ↓ Sensory stimulation Altered sleep–wake pattern ↑ Risk for depression

2. a. Motion
  b. Maintenance of posture
  c. Heat production
3. a. Point of origin: Attachment of a muscle to the more stationary bone
  b. Point of insertion: Attachment of a muscle to the more movable bone
4. a. The afferent nervous system conveys information from receptors in the periphery of the body to the central nervous system.

b. Nerve cells called neurons are responsible for conducting impulses from one part of the body to another.
  c. This information is processed by the central nervous system, and a response is decided on.
  d. The efferent system conveys the desired response from the CNS to skeletal muscles by way of the somatic nervous system.
5. a. Body alignment or posture: The alignment of body parts that permits optimal musculoskeletal

balance and operation and promotes healthy physiologic functioning

b. Balance: A body in correct alignment is balanced; its center of gravity is close to the base of support, the line of gravity goes through the base of support, and the object has a wide base of support.

c. Coordinated body movement: Using major muscle groups rather than weaker ones and taking advantage of the body's natural levers and fulcrums

6. Sample answers:

a. Develop a habit of maintaining erect posture and begin activities by broadening the base of support and lowering the center of gravity.

b. Use the weight of the body as a force for pulling or pushing by rocking on the feet or leaning forward or backward.

c. Slide, roll, push, or pull an object rather than lifting it to reduce the energy needed to move the weight against the pull of gravity.

d. Use the weight of the body to push an object by falling or rocking forward, and to pull an object by falling or rocking backward.

7. **a.** Aerobic exercises (running, swimming, tennis): Sustained muscle movements that increase blood flow, heart rate, and metabolic demand for oxygen over time, thereby promoting cardiovascular conditioning

b. Stretching exercises (warm-up and cool-down exercises): Movements that allow muscles and joints to be stretched gently through their full range of motion; increase flexibility

c. Strength and endurance exercises (weight training): Weight training, calisthenics, and specific isometric exercises can build both strength and endurance, increase the power of the musculoskeletal system, and improve the body.

d. Activities of daily living (shopping, cleaning): All activities of daily living have an effect on health and provide increased fitness that does not require a gym.

8. Sample answers:

a. Increased energy, vitality, and general well-being

b. Improved sleep

c. Improved self-concept

d. Increased positive health behaviors

9. **a.** Pillows: Pillows are used primarily to provide support or to elevate a part. Pillows of different sizes are useful for different body parts.

b. Mattresses: A mattress should be firm but should have sufficient "give" to permit good body alignment to be comfortable and supportive. A well-made and well-supported foam-rubber mattress retains a uniform firmness.

c. Adjustable bed: The head of an adjustable bed can be elevated to the desired degree, and the distance from the floor can be altered to allow the patient to get in and out of bed easier or to

allow healthcare workers to give care without back strain.

d. Bed side rails: They help to remind patients that they are not in their usual environment and keep them from falling out of bed.

e. Trapeze bar: This handgrip suspended from a frame near the head of the bed makes moving and turning considerably easier for many patients and facilitates transfers into and out of bed.

f. Cradle: A metal frame that keeps the top bedding off the patient's lower extremities while providing privacy and warmth.

g. Sandbags: Sandbags immobilize an extremity and support body alignment. They are not hard or firmly packed but should be placed so they do not create pressure on bony prominences.

h. Trochanter rolls: Used to support the hips and legs so that the femurs do not rotate outward.

i. Hand/wrist splints or rolls: A commercial plastic or aluminum splint is used to hold the thumb in place no matter what position the hand is in.

10. **a.** Quadriceps drills: Have the patient contract the muscles on the front of the thighs by pulling kneecaps toward hips; hold the position to the count of four; relax muscles for count of four. Frequency: two or three times each hour, four to six times a day.

b. Pushups: Sitting in bed: Instruct patient to lift hips off the bed by pushing down with hands on mattress. Lying on abdomen: Instruct patient to place hands near the outstretched body at shoulder level with palms down on the mattress and elbows bent sharply; then have patient straighten elbows while lifting head and shoulders off bed. Wheelchair: Instruct patient to place hands on arms of chair and raise body three or four times a day.

c. Dangling: Instruct the patient to sit on the edge of the bed with legs and feet dangling over the side. Rest the patient's feet on the floor or footstool. Have patient assume a marching position. (Remain with patient in case he/she feels faint.)

11. **a.** Physical assessment: The nurse would assess the following:

1. General ease of movement: Are body parts fluid and is voluntary movement controlled and coordinated?

2. Gait: Is head erect? Are the vertebrae straight, knees and feet forward, and arms swinging freely in alternation with leg swings?

3. Alignment—in standing position: Can a straight line be drawn from the ear through the shoulder and hip?

4. Joint structure and function: Are there any joint deformities or limitations in full range of motion?

5. Muscle mass tone and strength: Are they adequate to accomplish movement and work?

6. Endurance: Is patient able to turn in bed, maintain correct alignment when sitting and standing, ambulate, and perform self-care activities?

b. Diagnosis: Activity Intolerance related to decreased muscle mass, tone, and strength

c. Exercise program: Do range-of-motion exercises twice a day to build up muscles and joint capabilities. Use quadriceps drills two or three times an hour, four to six times a day. Do settings twice a day and pushups three or four times a day.

12. Sample answers:

a. General ease of movement: Normal: Body movements are voluntarily controlled, fluid, and coordinated.
Abnormal: Involuntary movements, tremors, tics, chorea, and so on.

b. Gait and posture: Normal: Head erect, vertebrae straight.
Abnormal: Spastic hemiparesis, scissors gait

c. Alignment: Normal: In the standing and sitting position, a straight line can be drawn from the ear through the shoulder and hip; in bed, the head, shoulders, and hips are aligned.
Abnormal: Abnormal spinal curvatures, inability to maintain correct alignment independently

d. Joint structure and function: Normal: Absence of joint deformities, full range of motion.
Abnormal: Limitations in the normal range of motion, increased joint mobility

e. Muscle mass, tone, and strength: Normal: Adequate muscle mass and tone. Abnormal: Atrophy, hypotonicity

f. Endurance: Normal: Ability to turn in bed, maintain correct alignment.
Abnormal: Weakness, pallor

APPLYING YOUR KNOWLEDGE

REFLECTIVE PRACTICE USING CRITICAL THINKING SKILLS

Sample Answers

1. What patient teaching might the nurse incorporate into the plan of care to help Kelsi's parents minimize the complications of immobility for their daughter? The nurse should review the nursing history to assess Kelsi's activity level prior to the accident and develop a teaching plan that maximizes her level of functioning. The nurse should communicate with Kelsi and her parents and explain what is happening to her and the reasoning behind the positioning and turning schedules and range-of-motion exercises. The parents could also be taught to assist with these interventions.

2. What would be a successful outcome for this patient? By next visit, Kelsi's parents will demonstrate range-of-motion exercises to help restore mobility to their daughter. By next visit, Kelsi will manifest appropriate muscle strength and freedom from skin alterations.

3. What intellectual, technical, interpersonal, and/or ethical/legal competencies are most likely to bring about the desired outcome?
Intellectual: knowledge of common problems associated with mobility and inactivity
Technical: ability to use correctly the protocols, products, and equipment necessary to promote body alignment and to prevent or treat complications related to immobility
Interpersonal: ability to demonstrate respect for a patient's human dignity and autonomy and to encourage patients and their caregivers to maximize their mobility and functional status
Ethical/Legal: ability to act as a patient advocate to promote the maximum level of patient functioning

4. What resources might be helpful for the Lester family? Home healthcare services, physical rehabilitation services, printed or AV materials on range-of-motion exercises

PATIENT CARE STUDY

1. Objective data are underlined; subjective data are in boldface.
Robert Witherspoon, a 42-year-old university professor, presents for a checkup shortly after his father's death. His father died of complications of coronary artery disease. Mr. Witherspoon is 5 foot 9 inches, weighs 235 lb, has a decided "paunch," and **reports that until now he has made no time for exercise because he preferred to use his free time reading or listening to classical music. He enjoys French cuisine, including rich desserts,** and has a cholesterol level of 310 mg/dL (normal is 150 to 250 mg/dL). **He admits being frightened by his father's death and is appropriately concerned about his elevated cholesterol level. "I guess I've never given much thought to my health before, but my Dad's death changed all that," he tells you. "I know coronary artery disease runs in families, and I can tell you that I'm not ready to pack it all in yet. Tell me what I have to do to fight this thing."** He admits that he used to tease a colleague—who lowered his own cholesterol from 290 to 200 mg/dL by diet and exercise alone—by accusing him of being a fitness freak. **"Now, I'm recognizing the wisdom of his health behaviors and wondering if diet and exercise won't do the trick for me. Can you help me design an exercise program that will work?"**

2. Nursing Process Worksheet
Health Problem: Altered health maintenance; lack of exercise program
Etiology: Low value placed on fitness and self-care behaviors in the past
Signs and Symptoms: 5 foot 9 inches tall; 235 lb; until now "no time" for exercise; "I've never given much thought to my health before"; "Tell me what I have to do to fight this thing," "Can you help me design an exercise program that will work?"

Expected Outcome: At next visit, 10/27/11, patient will report adherence to the exercise program developed 9/30/11 (additional goals will describe desired changes in weight and cholesterol level).

Nursing Interventions:

a. Explore the patient's fitness goals, interest, skills, exercise opportunities, and exercise capacity.

b. Assist the patient in obtaining medical clearance for exercise.

c. Explore feasible exercise activities with the patient, considering health benefits sought, time involved, need for special equipment, precautions, and risk.

d. Develop an exercise program that specifies warm-up and cool-down activities and three or four major exercise activities from which the patient can choose. Specify frequency, duration, and intensity.

e. Encourage the patient to complement the exercise program with everyday activities that require exercise.

f. Try to identify with the patient potential threats to the exercise program's successful implementation. Plan support strategies.

Evaluative Statement: 10/27/11: Goal partially met—patient reports that the second week into his program his "jogging buddy" got sick and that without the support of his friend he stopped exercising regularly; wants to resume. Revision: Explore new strategies to strengthen resolve/adherence. —*J. McKeough, RN*

3. Patient strengths: Patient is highly motivated to develop new self-care behaviors as a result of his father's death—asking for help.

Personal strengths: Good understanding of the relationship between self-care behaviors (exercise, nutrition) and health; experienced in designing exercise programs; knowledge of benefits/risks associated with exercise; strong interpersonal/counseling skills

4. 10/27/11: Whereas the patient left the last session "enthusiastic" about beginning an exercise program, he reported today that he "feels like a failure" since he wasn't faithful to the goals he set for himself. After losing his exercise buddy, he found it easy to "skip runs," and he hasn't found another racquetball partner. We identified and reinforced the progress he has made and developed new expected outcomes that are less dependent on external support.—*J. McKeough, RN*

CHAPTER 34

PRACTICING FOR NCLEX
MULTIPLE CHOICE QUESTIONS

1. b	**2.** a	**3.** d	**4.** b	**5.** a
6. d	**7.** c	**8.** d	**9.** b	**10.** c
11. b	**12.** b			

ALTERNATE-FORMAT QUESTIONS
Multiple Response Questions

1. a, c, e
2. d, e, f
3. a, d, f
4. b, d, e
5. c, d, f
6. a, b, c
7. b, c, e
8. a, e, f

Prioritization Question

1.

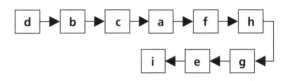

DEVELOPING YOUR KNOWLEDGE BASE
FILL-IN-THE-BLANKS

1. The reticular activating system (RAS) and bulbar synchronizing region
2. Delta sleep
3. Parasomnias
4. Insomnia
5. Hypersomnia
6. Narcolepsy

MATCHING EXERCISES

1. g	**2.** a	**3.** c	**4.** h	**5.** b
6. d	**7.** f	**8.** i	**9.** j	**10.** c
11. a	**12.** a	**13.** d	**14.** b	**15.** c, d
16. b	**17.** d	18. a		

CORRECT THE FALSE STATEMENTS

1. True
2. True
3. False—at stage I, NREM sleep
4. False—4 or 5
5. False—14 to 20
6. True
7. False—protein and carbohydrate
8. False—hinders
9. True
10. True
11. False—sleep apnea

SHORT ANSWER

1. a. Restores physical well-being
   b. Relieves stress and anxiety
   c. Restores the ability to cope and to concentrate on activities of daily living
2. a. Infants: 10 to 12 hours/day
   b. Growing children: 10 to 14 hours/day
   c. Adults: 7 to 9 hours/day
   d. Older adults: May require a longer time to go to sleep and wake earlier and more frequently during the night

3. **a.** Physical activity: Activity increases fatigue and promotes relaxation that is followed by sleep. It also increases both REM and NREM sleep.

b. Psychological stress: The person experiencing stress tends to find it difficult to obtain the amount of sleep he/she needs, and REM sleep decreases.

c. Motivation: A desire to be wakeful and alert helps overcome sleepiness and sleep; when there is minimal motivation to be awake, sleep generally follows.

d. Culture: Bedtime rituals, sleeping place, and pattern of sleep may vary according to culture.

e. Diet: Carbohydrates appear to have an effect on brain serotonin levels and promote feelings of calmness and relaxation; protein may actually increase brain energy alertness and concentration.

f. Alcohol and caffeine: Alcohol in moderation seems to help induce sleep in some people, but large quantities limit REM and delta sleep. Caffeine is a CNS stimulant and may interfere with the ability to fall asleep.

g. Smoking: Nicotine has a stimulating effect, and smokers usually have a more difficult time falling asleep.

h. Environmental factors: Most people sleep best in their usual home environments.

i. Lifestyle: Sleep disorders are the major problem associated with shift work, and developing a sleep pattern is especially difficult if the shift changes periodically. Sleep can be affected by watching some types of television shows, participating in stimulating activity, and level of activity or exercise.

j. Exercise: Moderate exercise is a healthy way to promote sleep, but exercise that occurs within 2 hours before normal bedtime can hinder sleep.

k. Illness: Illness is a physiologic and psychological stressor and, therefore, influences sleep.

l. Medications: Sleep quality is influenced by certain drugs that may decrease REM sleep.

4. The cause of the sleep disturbance, the related signs and symptoms, when it first began and how often it occurs, how it affects everyday living, the severity of the problem and whether it can be treated independently by nursing, how the patient is coping with the problem, and the success of any treatments attempted

5. **a.** Energy level
    b. Facial characteristics
    c. Behavioral characteristics
    d. Data suggestive of potential sleep problems

6. Make sure the patient has a comfortable bed, with bottom linens tight and clean. The upper linens should allow freedom of movement and not exert pressure. A quiet, darkened room with privacy, with proper ventilation and a comfortable temperature, should be provided.

7. Sample answers:
    a. Sleep Pattern Disturbance: Difficulty remaining asleep related to noise of hospital environment and need for periodic treatments
    b. Sleep Pattern Disturbance: Excessive daytime sleeping related to effects of biologic aging
    c. Sleep Pattern Disturbance: Altered sleep–wake patterns related to frequent rotations of shift
    d. Sleep Pattern Disturbance: Premature wakening related to alcohol dependency
    e. Sleep Pattern Disturbance: Difficulty falling asleep related to worries about family

8. **a.** Eyes: Dart back and forth quickly
    b. Muscles: Small muscle twitching, large muscle immobility
    c. Respirations: Irregular; sometimes interspersed with apnea
    d. Pulse: Rapid or irregular
    e. Blood pressure: Increases or fluctuates
    f. Gastric secretions: Increase
    g. Metabolism: Increases; body temperature increases
    h. Sleep cycle: REM sleep enters from stage II of NREM sleep and reenters NREM sleep at stage II; arousal from sleep difficult

9. Sample answers:
    a. Prepare a restful environment.
    b. Offer appropriate bedtime snacks and beverages.
    c. Promote comfort and relaxation.

10. Sample answers:
    a. Usual sleeping and waking times: Do you usually go to bed and wake up around the same time?
    b. Number of hours of undisturbed sleep: Do you have any difficulty falling asleep? Do you wake up during the night?
    c. Quality of sleep: Do you feel rested after the amount of sleep you get?
    d. Number and duration of naps: Do you find yourself falling asleep during the day?
    e. Energy level: Do you feel refreshed after a night's sleep?
    f. Means of relaxing before bedtime: Do you watch television or read before bedtime?
    g. Bedtime rituals: What do you do before going to bed?
    h. Sleep environment: What is your bedroom environment like?
    i. Pharmacologic aids: Do you ever take medications to help you fall asleep?
    j. Nature of sleep disturbance: What do you think is causing your sleep problem?
    k. Onset of a disturbance: When did you first notice that you had trouble falling asleep?
    l. Causes of a disturbance: Are you doing anything different before bedtime?
    m. Severity of a disturbance: Do you have breathing problems during the night?

n. Symptoms of a disturbance: Do you grind your teeth at night?

o. Interventions attempted and results: What measures have you taken to promote a comfortable sleep environment?

APPLYING YOUR KNOWLEDGE

REFLECTIVE PRACTICE USING CRITICAL THINKING SKILLS

Sample Answers

1. What nursing interventions might the nurse employ to help alleviate Mr. Bittner's sleep disturbances?

Nursing strategies for promoting rest and sleep in older adults include encouraging physical activity, discouraging napping, arranging an assessment for depression and treatment, reviewing medications, assessing for any side effects of sleep pattern disturbance, and decreasing fluids in the evening.

2. What would be a successful outcome for this patient?

At next visit, Mr. Bittner lists 3 strategies to follow to help alleviate his sleep disturbance.

In 3 weeks, Mr. Bittner reports obtaining 6 undisturbed hours of sleep at night.

3. What intellectual, technical, interpersonal, and/or ethical/legal competencies are most likely to bring about the desired outcome?

Intellectual: knowledge of the factors that affect rest and sleep, including developmental variables

Interpersonal: ability to assist older adults to develop methods to promote adequate sleep and cope with disturbed sleep patterns

Ethical/Legal: ability to practice in an ethically and legally defensible manner when providing care to patients experiencing disturbed sleep pattern

4. What resources might be helpful for Mr. Bittner?

Printed materials on sleep enhancement strategies, relaxation therapy, consultation with a sleep therapist

PATIENT CARE STUDY

1. Objective data are underlined; subjective data are in boldface.

Gina Cioffi, a 23-year-old graduate nurse, has been in her new position as a critical care staff nurse in a large tertiary-care medical center for 3 months. **"I was so excited about working three 12-hour shifts a week when I started this job, thinking I'd have lots of time for other things I want to do, but I'm not sure anymore," she says. "I've been doing extra shifts when we're short-staffed because the money is so good, and right now it seems I'm always tired and all I think about all day long is how soon I can get back to bed. Worst of all, when I do finally get into bed, I often can't fall asleep, especially if things have been busy at work and someone 'went bad.' Does everyone else feel like me?"** Looking at Gina, you notice dark circles under her eyes and are suddenly struck by the change in her appearance from when she first started working. At that time, she "bounced into work" looking fresh each morning, and her features were always animated. Now, her skin is pale, her hair and clothes look rumpled, and the "brightness" that was so characteristic of her earlier is strikingly absent. With some gentle questioning, you discover that **she frequently goes out with new friends she has made at the hospital when her shift is over, and sometimes goes for 48 hours without sleep. "I know I've gotten myself into a rut. How do I get out of it? I used to think my sleep habits were bad at school, but this is a hundred times worse because there never seems to be time to crash. I just have to keep on going."**

2. Nursing Process Worksheet

Health Problem: Sleep pattern disturbance: altered sleep–wake patterns

Etiology: Twelve-hour shift work and stress of new job

Signs and Symptoms: Works three 12-hour shifts plus two or three extra shifts per week; "right now it seems like I am always tired and all I think about all day long is how soon I can get back to bed; when I do finally get into bed I often can't fall asleep." Dark circles under eyes; pale skin; sometimes goes 48 hours without sleep; reports being less animated.

Expected Outcome: By this time next month (7/22/11), patient will report she is sleeping soundly for a minimum of 6 hours per night at least 6 days a week, as evidenced by her feeling less fatigued and more in control of sleep situation.

Nursing Interventions:

a. Instruct patient to keep a sleep diary for 7 days and analyze its contents at the end of the week.

b. Counsel patient about the need to reevaluate priorities (e.g., working extra shifts).

c. Develop stress management strategies, including relaxation exercises.

d. Identify and reduce (where possible) factors interfering with sleep.

Evaluative Statement: 10/6/11 Expected outcome met: Sleeping 7 to 8 hours per night and generally feels refreshed upon awakening.—N. McLoughlin, RN

3. Patient strengths: Strongly motivated to address this problem

Personal strengths: Comprehensive knowledge of the physiology of sleep and sleep requirements and patterns; familiarity with the stresses of clinical nursing, especially for the graduate nurse; strong interpersonal skills; creative problem solver

4. 10/6/11: Patient "bounced into the office" with the vigor and enthusiasm she displayed when she first started working. Her skin had regained its usual coloring and glow, and her face was animated. She expressed gratitude for "helping me recover my old self" and reported that she is sleeping 7 to 8 hours per night and usually wakes up refreshed and ready to tackle the new day. On questioning, she expressed an appreciation for the need to balance rest and activity and appears to have developed a workable plan for ensuring adequate rest.—N. McLoughlin, RN

CHAPTER 35

PREPARING FOR NCLEX
MULTIPLE CHOICE QUESTIONS

1. c	**2.** d	**3.** a	**4.** d	**5.** a
6. c	**7.** b	**8.** d	**9.** a	**10.** c
11. d	**12.** b	**13.** b	**14.** d	**15.** c
16. b	**17.** c			

ALTERNATE-FORMAT QUESTIONS
Multiple Response Questions

1. a, c, d
2. c, e, f
3. b, d, e
4. b, c, d
5. a, e, f
6. c, d, e

DEVELOPING YOUR KNOWLEDGE BASE

FILL-IN-THE-BLANKS

1. Nociceptive
2. Cutaneous
3. Visceral
4. Allodynia
5. Referred

MATCHING EXERCISES

1. e	**2.** k	**3.** f	**4.** j	**5.** a
6. c	**7.** g	**8.** b	**9.** d	**10.** h
11. c	**12.** d	**13.** b	**14.** a	**15.** c
16. a	**17.** b	**18.** c	**19.** j	**20.** b
21. d	**22.** k	**23.** a	**24.** i	**25.** c
26. f	**27.** h	**28.** g		

SHORT ANSWER

1. See table below. Sample answers:
   Situation A: Pain, acute migraine, related to unrelieved stress as manifested by furrowed brows, nausea, and anxiety
   Situation B: Pain related to animal scratch and fear, as manifested by pulling back from cat, swelling and redness around scratch, and exaggerated weeping
   Situation C: Pain, acute postoperative, related to cesarean section as manifested by refusal to move, muscle tension, and rigidity and helplessness
   Situation D: Chronic pain related to degenerative joint disease as manifested by grimacing, refusal to walk, increased blood pressure, and exaggerated restlessness

Situation	Behavioral	Physiological	Affective
A	Furrowed brows	Nausea	Anxiety
B	Crying	Swelling and redness on scratched area	Fear
C	Refusal to move	Muscle tension, rigidity	Helplessness
D	Grimacing, refusal to walk	Increased blood pressure	Exaggerated restlessness

2. The injured tissue releases chemicals that excite nerve endings. A damaged cell releases histamine, which excites nerve endings. Lactic acid accumulates in tissues injured by lack of blood supply and is believed to excite nerve endings and cause pain or lower the threshold of nerve endings to other stimuli. Bradykinin, prostaglandins, and substance P are also released.

3. Referred pain can be transmitted to a cutaneous site different from where it originated because afferent neurons enter the spinal cord at the same level as the cutaneous site to which the pain has been referred.

4. The gate control theory states that small-diameter nerve fibers conduct excitatory pain stimuli toward the brain, but nerve fibers of a large diameter inhibit the transmission of pain impulses from the spinal cord to the brain. A gating mechanism is believed to be located in the substantia gelatinosa of the dorsal horn of the spinal cord. The "gate" is believed to be capable of comparing the strength of excitatory and inhibitory signals entering this region to determine which impulses will travel toward the brain. When too much information arrives

at the gate, certain cells in the spinal cord are believed to interrupt the signal, closing the gate.

5. **a.** Acute pain: Generally rapid in onset, varying in intensity from mild to severe, and lasting from a brief period up to 6 months (e.g., surgery pain)
   b. Chronic pain: May be limited, intermittent, or persistent, but lasts for 6 months or longer and interferes with normal functioning (e.g., arthritis pain)
   c. Intractable pain: Pain that is resistant to therapy and persists despite a variety of interventions

6. Sample answers:
   a. Culture: In one culture, it may be acceptable to express pain vocally, whereas in another culture, such vocal expressions of pain are unacceptable.
   b. Ethnicity: An Italian man may respond to pain with cries, moans, complaints, and so on, whereas an Irish man may be calm and unemotional about his pain.
   c. Family, gender, or age: Spouses may reinforce pain behavior in their partners.
   d. Religious beliefs: In some religions, pain is viewed as suffering and as a means of purification to make up for individual or community sin.
   e. Environment and support people: Caring support people can help a patient cope with the strangeness of the healthcare environment.
   f. Anxiety and other stressors: Fear of the unknown may compound anxiety and aggravate pain.
   g. Past pain experience: A child may have no fear of pain because he has never experienced pain.

7. Answers will vary with student's experiences.

8. Sample answers:
   a. "You are the authority on your pain experience, and you must let your nurse know when you are in pain or when the medication isn't working anymore."
   b. "Physical addiction may occur with chronic opioid use, but this is not the same as the psychological dependence of addiction. Studies suggest that only half of 1% of all individuals with cancer pain and other severe types of pain will become addicted to opioids."
   c. "Opioid drugs can be used to manage your pain safely as long as we take the appropriate precautions and conscientiously assess any side effects."

9. Sample answers:
   a. Duration of pain: "For how long have you been experiencing this pain?"
   b. Quantity and intensity of pain: "How frequently do you get these attacks? On a scale of 1 to 10, how would you rate the intensity of this pain?"
   c. Quality of pain: "How would you describe the pain (sharp, intense, dull, throbbing, etc.)?"
   d. Physiologic indicators of pain: "Have you noticed any physical changes since you've been experiencing this pain?"

10. Answers will vary with the student's experiences and may include the following: If a patient suspects a plot to trick him/her into feeling better, the patient is unlikely to respect or appreciate the good intentions of the physicians and nurses involved.

11. **a.** A patient with a cognitive impairment: Many cognitively impaired patients cannot verbally report their pain or express concepts; therefore, nurses must rely on their own careful assessments, their empathetic qualities, and the expectation that this patient will experience pain if a verbal patient usually reports this event as painful.
    b. A 5-year-old patient: Children cannot always express their pain; the nurse must observe facial expressions, body positions, crying, and physiologic responses. Communication with parents or guardians is vital for accurate pain assessment.
    c. An older patient: Nurses should be aware that older patients fear that admitting pain may limit their independence; boredom, loneliness, and depression may affect an older person's perception of pain and willingness to report it. Also, their choice of terms in describing pain may be deceptive.

APPLYING YOUR KNOWLEDGE

REFLECTIVE PRACTICE USING CRITICAL THINKING SKILLS
Sample Answers

1. What nursing interventions might the nurse use to help minimize the effects of premenstrual syndrome on Ms. Potter?
   The nurse should investigate Ms. Potter's symptoms and pain history to determine what pharmaceutical or CAM measures might help relieve the pain and anxiety she is experiencing.
   The nurse should also keep in mind that stress and fatigue intensify the effects of pain.

2. What would be a successful outcome for this patient?
   By next visit, Ms. Potter vocalizes pain relief related to learned relaxation measures

3. What intellectual, technical, interpersonal, and/or ethical/legal competencies are most likely to bring about the desired outcome?
   Intellectual: knowledge of the pain experience, pain process, and factors influencing the pain experience, such as stress and fatigue
   Interpersonal: ability to communicate and interact effectively with patients experiencing pain

4. What resources might be helpful for Ms. Potter?
   Consultation with an experienced CAM practitioner, printed materials on PMS and relief measures

PATIENT CARE STUDY

1. Objective data are underlined; subjective data are in boldface.

   Tabitha Wilson is a <u>24-month-old infant with AIDS who is hospitalized with infectious diarrhea.</u> She is well-known to the pediatric staff, and there is real concern that she might not pull through this admission. She has suffered many of the complications of AIDS and is no stranger to pain. At the present time, <u>the skin on her buttocks is raw and excoriated, and tears stream down her face whenever she is moved. Her blood pressure also shoots up when she is touched.</u> The severity of her illness has left her <u>extremely weak and listless,</u> and **her foster mother reports that she no longer recognizes her child.** When alone in her crib, <u>she seldom moves, and she moans softly.</u> Several nurses have expressed great frustration caring for Tabitha because they find it hard to perform even simple nursing measures like turning, diapering, and weighing her when they see how much pain these procedures cause.

2. Nursing Process Worksheet

   Health Problem: Pain

   Etiology: Excoriated skin on buttocks and debilitating effects of illness

   Signs and Symptoms: Tears stream down face when moved and blood pressure shoots up; moans; skin on buttocks is raw and excoriated.

   Expected Outcome: By 2/15/11, patient's behaviors will indicate that pain is sufficiently relieved for patient to rest comfortably—even during clinical procedures.

   Nursing Interventions:

   a. Report pain assessment to MD and collaborate on designing effective pain management program.

   b. Ensure that the analgesia administration schedule produces consistent comfort.

   c. Collaborate with wound care specialist in implementing program for healing of lesions on buttocks.

   Evaluative Statement: 2/15/11: Expected outcome partially met—patient's behavior (absence of tears, decreased moaning, decreased BP) indicates some pain relief, but procedures that involve moving the patient still result in great discomfort. Revision: consult with physician again.—*E. Daniel, RN*

3. Patient strengths: Patient and her foster parents are greatly liked by the staff; parents show great willingness to be involved in care.

   Personal strengths: Knowledge of pain experience; experience in designing and monitoring pain management regimens; experience with pain management in infants and children; good rapport with wound and skin care specialist; strong interpersonal skills

4. Tabitha's response to procedures is markedly improved since the new analgesic regimen was implemented. However, although she no longer "tears up" when touched, and her blood pressure is more stable during procedures, she continues to cry during her bath and during procedures that involve more movement. Will speak with MD about modifying analgesic regimen.—*E. Daniel, RN*

CHAPTER 36

PRACTICING FOR NCLEX
MULTIPLE CHOICE QUESTIONS

1. d	**2.** a	**3.** b	**4.** c	**5.** a
6. d	**7.** a	**8.** b	**9.** d	**10.** c
11. b	**12.** a	**13.** c	**14.** b	**15.** d
16. a				

ALTERNATE-FORMAT QUESTIONS
Multiple Response Questions

1. c, d, f
2. a, d, e
3. b, c, d
4. a, b, d, f
5. b, e, f
6. a, c, d
7. d, e, f
8. c, d, e
9. a, c, d

Fill-in-the-Blank Questions

1. 27.5
2. 2,178
3. 50 to 100 grams
4. 10% to 20%
5. 50% to 60%
6. 115 lb
7. 154 lb

DEVELOPING YOUR KNOWLEDGE BASE
MATCHING EXERCISES

1. a	**2.** c	**3.** b	**4.** a	**5.** b
6. c	**7.** a	**8.** c	**9.** b	**10.** b
11. d	**12.** a	**13.** j	**14.** m	**15.** n
16. b	**17.** e	**18.** g	**19.** h	**20.** l
21. o	**22.** i	**23.** k	**24.** c	

25. d, milk, eggs, nuts
26. a, dairy products
27. g, salt
28. i, seafood
29. e, salt and processed foods
30. k, liver
31. m, fish and tea
32. f, wheat
33. o, liver and whole grains
34. b, milk products and soft drinks
35. h, liver
36. j, oysters
37. l, beans and fruit
38. n, whole grains

39. e	**40.** a	**41.** g	**42.** b	**43.** i
44. c	**45.** f	**46.** d		

SHORT ANSWER

1. Nitrogen balance is a comparison between catabolism and anabolism and can be measured by comparing nitrogen intake and nitrogen excretion. When catabolism and anabolism are occurring at the same rate, as in healthy adults, the body is in a state of neutral nitrogen balance.

2. **a.** Saturated fatty acids: Cannot bind additional hydrogen atoms (i.e., their carbon bonds are all saturated). Example: animal fats. Saturated fats raise cholesterol.

   b. Unsaturated fatty acids: Have one or more double bonds between carbon atoms. When double bonds are broken, carbons can bind with additional hydrogen atoms. Example: vegetable fats. Unsaturated fats lower serum cholesterol levels.

3. **a.** Certain age groups: Infants, adolescents, pregnant and lactating women, and the elderly

   b. Smoking, alcohol abuse, and long-term use of certain medications

   c. Chronic illnesses

   d. Poor appetite

4. **a.** Infancy: The period from birth to 1 year of age is the most rapid period of growth. Nutritional needs per unit of body weight are greater than at any other time in the life cycle.

   b. Toddlers and preschoolers. During this stage, the decrease in growth is dramatic. Mobility, autonomy, and coordination increase, as do muscle mass and bone density. This age group develops an attitude toward food. Appetite decreases and becomes erratic.

   c. School-aged children: Nutritional implications focus on health promotion. Increasing energy requirements should be balanced with foods of high nutritional value. The appetite improves but may still be irregular.

   d. Adolescents: Nutrient needs increase to support growth. Weight consciousness becomes compulsive in 1 of 100 teenage girls and results in an eating disorder.

   e. Adults: Growth ceases, and nutritional needs level off.

   f. Pregnant women: Nutrient needs increase to support growth and maintain maternal homeostasis, particularly during the second and third trimesters. Caloric needs are higher for lactation than pregnancy.

   g. Older adults: Because of the decreases in BMR and physical activity and loss of lean body mass, energy expenditure decreases. The calorie needs of the body decrease.

5. See table below.

Nutrient	Function	Recommended %
a. Carbohydrates	Supply energy (4 cal/g); also spares protein, helps burn fat efficiently, and prevents ketosis	50%–60%
b. Proteins	Maintain body tissues; support new tissue growth; component of body framework	10%–20%
c. Fats	Important component of cell membranes; synthesis of bile acids; precursor of steroid hormones and vitamin D; most concentrated source of energy (9 cal/g); aids in absorption of fat-soluble vitamins; provides insulation, structure, and body temperature control.	Saturated <10% Unsaturated <35%
d. Vitamins	Metabolism of carbohydrates, protein, and fat	
e. Minerals	Key components of body structures; regulation of body processes	
f. Water	Essential for all biochemical reactions; participates in many biochemical reactions; helps regulate body temperature, helps lubricate body joints; needed for adequate mucous secretions	2,000–3,000 mL/day

6. Sample answers:
   a. Eat a variety of high-fiber foods daily.
   b. Drink six to eight glasses of water daily.
   c. Substitute high-fiber foods for lower-fiber foods.
   d. Add bran to diet slowly to decrease likelihood of flatus and distention.
7. a. Anorexia nervosa: Characterized by denial of appetite and bizarre eating patterns; may result in extremely dangerous amount of weight loss; can be fatal. Typical individual is adolescent girl from middle or upper socioeconomic class; competitive; obsessive; distorted body image.
   b. Bulimia: Characterized by episodes of gorging followed by purging. Typical individual is college student who fears gaining weight but is overwhelmed by periods of intense hunger.
8. a. Sex: Men have higher caloric and protein requirements than women because of their larger muscle mass.
   b. State of health: The alteration in nutrient requirements that results from illness and trauma varies with the intensity and duration of stress.
   c. Alcohol abuse: Alcohol can alter the body's use of nutrients and thereby its nutrient requirements by numerous mechanisms.
   d. Medications: Nutrient absorption may be altered by drugs that change the pH of the gastrointestinal tract, increase gastrointestinal motility, damage the intestinal mucosa, or bind with nutrients, rendering them unavailable to the body.
   e. Megadoses of nutrient supplements: An excess of one nutrient can lead to a deficiency of another.
   f. Religion: Nurses need to be aware of dietary restrictions associated with religions that might affect a patient's nutritional requirements.
   g. Economics: A person's food budget affects dietary choices and patterns.
9. a. Food diaries: The patient records all food and beverages consumed in a specified time period (3 to 7 days).
   b. Diet history: 24-hour recall, food frequency record, plus interview designed to determine past and present food intake and habits
10. Sample answer:
    The nurse should explain the diet order to the patient, screen patients at home who are at nutritional risk, observe intake and appetite, evaluate patient's tolerance for specific types of foods, assist the patient with eating, address potential for harmful drug–nutrient interactions, and teach nutrition.
11. Sample answers:
    a. Provide simple verbal instructions; include family members when appropriate.
    b. Advise the patient to eliminate any foods that are not tolerated.
    c. Offer support and encouragement.

12. a. Clear liquid diet: Only foods that are clear liquids at room temperature, such as gelatins, fat-free bouillon, ice pops, clear juices, and so on; inadequate in calories, proteins, and most nutrients
    b. Full liquid diet: All liquids that can be poured at room temperature, such as clear liquids plus milk, plain frozen desserts, pasteurized eggs, cereal gruels; high-calorie, high-protein supplements are recommended if used for more than 3 days
    c. Soft diet: Regular diets that have been modified to eliminate foods that are hard to digest and chew, including those that are high in fiber and fat, adequate in calories and nutrients, and can be used long term
13. a. Nasogastric feeding tube: Inserted through nose and into stomach. Advantage: Allows stomach to be used as natural reservoir, regulating amount of food that enters intestine. Disadvantage: Introduces risk for aspiration of tube feeding solution into lungs.
    b. Nasointestinal feeding tube: Passed through the nose into the upper portion of the small intestine. Advantage: Minimal risk for aspiration. Disadvantage: Dumping syndrome may develop.
14. a. Patient's progress toward meeting nutritional goals
    b. Patient's tolerance of and adherence to the diet when appropriate
    c. Patient's level of understanding of the diet and need for further diet instruction
    d. Findings should be communicated to other healthcare team members.
    e. Plan should be revised or terminated as needed.

APPLYING YOUR KNOWLEDGE

REFLECTIVE PRACTICE USING CRITICAL THINKING SKILLS

Sample Answers

1. What patient teaching might the nurse provide to help Mr. Johnston meet his nutritional and exercise needs?
   The nurse should assess Mr. Johnston's eating habits by conducting a diet history. A diet plan could then be devised that would contain foods low in fat and cholesterol, enabling him to lose 1 to 2 pounds/week. The nurse should also set up an exercise program for Mr. Johnston that he could adapt to his busy lifestyle. For the greatest chance of success, the nurse should tailor diet instructions individually to Mr. Johnston's lifestyle, culture, intellectual ability, and level of motivation.
2. What would be a successful outcome for this patient?
   By the end of the visit, Mr. Johnston lists recommended allowances of grains, vegetables, fruits, milk, and meat and beans as seen in the MyPyramid Food Guide

By next visit, Mr. Johnston manifests a weight loss of 2 pounds and has lower blood pressure and cholesterol levels

3. What intellectual, technical, interpersonal, and/or ethical/legal competencies are most likely to bring about the desired outcome?

Intellectual: knowledge of nutrients and nutritional requirements for patients across the life span. Knowledge of hypertension and high cholesterol and strategies for managing these conditions through dietary restrictions

Interpersonal: special interpersonal competencies to help the executive see the value in making lifestyle changes necessary to improve his nutritional status

Ethical/Legal: ability to act as a trusted and effective patient advocate

4. What resources might be helpful for Mr. Johnston? Consultation with a nutritionist, printed materials on hypertension and high cholesterol, exercise programs

PATIENT CARE STUDY

1. Objective data are underlined; subjective data are in boldface.

Mr. Church, a 74-year-old white man, is being admitted to the geriatric unit of the hospital for a diagnostic workup. He was diagnosed with Alzheimer's disease 4 years ago, and 1 year ago, he was admitted to a long-term care facility. His wife of 49 years is extremely devoted and informs the nurse taking the admission history that she instigated his admission to the hospital because she **was alarmed by the amount of weight he was losing.** Assessment reveals a 6-foot, 1-inch tall, emaciated man who weighs 149 pounds. His wife reports he has lost 20 pounds in the past 2 months. The staff at the long-term care facility report that he was eating his meals and his wife validated that this was the case. No one seems sure, however, of the caloric content of his diet. **Mrs. Church nods her head vigorously when asked if her husband had seemed more agitated and hyperactive recently.** Mr. Church has dull, sparse hair; pale, dry skin; and dry mucous membranes.

2. Nursing Process Worksheet

Health Problem: Altered nutrition: less than body requirements

Etiology: Imbalance between energy expenditure and caloric intake

Signs and Symptoms: 6 feet tall, 149 lb; appears "emaciated"; 20-lb weight loss over 2 months; is eating meals; more hyperactive and agitated than usual; dull, sparse hair; pale, dry skin; dry mucous membranes

Expected Outcome: In 1 month (1/20/11), patient will demonstrate signs of ingesting enough calories to meet energy needs, as evidenced by a 5- to 10-lb weight gain.

Nursing Interventions:

a. Do a 72-hour diet history to determine the average number of calories he ingests daily.

b. Provide whatever assistance he needs with feeding. Add high-calorie snacks to his diet, increasing calories progressively until the pattern of weight loss is replaced by weight gain.

c. Until the desired weight is regained and maintained, weigh the patient daily and keep an accurate fluid I&O and calorie intake record.

d. Explore nursing strategies to reduce agitation and hyperactivity, such as music, balance between solitude and social interaction, rest periods, and so on.

Evaluative Statement: 1/20/11: Expected outcome met—patient gained 8 lb over past month and seems to enjoy high-calorie snacks.—*M. Bendyma, RN*

3. Patient strengths: Patient has a very supportive wife.

Personal strengths: Sound knowledge of nutrition and Alzheimer's disease; experienced in working with persons with Alzheimer's disease and their families; experienced gerontologic nurse

4. Over the past month, the patient's intake has increased by 2,000 cal/day. He enjoys high-calorie snacks of peanut butter and jelly sandwiches, milkshakes, dried fruit and nuts, pasta salads, and an occasional Snickers bar. He has regained 8 of the 20 pounds he lost, and his wife is delighted. He remains hyperactive, but scheduled walks have decreased some of his agitation. Will continue to monitor his nutritional needs.—*M. Bendyma, RN*

CHAPTER 37

PRACTICING FOR NCLEX
MULTIPLE CHOICE QUESTIONS

1. a	**2.** b	**3.** d	**4.** a	**5.** c
6. d	**7.** a	**8.** b	**9.** c	**10.** a
11. d	**12.** d			

ALTERNATE-FORMAT QUESTIONS
Multiple Response Questions

1. b, e, f
2. a, d, f
3. a, e
4. b, c, e, f
5. a, c, e, f
6. b, d, e
7. a, c, e
8. a, b, d, e

Hot Spot Questions
Refer to figures.
1. Urethra positions.

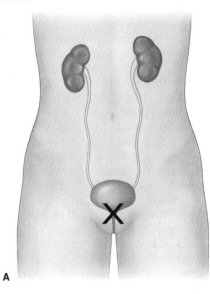

A

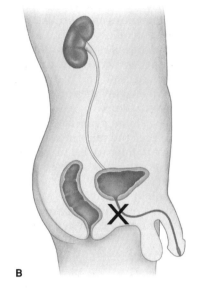

B

2. External sphincter location.

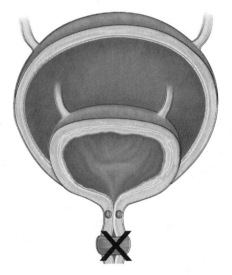

3. Bladder location and size (male).

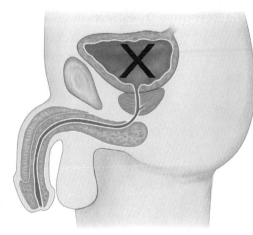

4. Suprapubic catheter position.

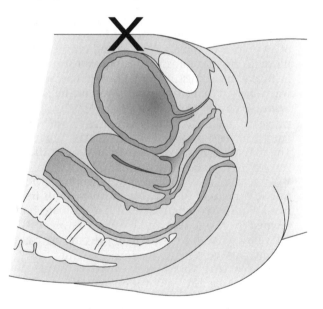

DEVELOPING YOUR KNOWLEDGE BASE

MATCHING EXERCISES

1. f	**2.** h	**3.** k	**4.** a	**5.** d
6. c	**7.** j	**8.** l	**9.** e	**10.** g
11. i	**12.** d	**13.** a	**14.** c	**15.** c
16. b	**17.** d	**18.** e		

SHORT ANSWER

1. a. Developmental considerations: Infants are born with no urinary control. Most children develop urinary control between the ages of 2 and 5 years.

Physiologic changes that accompany normal aging may affect urination in the older adult.

b. Food and fluid: The kidneys should preserve a careful balance of fluid intake and output. Caffeine-containing beverages have a diuretic effect and increase urine production. Alcohol produces the same effect by inhibiting the release of antidiuretic hormone. Foods high in water may increase urine production. High-sodium foods and beverages cause sodium and water reabsorption and retention.

c. Psychological variables: Individuals experiencing stress often find themselves voiding smaller amounts of urine at more frequent intervals. Stress can also interfere with the ability to relax perineal muscles and the external urethral sphincter.

d. Activity and muscle tone: Exercise increases metabolism and optimal urine production and elimination. With prolonged periods of immobility, decreased bladder and sphincter tone can result in poor urinary control and urinary stasis.

e. Pathologic conditions: Certain renal or urologic problems can affect both the quantity and quality of urine produced.

f. Medications: Medications have numerous effects on urine production and elimination. Nephrotoxic drugs are a serious concern. Abuse of analgesics can result in nephrotoxicity. Certain drugs cause urine to change color.

2. a. The child should be able to hold urine for 2 hours.

b. The child should recognize bladder fullness.

c. The child should be able to express the need to void and control urination until reaching the toilet.

3. a. Infants and young children: It is important to assess whether the child has achieved bladder control and whether a toileting schedule has been established for the child. It is also important to identify the words the child uses to indicate the need to void.

b. Older adults: Decreased bladder tone may be a problem. The nursing history should note how the person handles these problems and the adequacy of the solution.

c. Patients with limited or no bladder control or urinary diversions: The procedures and equipment used should be assessed to make sure they follow accepted guidelines and are not predisposing the person to infection or other risk.

4. a. Kidneys: The right kidney may at times be palpated by the nurse by pushing down on the diaphragm as the patient inhales. The left kidney is palpated similarly. The contour and size of the kidneys are noted, as are any tenderness or lumps. A check for costovertebral tenderness should be performed.

b. Bladder: The bladder cannot be assessed by the nurse when it is empty. When it is distended, the nurse observes the lower abdominal wall, noting any swelling, and palpates the area for tenderness, noting the smoothness and roundness of the bladder.

c. Urethral orifice: This is inspected for any signs of inflammation or discharge. Foul odors should be noted.

d. Skin integrity and hydration: The skin should be carefully assessed for color, texture, turgor, and the excretion of wastes. The integrity of the skin in the perineal area should also be assessed.

e. Urine: Each time a patient's urine is handled, it should be assessed for color, odor, clarity, and the presence of sediment. Abnormalities should be noted.

5. Urine is placed in a cylindrical container, and the urinometer is inserted in a circular motion without touching the bottom or side of the container. The reading should be made at eye level at the bottom of the meniscus formed by the urine. The density of the urine supports the urinometer. If urine is concentrated, the urinometer will be buoyed high; if urine is dilute, the urinometer will be supported low in the urine.

6. Sample answers:
a. The patient will produce urine output about equal to fluid intake.
b. The patient will maintain fluid and electrolyte balance.
c. The patient will report ease of voiding.
d. The patient will maintain skin integrity.

7. a. Schedule: Some patients report voiding on demand in no apparent pattern; others have inflexible patterns that have developed over the years and become anxious if these are interrupted.

b. Privacy: Many adults and children cannot void in the presence of another person; privacy should be offered in the healthcare and home setting.

c. Position: Helping patients assume normal voiding positions may be all that is necessary to resolve an inability to void.

d. Hygiene: Patients confined to bed will find it difficult to perform their usual genital hygiene. The nurse should place these patients on a bedpan and pour warm soapy water over the perineal area, followed by clear water.

8. Sample answers:
a. To relieve urinary retention
b. To obtain a sterile specimen from a woman
c. To empty the bladder before, during, and after surgery

9. Sample answers:
a. The patient will explain the cause for the urinary diversion and the rationale for treatment.
b. The patient will demonstrate self-care behaviors and manage the diversion effectively.

APPLYING YOUR KNOWLEDGE

REFLECTIVE PRACTICE USING CRITICAL THINKING SKILLS

1. How might the nurse respond to Mrs. Morita's remarks regarding her husband's home care?
Mr. Morita has the right to a urinary assessment to determine if there are any underlying causes either physical or psychological for the incontinence. The nurse should speak to the couple to assess their feelings regarding the incidents. Nursing strategies could be implemented to promote urinary continence prior to inserting a urinary catheter. If these measures fail, the nurse might suggest using a condom catheter for Mr. Morita as a possible alternative, rather than an indwelling catheter, which would increase his risk for infection. The nurse could also look into home healthcare personnel for the couple to assist with toileting and/or light housekeeping.

2. What would be a successful outcome for this patient?
By next visit, Mr. Morita states two methods to promote urinary continence.
By next visit, Mrs. Morita expresses satisfaction with urinary strategies to promote continence and receives outside help in the home.

3. What intellectual, technical, interpersonal, and/or ethical/legal competencies are most likely to bring about the desired outcome?
Intellectual: knowledge of the anatomy and physiology of the urinary systems and developmental variables that influence urination
Technical: ability to use the equipment and protocols necessary to diagnose and treat urinary problems
Ethical/Legal: strong sense of accountability for the health and well-being of patients experiencing urinary problems

4. What resources might be helpful for the Morita family?
Home healthcare services, printed information on urinary incontinence and care of urinary catheters

PATIENT CARE STUDY

1. Objective data are underlined; subjective data are in boldface.
Mr. Eisenberg, age 84, was admitted to a nursing home when his wife of 62 years died. He has two adult children, neither of whom feels prepared to care for him the way his wife did. **"We don't know how Mom did it year after year,"** his son says. **"After he retired from his law practice, he was terribly demanding, and it just seemed nothing she did for him pleased him. His Parkinson's disease does make it a bit difficult for him to get around, but he's able to do a whole lot more than he is letting on. He's always been this way."** The aides have reported to you that Mr. Eisenberg is frequently incontinent of both urine and stool during the day as well as during the night. He is alert and appears capable of recognizing the need to void or defecate and signaling for any assistance. His son and daughter report that this was never a problem at home and that he was able to go into the bathroom with assistance. He has been depressed about his admission to the home and seldom speaks, even when directly approached. He has refused to participate in any of the floor social events since his arrival.

2. Nursing Process Worksheet
Health Problem: Toileting self-care deficit
Etiology: Depression on entering nursing home and decreased will to live
Signs and Symptoms: Incontinent of both urine and stool during the day and night (need to determine the frequency); alert and capable of recognizing and signaling the need to void/defecate; able to walk to bathroom with assistance
Expected Outcome: Within 2 weeks (6/17/11), patient will communicate the need to void/defecate appropriately, as evidenced by reduction in incontinent episodes to one "accident" daily.
Nursing Interventions:
   a. Initiate a regular toileting schedule with the patient in which he is assisted to the bathroom; use these interactions to reinforce the importance of his maintaining his independence.
   b. Refrain from using adult incontinent pads or in any way communicating that incontinence is "OK."
   c. Call an interdisciplinary conference to develop a strategy to ease his transition to the home.
Evaluative Statement: 6/17/11: Expected outcome partially met—when assisted to the bathroom, the patient voids/defecates; but if the staff neglects to offer assistance, the patient will not use his call light to request it, and incontinent episodes recur (more than one a day on some days). Revision: Continue to counsel regarding transition to the home and importance of independence.
—P. Wu, RN

3. Patient strengths: Patient is alert and capable of expressing his needs for assistance. Mobile with assistance.
Personal strengths: Good knowledge of gerontologic nursing and experience in caring for the elderly; experienced counselor and teacher of appropriate self-care measures

4. 6/15/11: A review of the patient's record reveals three incontinent episodes in the past 24 hours (two urine, one stool). When asked why he did not ask for assistance to get to the bathroom, the patient refused to answer. Generally, he cooperates with the toileting regimen, and when taken to the bathroom voids/defecates as needed. Will continue to counsel regarding the importance of his independently managing his toileting needs. Will reevaluate his ability to recognize the need to void/defecate and ask for assistance.—P. Wu, RN

CHAPTER 38

PRACTICING FOR NCLEX
MULTIPLE CHOICE QUESTIONS

1. d   **2.** c   **3.** b   **4.** b   **5.** a
6. d   **7.** b   **8.** c

ALTERNATE-FORMAT QUESTIONS
Multiple Response Questions

1. a, c, d, f
2. b, c, f
3. c, d, f
4. b, e, f
5. a, c, d, e
6. b, d, e
7. c, d, e
8. a, c
9. b, d, f

Prioritization Questions
1.

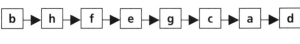

2.

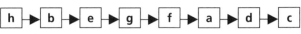

DEVELOPING YOUR KNOWLEDGE BASE

IDENTIFICATION

1. a. Rectum
   b. Internal anal sphincter
   c. External anal sphincter
   d. Anal valve
   e. Anal canal
2. a. Sigmoid colostomy—formed
   b. Descending colostomy—formed
   c. Transverse (single B) colostomy—soft
   d. Ascending colostomy—soft to liquid
   e. Ileostomy—liquid

MATCHING EXERCISES

1. h   **2.** a   **3.** d   **4.** f   **5.** c
6. e   **7.** b   **8.** g   **9.** a   **10.** d
11. c   **12.** e   **13.** b, f   **14.** g   **15.** a
16. h   **17.** b   **18.** d   **19.** i   **20.** c
21. e   **22.** k   **23.** g   **24.** f   **25.** a
26. m   **27.** h   **28.** b   **29.** n   **30.** c
31. i   **32.** q   **33.** o   **34.** r   **35.** d
36. l   **37.** p   **38.** e   **39.** k   **40.** j

SHORT ANSWER

1. a. Completion of absorption
   b. Manufacture of certain vitamins
   c. Formation of feces
   d. Expulsion of feces from the body
2. a. One is situated in the medulla.
   b. A subsidiary center is situated in the spinal cord.

3. a. Direct manipulation of the bowel during surgery inhibits peristalsis, causing a condition termed paralytic ileus. This temporary stoppage lasts 24 to 48 hours.
   b. Inhalation of anesthetic agents inhibits peristalsis by blocking parasympathetic impulses to the intestinal musculature.
4. a. Inspection: The nurse observes the contour of the abdomen, noting any masses or areas of distention.
   b. Auscultation: The nurse uses a warmed stethoscope to listen for bowel sounds in a systematic, clockwise manner in all abdominal quadrants.
   c. Percussion: The nurse percusses all quadrants of the abdomen in a systematic, clockwise manner to identify any masses, fluid, or air.
   d. Palpation: Light and deep palpations in each quadrant are performed; tenderness, muscular resistance, enlargement of organs, and masses are noted.
5. a. Developmental considerations: The stool characteristics of an infant depend on whether the infant is being fed breast milk or formula.
   b. Daily patterns: A change in a person's daily routine may lead to constipation.
   c. Food and fluids: Both the type and the amount of foods eaten affect elimination.
   d. Activity and muscle tone: Regular exercise improves gastrointestinal motility.
   e. Lifestyle: A person's daily schedule, occupation, and leisure activities may contribute to a habit of defecating at regular times or to an irregular pattern.
   f. Psychological variables: In some people, anxiety may have a direct effect on gastrointestinal motility, and diarrhea accompanies periods of high anxiety.
   g. Medications: Medications may influence the appearance of the stool—for instance, iron salts result in a black stool from the oxidation of iron.
   h. Diagnostic studies: Patients may need to fast for tests, which may alter elimination patterns.
6. Sample answer:
   When were you first diagnosed with diverticular disease? How long have you had the pain? Have you ever had this pain before? How often do you move your bowels? What do your stools look like? Have you noticed any changes in stool lately? What is your regular diet like? Are there any foods you avoid? Are there any foods that help relieve the pain?
7. a. Daily fluid intake of 2,000 to 3,000 mL
   b. Increased intake of high-fiber foods
   c. Regular exercise
   d. Acceptance of bowel elimination as a normal process of life

8. a. Constipating: Processed cheese, lean meat, eggs, pasta
   b. Laxative: Certain fruits and vegetables, bran, chocolate
   c. Gas-producing: Onions, cabbage, beans, cauliflower

9. a. The patient will have a soft, formed bowel movement every 1 to 3 days without discomfort.
   b. The patient will explain the relation between bowel elimination and dietary fiber, fluid intake, and exercise.
   c. The patient will relate the importance of timing, positioning, and privacy to healthy bowel elimination.

10. a. Constipation: Increase intake of high-fiber foods and fluid.
   b. Diarrhea: Prepare and store food properly, avoid highly spiced foods or laxative-type foods, increase intake of low-fiber foods, and replace lost fluids.
   c. Flatulence: Avoid gas-producing foods such as beans, cabbage, onions, cauliflower, and beer.
   d. Ostomies: A low-fiber diet is usually recommended, although patients may experiment with their diet to determine how much fiber they can tolerate.

11. a. Abdominal settings: Lying in a supine position, tighten and hold the abdominal muscles for 6 seconds and then relax them. Repeat several times every waking hour.
   b. Thigh strengthening: Flex and contract the thigh muscles by slowly bringing the knees up to the chest—one at a time—and then lowering them to the bed. Perform several times for each knee, each waking hour.

12. a. To relieve constipation or fecal compaction
   b. To prevent involuntary escape of fecal material during surgical procedures
   c. To promote visualization of the intestinal tract by radiographic or instrument examination
   d. To help establish regular bowel function during a bowel training program

13. a. Ileostomy: Allows liquid fecal content from the ileum of the small intestine to be eliminated through the stoma
   b. Colostomy: Permits formed feces from the colon to exit through the stoma

14. a. Timing: Patients should be allowed to heed the natural urge to defecate.
   b. Positioning: The squatting position best facilitates defecation.
   c. Privacy: Most patients consider elimination a private act, and nurses should provide privacy for their patients.
   d. Nutrition: Patients with elimination problems may need a dietary analysis to determine which foods and fluids are contributing to their problem.
   e. Exercise: Regular exercise improves gastrointestinal motility and aids in defecation.

APPLYING YOUR KNOWLEDGE

REFLECTIVE PRACTICE USING CRITICAL THINKING SKILLS
Sample Answers

1. What nursing interventions might the nurse implement for this patient?
The nurse should address methods to counteract the constipating effects of the medication on Mr. Cobb's gastrointestinal system. The nurse could then prepare a teaching plan for Mr. Cobbs that lists the foods that he should eat to stimulate peristalsis. Nursing interventions to remove the fecal impaction in a competent manner should also be initiated.

2. What would be a successful outcome for Mr. Cobbs?
By next visit, Mr. Cobbs lists three foods to include in his diet to prevent constipation
By next visit, Mr. Cobbs verbalizes having regular, pain-free bowel movements

3. What intellectual, technical, interpersonal, and/or ethical/legal competencies are most likely to bring about the desired outcome?
Intellectual: knowledge of the anatomy and physiology of bowel elimination and variables, such as medications, that influence bowel elimination
Technical: ability to perform digital extraction of fecal matter in a safe and competent manner
Interpersonal: ability to interact in a nonjudgmental and professional manner when interacting in situations involving bowel elimination, a typically private matter
Ethical/Legal: adherence to safety and quality when performing nursing interventions to promote bowel elimination

4. What resources might be helpful for Mr. Cobbs?
Consultation with a dietitian, printed or AV materials discussing the effect of medications on the gastrointestinal system and appropriate interventions

PATIENT CARE STUDY

1. Objective data are underlined; subjective data are in boldface.
Ms. Elgaresta, <u>age 54, a single Hispanic woman</u>, is being followed by a cardiologist who monitors her arrhythmia. <u>Last month, she started taking a new heart medication</u>. At this visit, she says to the nurse practitioner who works with the cardiologist: **"Right after I started taking that medication, I got terribly constipated, and nothing seems to help. I'm desperate and about ready to try dynamite unless you can think of something else!" She reports a change in her bowel movements from one soft stool daily to one or two hard stools weekly, stools that cause much straining.** The nurse practitioner realizes that regulating Ms. Elgaresta's heart is difficult and that her best cardiac response to date has been with the medication that is now causing constipation. Reluctant to suggest substituting another medication too quickly, she asks more questions, and Ms. Elgaresta responds,

"I've never been much of a drinker, two cups of coffee in the morning and maybe a glass of wine at night. Water? Almost never. And I don't drink juices or soft drinks." Analysis of her diet reveals a <u>diet low in fiber</u>: "I never was one much for vegetables, and they can just keep all this bran stuff that's out on the market! Coffee and a cigarette. That's for me!" Ms. Elgaresta is a workaholic computer programmer and spends what little spare time she has watching TV. She reports **tiring after walking one flight of stairs and says she avoids all forms of vigorous exercise.**

2. Nursing Process Worksheet
   Health Problem: Constipation
   Etiology: New medication, deficient fiber and fluid intake, and insufficient exercise
   Signs and Symptoms: Change in bowel habits from one soft, formed stool daily to one or two hard stools per week and straining
   Expected Outcome: One month after new regimen begins (5/4/11), patient reports one soft, formed stool every 1 to 2 days
   Nursing Interventions:
   a. Counsel patient about the relationship between diet (fiber intake and fluids) and bowel elimination, and exercise and bowel elimination.
   b. Assess patient's willingness and motivation to make lifestyle changes and develop a workable plan.
   c. Reinforce importance of continuing medication.
   Evaluative Statement: Expected outcome met— patient now passing a soft, formed stool almost every day.—*B. Shevorkis, RN*

3. Patient strengths: Patient is highly motivated to learn new self-care behaviors.
   Personal strengths: Knowledge of the physiology of elimination; experienced patient educator and counselor; excellent role model of healthy self-care behaviors

4. 5/4/11: Patient in for 1-month follow-up. Expressed delight with effects of new self-care behaviors: (1) decreased fat consumption and increased fiber in diet, (2) increased fluid intake—especially water, (3) increased exercise—four 30-minute periods of aerobic exercise per week. Constipation problem is resolved—passes soft stool almost every day—and reports having much more energy for work. Progress reinforced.—*B. Shevorkis, RN*

CHAPTER 39

PRACTICING FOR NCLEX
MULTIPLE CHOICE QUESTIONS

1. d	**2.** a	**3.** b	**4.** d	**5.** b
6. c	**7.** c	**8.** a	**9.** d	**10.** c
11. b	**12.** b	**13.** d	**14.** a	**15.** d
16. b	**17.** d			

ALTERNATE-FORMAT QUESTIONS
Multiple Response Questions

1. a, b, e
2. b, c, e
3. a, d, e
4. c, d, e
5. a, b, e
6. b, e, f
7. a, c, e
8. a, d, e
9. b, c, e

Prioritization Questions

1.

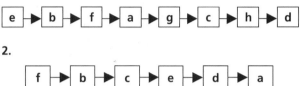

2.

f → b → c → e → d → a

DEVELOPING YOUR KNOWLEDGE BASE
IDENTIFICATION

1.
   a. Frontal sinus
   b. Nasal cavity
   c. Epiglottis
   d. Right lung
   e. Right bronchus
   f. Terminal bronchiole
   g. Diaphragm
   h. Mediastinum
   i. Left lung
   j. Trachea
   k. Esophagus
   l. Larynx and vocal cords
   m. Laryngeal pharynx
   n. Oropharynx
   o. Nasopharynx
   p. Sphenoidal sinus
2. Cuffed tracheostomy set

MATCHING EXERCISES

1. b	**2.** f	**3.** i	**4.** k	**5.** a
6. e	**7.** d	**8.** g	**9.** h	**10.** j
11. c	**12.** e	**13.** b	**14.** f	**15.** a
16. h	**17.** d			

SHORT ANSWER

1.
   a. The integrity of the airway system to transport air to and from the lungs
   b. A properly functioning alveolar system in the lungs to oxygenate venous blood and remove carbon dioxide from the blood
   c. A properly functioning cardiovascular system to carry nutrients and wastes to and from body cells
2.
   a. Upper airway: The upper airway comprises the nose, pharynx, larynx, and epiglottis. Its main function is to warm, filter, and humidify inspired air.

b. Lower airway: The lower airway comprises the trachea, right and left mainstem bronchus, segmental bronchi, and terminal bronchioles. The major functions are conduction of air, mucociliary clearance, and production of pulmonary surfactant.

3. According to Boyle's law, the volume of a gas at a constant temperature varies inversely with the pressure. Pressure in the lungs is lower than atmospheric pressure; this condition facilitates the movement of air into the lungs.

4. a. Any change in the surface area available for diffusion will have a negative effect on diffusion.

b. Incomplete lung expansion or lung collapse (atelectasis) prevents pressure changes and exchange of gases by diffusion in the lungs.

c. Any disease or condition that results in thickening of the alveolar–capillary membrane makes diffusion more difficult.

d. The solubility and molecular weight of the gases are factors in diffusion.

5. a. It is dissolved in plasma.

b. Most oxygen (97%) is carried in the body by red blood cells in the form of oxyhemoglobin.

6. a. Infant: Respiratory activity is abdominal. The chest wall is so thin that the ribs, sternum, and xiphoid process are easily identified.

b. Preschool and school-aged child: Some subcutaneous fat is deposited on the chest wall, so landmarks are less prominent than in an infant; preschool child's eustachian tubes, bronchi, and bronchioles are elongated and less angular than in an infant, so the number of routine colds and infections decreases until the child enters school.

c. Older adult: Bony landmarks are more prominent; kyphosis contributes to appearance of leaning forward; barrel chest deformity may result; senile emphysema may be present; power of respiratory and abdominal muscles is reduced.

7. a. Thoracic excursion: This is measured by placing one's hands on the patient's posterior thorax at the level of the 10th rib, with both thumbs almost touching the vertebrae. While patient takes a few deep breaths, the nurse's thumbs should move 5 to 8 cm symmetrically at maximal inspiration.

b. Tactile fremitus: The nurse should place the palm's surface on each side of the patient's chest wall, avoiding bony areas; the nurse should detect equal vibrations as the patient says a multisyllable word.

8. Before: Collect baseline data; instruct patient to remain still.
During: Observe patient for reactions; report any deviation from normal color, pulse, and respiratory rates to physician.

After: Observe patient for changes in respirations; chest x-ray.

9. The inhalation of cigarette smoke increases airway resistance, reduces ciliary action, increases mucus production, causes thickening of the alveolar–capillary membrane, and causes bronchial walls to thicken and lose their elasticity.

10. a. Deep breathing: The nurse instructs the patient to make each breath deep enough to move the bottom ribs. The patient should start slowly, inspiring deeply through the nose and expiring slowly through the mouth.

b. Incentive spirometry: The patient takes a deep breath and observes the results of his/her efforts as they register on the spirometer as the patient sustains maximal inspiration.

c. Abdominal breathing: The patient places one hand on the stomach and the other on the middle of the chest. He/she then breathes slowly in through the nose, letting the abdomen protrude, then out through pursed lips while contracting the abdominal muscles. One hand should be pressing inward and upward on the abdomen. These steps should be repeated for 1 minute, followed by a 2-minute rest.

11. a. Avoid open flames in the patient's room.

b. Place "No Smoking" signs in conspicuous places in the patient's room.

c. Check to see that electric equipment is in good working order.

d. Avoid wearing and using synthetic fabrics, which build up static electricity.

e. Avoid using oils in the area.

12. a. Oropharyngeal/nasopharyngeal airway: Semicircular tube of plastic or rubber inserted into the back of the pharynx through the mouth or nose in a spontaneously breathing patient; used to keep the tongue clear of the airway and to permit suctioning of secretions

b. Endotracheal tube: Polyvinylchloride tube that is inserted through the nose or mouth into the trachea, using a laryngoscope as guide; used to administer oxygen by mechanical ventilator, to suction secretions easily, or to bypass upper airway obstructions

c. Tracheostomy tube: An artificial opening made into the trachea. The curved tracheostomy tube is inserted into this opening to replace an endotracheal tube, provide a method to mechanically ventilate the patient, bypass an upper airway obstruction, or remove tracheobronchial secretions.

13. a. A: Airway: Tip the head and check for breathing.

b. B: Breathing: If the victim does not start to breathe spontaneously after the airway is opened, give two slow, full breaths.

c. C: Circulation: Check the pulse. If the victim has no pulse, artificial circulation must be started with breathing.

14. The nurse is responsible for collecting the baseline data before the examination. Pain medication should be administered before the test if requested. During the procedure, the nurse should observe the patient for reactions. The patient's color, pulse, and respiratory rates should be observed and any deviation from the norm reported to the physician immediately. After the procedure, the nurse should observe the patient for changes in respirations. A chest x-ray is usually done to verify the absence of complications.

15. a. Help the patient assume a position that allows free movement of the diaphragm and expansion of the chest wall to promote ease of respiration.
    b. Keep the patient's secretions thin by asking the patient to drink 2 to 3 quarts of clear fluids daily.
    c. Provide humidified air.
    d. Perform cupping on the patient's lungs to loosen pulmonary secretions.
    e. Use vibration to help loosen respiratory secretions.
    f. Provide postural drainage.
    g. Help patient maintain good nutrition.

APPLYING YOUR KNOWLEDGE

REFLECTIVE PRACTICE USING CRITICAL THINKING SKILLS

Sample Answers

1. How might the nurse respond to Ms. McIntyre's request for a DNR order while taking into consideration the wishes of her daughter?
   The nurse could check Ms. McIntyre's chart for advance directives or a living will and if one is not executed, the nurse could help Ms. McIntyre fill one out. The nurse should consult with the daughter and inform her of her mother's wishes for a DNR order. A counselor could be called in to facilitate the process. When planning patient care, the nurse should take into consideration age-related changes that may be increasing Ms. McIntyre's symptoms and may respond to appropriate treatment and therapy.

2. What would be a successful outcome for this patient?
   By next visit, Ms. McIntyre vocalizes understanding of, and signs, an advance directive to direct her future care and protect her rights as a patient.

3. What intellectual, technical, interpersonal, and/or ethical/legal competencies are most likely to bring about the desired outcome?

Intellectual: knowledge of developmental variables affecting respiratory function
Technical: ability to use the equipment and protocols necessary to diagnose and treat respiratory problems
Ethical/Legal: knowledge of patients' and families' rights related to refusal of care

4. What resources might be helpful for Ms. McIntyre?
   Legal counseling, family counseling, advance directives and living wills

PATIENT CARE STUDY

1. Objective data are underlined; subjective data are in boldface.
   Toni is a 14-year-old girl who is in the adolescent mental health unit following a suicide attempt. Her chart reveals that on several occasions when her mother was visiting, she began hyperventilating (respiratory rate of 42 and increased depth). Gasping for breath on these occasions, she nevertheless pushed away all who approached her to assist. Her mother confided that she and her husband are in the midst of a divorce and that it hasn't been easy for Toni at home: **"I know she's been having a rough time at school, and I guess I've been too caught up in my own troubles to be there for her."** When you attempt to discuss this with Toni and mention her mother's concern, she begins hyperventilating again.

2. Nursing Process Worksheet
   Health Problem: Ineffective breathing patterns
   Etiology: Anxiety
   Signs and Symptoms: Periods of hyperventilation (increased RR [42] and increased depth) associated with stressful situations (visits by mother)
   Expected Outcome: By her second week in the unit (3/22/11), Toni will demonstrate an effective respiratory rate and rhythm (not to exceed 24) during her mother's visits.
   Nursing Interventions:
   a. Use interview questions directed to Toni and her mother to determine the nature of the problem, its probable cause, and its effect on her lifestyle.
   b. Demonstrate consciously controlled breathing and encourage her to use it during periods of anxiety or activity.
   c. Maintain an emotionally "safe" environment. The same nurses should always work with this patient and maintain eye contact during conversations with her.
   d. If fear is the cause of her anxiety, encourage her to express concerns. Reduce cause of fear, if feasible.
   e. If there is a strong emotional component, discuss with the patient the possibility of developing effective coping skills with professional counseling.

Evaluative Statement: 3/22/11: Expected outcome partially met—on two occasions, Toni remained in control of her breathing during her mother's visits. On at least one occasion, she hyperventilated.
—*K. O'Leary, RN*

3. Patient strengths: The patient's strengths still need to be identified; mother seems to be gaining an appreciation of her needs.
Personal strengths: Good understanding of the effects of stress and experienced in helping patients replace maladaptive coping strategies with adaptive strategies.

4. 3/22/11: This morning, Toni began talking about the difficult situation at home. When asked about her relationship with her mother, she began gulping for air but "caught herself" and quickly reestablished control of her breathing, consciously decreasing her rate and depth. Whereas she has shown no signs of hyperventilation on two of her mother's last visits, she had one episode in which she hyperventilated and totally "lost control" and needed sedation. She stated, she feels like she is making progress but still has a long way to go before she will feel comfortable at home and in control of simple, everyday things like breathing.
—*K. O'Leary, RN*

CHAPTER 40

PRACTICING FOR NCLEX
MULTIPLE CHOICE QUESTIONS

1. c	2. a	3. b	4. b	5. c
6. d	7. a	8. d	9. b	10. d
11. a	12. b	13. b		

ALTERNATE-FORMAT QUESTIONS
Multiple Response Questions

1. c, d, f
2. a, b, d, f
3. b, d, f
4. d, e, f
5. a, b, c
6. b, d, f
7. a, b, e
8. c, d, e
9. b, c, e

Chart/Exhibit Questions

1. c
2. a
3. d
4. a
5. b
6. See table below.

pH	PaCO$_2$	HCO$_3^-$	Nature of Disturbance	Comp. Present?		If Yes		If Yes	
				Yes	No	Renal	Respiratory	Partial	Complete
7.28	63	25	respiratory acidosis		×				
7.20	40	14	metabolic acidosis		×				
7.52	40	35	metabolic alkalosis		×				
7.16	82	30	respiratory acidosis	×		×		×	
7.36	68	35	respiratory acidosis	×		×			×
7.56	23	26	respiratory alkalosis		×				
7.40	40	26	none						
7.56	23	26	respiratory alkalosis		×				
7.26	70	25	respiratory acidosis		×				
7.52	44	38	metabolic alkalosis		×				
7.32	30	18	metabolic acidosis	×			×	×	
7.49	34	26	respiratory alkalosis		×				

Hot Spot Questions

1. See figure below for PICC placement.

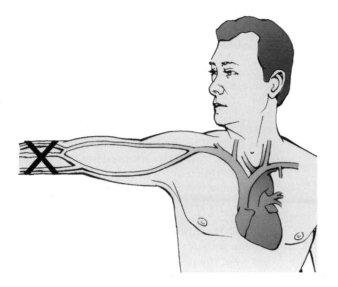

2. See figure below for triple-lumen nontunneled percutaneous central venous catheter placement.

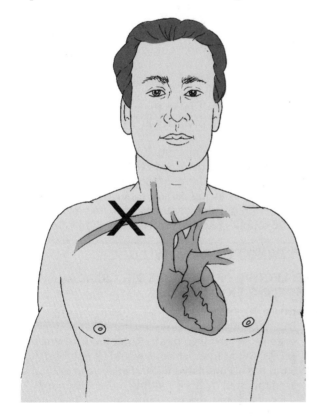

DEVELOPING YOUR KNOWLEDGE BASE

MATCHING EXERCISES

1. b	**2.** c	**3.** a	**4.** a	**5.** d
6. c	**7.** b	**8.** d	**9.** a	**10.** c
11. a	**12.** d	**13.** b	**14.** c	**15.** a
16. b	**17.** a	**18.** d	**19.** c	**20.** c
21. f	**22.** p	**23.** b	**24.** o	**25.** l
26. h	**27.** a	**28.** d	**29.** e	**30.** j
31. m	**32.** n	**33.** g	**34.** k	

CORRECT THE FALSE STATEMENTS

1. True
2. False—electrolytes
3. False—hypotonic solution
4. True
5. False—hydrogen
6. False—alkali
7. False—alkaline
8. False—lungs
9. True
10. False—hypernatremia
11. False—disproportionate
12. True

SHORT ANSWER

1. **a.** Osmosis: The solvent water passes from an area of lesser solute concentration to an area of greater solute concentration until an equilibrium is established.
   b. Diffusion: The tendency of solutes to move freely throughout a solvent. The solute moves from an area of higher concentration to an area of lower concentration until an equilibrium is established.
   c. Active transport: A process that requires energy for the movement of substances through a cell membrane from an area of lesser concentration to an area of higher concentration.
2. **a.** Ingested liquids: Fluid intake is regulated by the thirst mechanism and is stimulated by intracellular dehydration and decreased blood volume.
   b. Food: The amount of water depends on the food (e.g., melons have a higher water content than bread).
   c. Metabolic oxidation: Water is an end product of oxidation that occurs during the metabolism of food.
3. Water is lost:
   a. through the kidneys as urine
   b. through the skin as perspiration
   c. through insensible water loss
4. **a.** Kidneys: Approximately 170 L of plasma is filtered daily in the adult, while only 1.5 L of urine is excreted. They selectively retain electrolytes and water and excrete wastes.

b. Cardiovascular system: The heart and blood vessels are responsible for pumping and carrying nutrients and water throughout the body.

c. Lungs: The lungs regulate oxygen and carbon dioxide levels of the blood.

d. Thyroid: Thyroxine, released by the thyroid gland, increases blood flow in the body. This in turn increases renal circulation, which results in increased glomerular filtration and urinary output.

e. Parathyroid glands: The parathyroid glands secrete parathyroid hormone, which regulates the level of calcium in ECF.

f. Gastrointestinal tract: The GI tract absorbs water and nutrients that enter the body through this route.

g. Nervous system: The nervous system acts as a switchboard and inhibits and stimulates mechanisms that influence fluid balance.

5. a. Acidosis: Characterized by a high concentration of hydrogen ions in ECF, which causes the pH to fall below 7.35

b. Alkalosis: Characterized by a low concentration of hydrogen ions in ECF, which causes the pH to exceed 7.45

6. a. Respiratory acidosis: An excess of carbonic acid in ECF caused by decreased alveolar ventilation and resulting in the retention of carbon dioxide. The lungs cannot compensate for the rise in carbonic acid levels. As the carbonic acid concentration increases, the kidneys retain more bicarbonate and increase their excretion of hydrogen.

b. Respiratory alkalosis: A deficit of carbonic acid in ECF caused by increased alveolar ventilation and resulting in a decrease in carbon dioxide. Respiratory rate and depth increase because carbon dioxide is being excreted faster than normal; depression or cessation of respirations can occur. The kidneys attempt to alleviate this imbalance by increasing bicarbonate excretion and hydrogen retention.

c. Metabolic acidosis: A deficit of bicarbonate in ECF resulting from an increase in acidic components or an excessive loss of bicarbonate. The lungs attempt to increase the rate of carbon dioxide excretion by increasing the rate and depth of respirations; the kidneys attempt to compensate by retaining bicarbonate and excreting more hydrogen. May result in loss of consciousness and death.

d. Metabolic alkalosis: An excess of bicarbonate in ECF resulting from loss of acid or ingestion or retention of base. The body attempts to compensate by retaining carbon dioxide. Respirations become slow and shallow, and periods of apnea may occur. The kidneys excrete potassium and sodium along with excess bicarbonate and retain hydrogen within carbonic acid.

7. a. Increased hematocrit: Severe dehydration and shock (when hemoconcentration rises considerably)

b. Decreased hematocrit: Acute, massive blood loss; hemolytic reaction following transfusion of incompatible blood

c. Increased hemoglobin: Hemoconcentration of the blood

d. Decreased hemoglobin: Anemia, severe hemorrhage, and following a hemolytic reaction

8. a. Urine pH and specific gravity: Specific gravity is a measure of the kidney's ability to concentrate urine. Normal range: 1.005 to 1.030. Both may be obtained by dipstick measurement on a fresh voided specimen or through lab analysis.

b. Serum electrolytes: Indicates plasma levels of select electrolytes

c. Arterial blood gases: Indicate the adequacy of oxygenation and ventilation and acid–base status

9. a. Note the patient's fluid and food intake, and learn what the patient's previous eating and drinking patterns have been.

b. Note whether thirst is excessive or whether patient experiences little or no thirst.

c. Note excessive losses of fluid from the body and attempt to prevent losses when possible.

d. Physiologic changes that accompany the aging process may affect the patient's ability to maintain fluid balance.

10. a. Select a vein large enough to accommodate the needle.

b. Select a site that is naturally splinted by bone, such as the back of the hand or the forearm.

c. Select a site distal to the heart and move proximally, as necessary, to find the appropriate injection site.

d. Select a site while moving toward the heart and away from a damaged vein.

11. Handling all equipment, performing dressing changes, assessing patient for evidence of infection or other complications, and maintaining the supplies necessary to continue home infusion

APPLYING YOUR KNOWLEDGE

REFLECTIVE PRACTICE USING CRITICAL THINKING SKILLS

Sample Answers

1. Based on the data in this scenario, what body systems are involved in Mr. Park's fluid volume excess? What interventions would be appropriate? Fluid has accumulated in Mr. Park's heart and lungs as manifested by his bounding pulse, distended neck veins, and abnormal lung sounds. The nurse should make careful assessments of Mr. Park's IV infusion to ensure the proper flow rate. The nurse should also be aware that fluid restriction may be ordered and prepare the patient by explaining the reason for the restriction and what foods to avoid

(dry, salty, or sweet foods or fluids). The nurse could then work with the patient to develop short-term outcomes for accomplishing the overall task and discuss with the patient the time intervals at which fluids will be served. Fluids could be served in small cups to make the cup appear to contain more liquid and ice chips could be offered at intervals. The nurse should provide oral hygiene at regular intervals so that the patient's mouth remains clean and moist and lubricate the lips and mucous membranes as indicated.

2. What would be a successful outcome for Mr. Park? By end of shift, Mr. Park lists the reasons for fluid restrictions and states that he is breathing more easily following implementation of treatment regimen.

3. What intellectual, technical, interpersonal, and/or ethical/legal competencies are most likely to bring about the desired outcome?
Intellectual: knowledge of how to promote and maintain fluid, electrolyte, and acid–base balance
Technical: ability to use the equipment and protocols necessary to maintain and restore fluid, electrolyte, and acid–base balance
Ethical/Legal: strong sense of accountability for the health and well-being of patients and willingness to hold colleagues accountable for safe quality practice

4. What resources might be helpful for Mr. Park? Patient teaching plan, printed materials on overhydration

PATIENT CARE STUDY

1. Objective data are underlined; subjective data are in boldface.
Rebecca is a college freshman who had her wisdom teeth removed yesterday morning. She had a sore throat several days before the extraction but did not mention this to the oral surgeon. **Because of her sore throat, she had greatly decreased both her food and fluid intake.** The night of the surgery, she had an oral temperature of 39.5°C (103.1°F). Friends gave her some Tylenol, which brought her temperature down, and encouraged her to drink more fluids. When they checked on her this morning, her temperature was elevated again, and she said **she had felt too weak during the night to drink.** They took her to the student health service, where the admitting nurse noticed her dry mucous membranes, decreased skin turgor, and rapid pulse. At 5 feet 2 inches and 98 pounds, **Rebecca had lost 4 pounds in the past week.**

2. Nursing Process Worksheet
Health Problem: Fluid volume deficit
Etiology: Decreased fluid intake (sore throat and weakness) and loss of water and electrolytes in fever
Signs and Symptoms: Elevated temperature (39.5°C), 4-lb weight loss in 1 week, dry mucous membranes, decreased skin turgor, and rapid pulse
Expected Outcome: By 3/19/11, patient will demonstrate corrected fluid volume deficit by (1) balanced fluid intake and output, averaging 2,500 mL

fluid/day; (2) urine specific gravity within normal range (1.010 to 1.025); (3) moist mucous membranes and adequate skin turgor; and (4) pulse returned to baseline.
Nursing Interventions:
a. Assess for worsening of fluid volume deficit.
b. Give oral fluids that are nonirritating, as tolerated.
c. If oral fluids are not tolerated, confer with MD regarding IV replacement therapy.
d. Monitor response to fluid therapy: vital signs, urine volume and specific gravity, increased skin turgor, moist mucous membranes, increased body weight.
Evaluative Statement: 3/19/11: Goals met—patient has corrected fluid volume deficit; fluid intake and output average 2,700 mL fluid/day; pulse returned to baseline; skin turgor improved; mucous membranes are moist.—*J. Barclay, RN*

3. Patient strengths: Previously healthy; concerned friends; highly motivated to correct deficit
Personal strengths: Strong knowledge of fluid, electrolyte, and acid–base balance; good interpersonal skills

4. 3/19/11: Patient tolerating oral replacement fluids and understands importance of increasing fluids until the deficit is corrected. Friends remind her to drink at frequent intervals. Pulse returned to baseline. Yesterday's fluid intake was 2,900 mL fluid, output 2,500 mL. Improved skin turgor and moist mucous membranes. Gained 2 lb.—*J. Barclay, RN*

CHAPTER 41

PRACTICING FOR NCLEX
MULTIPLE CHOICE QUESTIONS

1. b 2. a 3. b 4. c 5. d
6. c 7. c 8. a 9. a

ALTERNATE-FORMAT QUESTIONS
Multiple Response Questions

1. b, c, f
2. a, d, e
3. a, b, d

DEVELOPING YOUR KNOWLEDGE BASE
FILL-IN-THE-BLANKS

1. Self-actualization
2. Self-concept
3. Global self
4. Ideal self
5. False self
6. Personal identity

MATCHING EXERCISES

1. a 2. d 3. h 4. e 5. f
6. c 7. g 8. d 9. b 10. c
11. a 12. d 13. b 14. c 15. d
16. a

SHORT ANSWER

1. Sample answer:
   Nurses interacting with older adults need to take simple measures such as addressing older patients respectfully, communicating that you take their concerns seriously, noticing and affirming their personal strengths, and interacting with them as individuals.
2. Answers will vary with student's experiences.
3. Sample answers:
   a. Significance: Do you feel loved and appreciated by the key people in your life?
   b. Competence: Does anything interfere with your ability to do your life work?
   c. Virtue: How would you describe your ability to follow your moral code?
   d. Power: Do you feel you are in control of your life?
4. Sample answers:
   a. Developmental considerations: A teenager needs to be trusted and guided to make good choices that affect his/her life.
   b. Culture: As a child internalizes the values of parents and peers, culture begins to influence his/her sense of self.
   c. Internal and external resources: The amount of money a person earns may influence his/her self-concept.
   d. History of success or failure: A child who repeatedly fails in school may have difficulty succeeding in life.
   e. Stressors: Self-concept determines the way a person perceives stressors in his/her life and reacts to them.
   f. Aging, illness, or trauma: A paralyzing injury will most likely affect self-concept.
5. Sample answers:
   a. Dispel the myth that it is necessary to know all there is to know about nursing to be a good nurse: Nurses must accept the fact that they must constantly learn new theories and procedures to keep up with medicine.
   b. Realistically evaluate strengths and weaknesses: A periodic review of a nurse's skills, strengths, and weaknesses should be built into the practice.
   c. Accentuate the positive: Nurses should not dwell on one mistake they may have made but should recall what they did right and learn from their mistakes.
   d. Develop a conscious plan for changing weaknesses into strengths: If a nurse has weak technical skills in one area, he/she should focus on this area and strengthen his/her knowledge and competency through research, study, and practice.
   e. Work to develop team self-esteem: Congratulate colleagues and celebrate when the nursing team is successful.

f. Actively demonstrate your commitment to nursing and concern about the nursing profession's public image: Nurses should be aware of their impact on society, and the image they project should be positive.

6. Answers will vary with student's experiences.
7. Sample answers:
   a. Personal identity: How would you describe yourself to others?
   b. Patient strengths: What special talents and abilities do you have?
   c. Body image: What are your positive physical attributes?
   d. Self-esteem: What do you like most about yourself?
   e. Role performance: What major roles describe you?
8. Sample answers:
   a. Diagnosis: Anxiety related to unwelcome change in body image (mastectomy)
      Patient goal: Patient will express satisfaction with ability to live with altered body image.
   b. Diagnosis: Anxiety related to inability to accept or manage new role
      Patient goal: Patient reports feeling less anxious about being pregnant.
   c. Diagnosis: Altered Health Maintenance related to low self-esteem and inability to cope with grief
      Patient goal: Patient will acknowledge his own self-worth and express a desire to take care of himself despite his grief.
   d. Diagnosis: Knowledge Deficit: how to help child develop self-esteem, related to lack of experience with parenting
      Patient goal: Patient will describe methods of developing self-esteem in children.
   e. Diagnosis: High Risk for Violence, domestic abuse, related to low self-esteem and sense of hopelessness
      Patient goal: Patient will verbalize that she is liked and deserves to live without fear of abuse.
   f. Diagnosis: Altered Sexuality Patterns related to changed body image, disturbance in self-concept
      Patient goal: Patient will describe self realistically, identifying strengths that make her desirable to husband
9. a. Encourage patients to identify their strengths.
   b. Notice and reinforce patient strengths.
   c. Encourage patients to will for themselves the strengths they desire and to try them on.
10. a. Using looks, touch, and speech to communicate worth
    b. Speaking respectfully to the patient and addressing the patient by preferred name
    c. Moving the patient's body respectfully if the patient cannot move on his/her own

11. Sample answers:

  a. Help her find meaning in the experience, regain mastery to the extent that this is possible, and realistically evaluate the adequacy of her coping strategy. Teach her to develop a "game plan" for confronting anxiety-producing situations. Identify and secure interventions for treatable depression. Remedy treatable causes of self-identity disturbances, such as pain or substance abuse.

  b. Notice and affirm positive physiologic characteristics of the patient. Teach preventive self-care measures that reduce uncomfortable signs of aging. Explore new activities (which may include old hobbies) that are within the changing physical abilities of the patient.

  c. Help patient identify and use personal strengths. Let him know that you value him simply for who he is. Use the name he prefers. Ask him questions about his life, interests, and values. Engage him in activities in which he can be successful. Empower him to meet his needs. Provide necessary knowledge, teach new behaviors, and instill in him the belief that he can change.

  d. Explore with patient the many roles she has fulfilled throughout her lifetime. Encourage her to reminisce. Facilitate grieving over valued roles that she can no longer perform.

APPLYING YOUR KNOWLEDGE

REFLECTIVE PRACTICE USING CRITICAL THINKING SKILLS

1. What interventions might the nurse employ to try to resolve Mr. Santorini's self-image disturbance? The nurse would need to assess Mr. Santorini's self-knowledge, self-expectations, and self-evaluation for each component of self-concept to determine if he will still be able to fulfill his role expectation to function as a complete, intact man. The nurse should keep in mind that major stressors place anyone at relative risk for maladaptive responses, such as withdrawal, isolation, depression, extreme anxiety, substance abuse, or exacerbation of physical illness. How Mr. Santorini perceives the amputation and his ability to mobilize personal strengths and other resources are determined largely by his self-concept, which, in turn, is influenced by the response he chooses. Following a complete history and assessment, the nurse could work with Mr. Santorini and assist with adapting to the loss of his leg. Patient teaching involving the use of a prosthesis may be helpful as he begins to adapt to his body change.

2. What would be a successful outcome for Mr. Santorini?
By next visit, Mr. Santorini lists three positive aspects of his self-image.
By next visit, Mr. Santorini reports acceptance of his amputation and successful use of his new prosthesis.

3. What intellectual, technical, interpersonal, and/or ethical/legal competencies are most likely to bring about the desired outcome?
Intellectual: knowledge of measures to modify a negative self-concept for a middle-aged man with a new amputation
Interpersonal: strong interpersonal skills to establish a trusting relationship with a middle-aged man with an amputation
Ethical/Legal: a commitment to patient advocacy, including getting Mr. Santorini the help needed to achieve his health goals

4. What resources might be helpful for Mr. Santorini?
Counseling services, printed or AV materials on the use of prostheses

PATIENT CARE STUDY

1. Objective data are underlined; subjective data are in boldface.

An English teacher asks you, the school nurse, to see one of her students, Julie, whose grades have recently dropped and who no longer seems to be interested in school or anything else. "She was one of my best students, and I can't figure out what's going on," the teacher says. "She seems reluctant to talk about this change." When Julie, a 16-year-old junior, walks into your office, you are immediately struck by her stooped posture, unstyled hair, and sloppy appearance. Julie is attractive, but at 5 foot 3 and 150 pounds, she is overweight. Julie is initially reluctant to talk, but she breaks down at one point and confides that for the first time in her life she feels **"absolutely awful"** about herself. **"I've always concentrated on getting good grades and achieved this easily. But now, this doesn't seem so important. I don't have any friends.** All I hear the girls talking about is boys, and I was never even asked out by a boy, which I guess isn't surprising. Look at me." After a few questions, it becomes clear that Julie has new expectations for herself based on what she observes in her peers, and she finds herself falling far short of her new, ideal self. Julie admits **that in the past, once she set a goal for herself, she was always able to achieve it because she is strongly self-motivated.** Although she has withdrawn from her parents and teachers, she admits that she does know adults she can trust who have been a big support to her in the past. She says, "If only I could become the kind of teenager other kids like and have lots of friends!"

2. Nursing Process Worksheet
Health Problem: Situational low self-esteem
Etiology: Perceived inability to meet newly accepted peer standards regarding socialization/dating
Signs and Symptoms: Feels "absolutely awful" about herself; 5 foot 3, 150 lb; "I don't have any friends"; never dated; grades have dropped recently; new lack of interest/vitality; stooped posture; unstyled hair; sloppy appearance

Expected Outcome: In 1 month, by 10/10/12, patient will report that she feels better about herself, based on new socialization experiences with peers and improved body image.

Nursing Interventions:

a. Help patient develop workable self-care strategies to lose weight and enhance physical appearance.

b. Explore patient's interest in activities that will serve two goals: (1) enable patient to develop friendships and (2) improve her body image (e.g., sports, dancing, hiking clubs).

c. Counsel patient about peer relationships, sexuality, and dating.

Evaluative Statement: 10/10/12: Goal partially met—patient states that she feels "great" about losing weight (150 pounds, down to 145 pounds) and likes her "new look" but still feels shy with peers and is not dating. Revision: Celebrate new self-care behaviors and reevaluate efforts to enhance peer relationships.—*M. Stenulis, RN*

3. Patient strengths: Physically attractive; past history of achieving personal goals; strongly self-motivated; has trusting relationships with adults (parents and teachers).

   Personal strengths: Ability to establish trusting nurse–patient relationships with high school students; knowledge of teen social "norms"; successful history of motivating teens to develop and take pride in health self-care behaviors

4. 10/10/12: Met with patient 1 month after initial meeting. In that time, she lost 5 pounds, which she attributes to decreased snacking and increased activity (joined field hockey team). She walked into the office with erect posture and exhibited more interest/vitality than at last meeting. She reports still feeling very shy with her peers and is uncomfortable with boys. She is very interested, however, in participating in group activities in which she can overcome her shyness and hopes to make new friends.—*M. Stenulis, RN*

CHAPTER 42

PRACTICING FOR NCLEX
MULTIPLE CHOICE QUESTIONS

1. a	**2.** c	**3.** b	**4.** b	**5.** a
6. d	**7.** c	**8.** c	**9.** a	**10.** a
11. d	**12.** a	**13.** b		

ALTERNATE-FORMAT QUESTIONS
Multiple Response Questions

1. b, d, f
2. a, d, e
3. c, e, f
4. c, d, f
5. a, e, f

Prioritization Question
1.

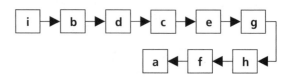

DEVELOPING YOUR KNOWLEDGE BASE
FILL-IN-THE-BLANKS

1. Stressor
2. Local adaptation
3. Inflammatory
4. Fight-or-flight
5. Psychosomatic
6. Anxiety
7. Coping mechanisms
8. Caregiver burden

MATCHING EXERCISES

1. c	**2.** i	**3.** l	**4.** f	**5.** b
6. e	**7.** a	**8.** d	**9.** g	**10.** h
11. j	**12.** c	**13.** i	**14.** b	**15.** h
16. a	**17.** e	**18.** f	**19.** g	

SHORT ANSWER

1. a. Mind–body interaction: Humans react to threats of danger as if they were real. The person perceives the threat on an emotional level, and the body prepares itself either to resist it or turn away and avoid the danger. For example: An executive has an important presentation to make in the morning and is restless the night before, cannot eat breakfast, and feels apprehensive and has a rapid heartbeat before the presentation.

   b. Local adaptation syndrome: A localized response of the body to stress. It does not involve the entire body, only a body part. LAS is an adaptive response, primarily homeostatic and short term. For example: Reflex pain response and inflammatory response.

   c. General adaptation syndrome: A biochemical model of stress developed by Hans Selye that describes the body's general response to stress and serves as part of the knowledge base essential to all areas of nursing care. For example: Alarm reaction—various defense mechanisms are activated; resistance—body attempts to adapt to the stressor; exhaustion—the body either rests and mobilizes its defenses to return to normal or reaches total exhaustion and dies.

2. a. Bleeding is controlled initially by vasoconstriction of blood vessels at the injury site. Histamines are released and capillary permeability increases, allowing increased

blood flow and bringing increased white blood cells to the area; blood flow returns to normal.

b. Exudate is released from the wound; amount depends on size, location, and severity of wound.

c. Damaged cells are repaired by either regeneration or formation of scar tissue.

3. a. Severity and duration of the stressor

b. Previous health of the person

c. Immediacy and effectiveness of healthcare interventions

4. a. Mild anxiety: Present in day-to-day living; increases alertness and perceptual fields and motivates learning and growth

b. Moderate anxiety: Narrows a person's perceptual fields so that the focus is on immediate concerns, with inattention to other details

c. Severe anxiety: Creates a very narrow focus on specific detail; causes all behavior to be geared toward relief

d. Panic: Causes the person to lose control and experience dread and terror; characterized by increased physical activity, distorted perceptions and relations, and loss of rational thought

5. Answers will vary with student's experiences.

6. Sample answers:

a. Stressors in health facilitate normal growth and development.

b. Fear of developing cardiovascular disease can motivate a person to exercise regularly.

c. Fear of failure in business can motivate a person to attend classes.

7. Sample answers:

a. Developmental stress: An infant learns that his hunger will be taken care of in a timely manner; a school-aged child learns the rewards of studying; an elderly man accepts the limitations of age on his social life.

b. Situational stress: A child contracts a life-threatening illness; a spouse loses her job; a spouse asks for a divorce.

8. Sample answers:

a. "It must have been frightening being in an automobile accident."

b. "I notice that you seem distracted; would you care to talk about it?"

9. Sample answers:
Confront the mother in an understanding manner and question her about her daily schedule and ability to do all the things necessary to take care of her family. Refer the mother to outside agencies (e.g., daycare programs), supportive friends and family members, or resources for hired help to give her a break from her responsibilities. Help the mother arrange her daily care to schedule some time for herself, if possible.

10. a. Exercise: The benefits of exercise include an improved musculoskeletal system, more effective cardiovascular function, weight control, and relaxation. It improves one's sense

of well-being, relieves tension, and enables one to cope with life better.

b. Rest and sleep: Allows the body to maintain homeostasis and restore energy levels; provides insulation against stress

c. Nutrition: Plays an active role in maintaining the body's homeostatic mechanisms and in increasing resistance to stress

11. a. Identify the problem.

b. List alternatives.

c. Choose from among the alternatives.

d. Implement a plan.

e. Evaluate the outcome.

12. a. Age affects the ability to adapt.

b. Nutrition affects stress levels.

c. Sleep affects stress levels.

d. Social factors and life events affect stress level.

13. a. Provide social support.

b. Provide emotional and physical support.

c. Help with problem-solving and teaching–learning activities.

APPLYING YOUR KNOWLEDGE

REFLECTIVE PRACTICE USING CRITICAL THINKING SKILLS

Sample Answers

1. What might be the cause of the flare-up of Ms. Rogerrios's inflammatory bowel disease? What nursing interventions would be beneficial for this patient?
The stress of having to return to work for financial reasons following a 15-year absence may have exacerbated Ms. Rogerrio's inflammatory bowel disease. The nurse could teach Ms. Rogerrio coping mechanisms to minimize this effect of stress. Examples of interventions appropriate for this patient include patient teaching regarding meditation and/or relaxation techniques, and maintaining a proper diet and exercise program.

2. What would be a successful outcome for this patient?
By next visit, Ms. Rogerrio lists three benefits of using stress-reduction strategies and their effect on relieving diarrhea related to her inflammatory bowel disease.

3. What intellectual, technical, interpersonal, and/or ethical/legal competencies are most likely to bring about the desired outcome?
Intellectual: knowledge about the physiologic and psychological responses to stress
Interpersonal: strong interpersonal skills to establish a trusting relationship with a woman returning to the workforce; ability to assist patients to develop positive coping mechanisms to deal with stress
Ethical/Legal: familiarity with agency policy and role responsibilities related to stress management

4. What resources might be helpful for Ms. Rogerrio?
Exercise classes, printed or AV materials on stress-reduction techniques.

PATIENT CARE STUDY

1. **a.** On a scale of 1 to 10, with 10 being most able to control this situation, how would you rate yourself at this time? What does that number mean to you?
   b. Who do you talk to when you feel sad or nervous?
   c. What has helped you handle stressful situations in the past? (Also, see samples of questions in text.)
2. Heart palpitations, dry mouth, difficulty breathing, increased perspiration, nausea, tremors, increased pulse rate, increased blood pressure, crying, sleep disturbances, eating disturbances.
3. **a.** Anxiety related to multiple stressors occurring in relatively short period of time
   b. Altered Thought Processes related to severe anxiety
   c. Risk for Altered Nutrition: Less Than Body Requirements related to decreased food intake
   d. Risk for Social Isolation related to perceived need to be family caregiver
4. **a.** Verbalize a decrease in anxiety with increased feelings of comfort.
   b. Develop effective coping skills through problem-solving and anxiety-reducing techniques.
   c. Maintain or slightly increase body weight.
   d. Actively participate in at least one social activity outside the home each week.
5. A crisis occurs when previous coping and defense mechanisms are no longer effective. This failure causes high levels of anxiety, disorganized behavior, and an inability to function adequately.
6. Identify the problem, list alternatives, choose from among alternatives, implement a plan, and evaluate the outcome.
7. Exercise: Exercise helps maintain physical and emotional health; it also improves ability to cope with stressors. Recommend an exercise program of 30 to 45 minutes of enjoyable exercise three or four times a week.
   Rest and sleep: Rest and sleep restore energy levels and provide insulation against stress. Relaxation techniques are often helpful in inducing sleep. Nutrition: Nutrition plays an active role in increasing resistance to stress. Follow recommended guidelines for amounts and types of foods to eat. (See Chapter 36 for more information about nutrition.)
8. Mrs. Brent will meet expected outcomes if she verbalizes the causes of stress and anxiety, identifies and uses sources of support, uses problem-solving techniques to reduce the number of stressors, practices healthy lifestyle habits, and verbalizes a decrease in anxiety and an increase in comfort.

CHAPTER 43

PRACTICING FOR NCLEX
MULTIPLE CHOICE QUESTIONS

1. c   **2.** d   **3.** b   **4.** c   **5.** a
6. d   **7.** b   **8.** a

ALTERNATE-FORMAT QUESTIONS
Multiple Response Questions

1. a, b, d
2. a, c, f
3. c, e, f
4. a, c, d
5. a, d, e, f
6. b, d, e, f

DEVELOPING YOUR KNOWLEDGE BASE

FILL-IN-THE-BLANKS

1. Perceived
2. Bereavement
3. Outcome
4. Dysfunctional
5. Irreversible cessation of all functions of the entire brain, including the brainstem
6. Palliative

MATCHING EXERCISES

1. h   **2.** e   **3.** a   **4.** g   **5.** b
6. d   **7.** c   **8.** d   **9.** a   **10.** e
11. b   **12.** c   **13.** f

CORRECT THE FALSE STATEMENTS

1. False—unresolved grief
2. False—anger
3. True
4. False—durable power of attorney for healthcare
5. True
6. False—no-code or do-not-resuscitate
7. True
8. False—mortician
9. False—nurse

SHORT ANSWER

1. **a.** Care of the body: Place body in normal anatomic position; remove soiled dressings and tubes (unless an autopsy is being performed); place ID tags on shroud, ankle, and prostheses.
   b. Care of the family: Be an attentive listener; attend funeral (if family permits); make follow-up call to assess family's well-being.
   c. Discharging legal responsibilities: Ensure death certificate has been signed by physician; review organ donation arrangements.
2. **a.** Denial and isolation: The patient denies that he or she will die, may repress what is discussed, and may isolate self from reality.
   b. Anger: The patient expresses rage and hostility and adopts a "why me?" attitude.

c. Bargaining: The patient tries to barter for more time.

d. Depression: The patient goes through a period of grief before death.

e. Acceptance: The patient feels tranquil; he/she has accepted death and is prepared to die.

3. As soon as possible, the patient should be told her diagnosis and prognosis, how the disease is likely to progress, and what this will mean for her.

4. Answers will vary with student's experiences.

5. Nursing's role is to participate in the decision-making process by offering helpful information about the benefits and burdens of continued ventilation and description of what to expect if it is initiated. Supporting the patient's family and managing sedation and analgesia are critical nursing responsibilities.

6. Sample answers:

a. Communicate openly with patients about their losses and invite discussion of the adequacy of their coping mechanisms.

b. Respond genuinely to the concerns and feelings of dying patients and their families; do not be afraid to cry with the patient and to allow feelings to show.

c. Value time spent with patients and family members in which supportive presence is the primary intervention.

7. Sample answers:

a. The patient shall make healthcare decisions reflecting his values and goals.

b. The patient shall experience a comfortable and dignified death.

c. The patient and family shall accept need for help as appropriate and use available resources.

8. Sample answers:

a. In favor of: It is a beneficent and compassionate act. It takes the matter outside the reach of "medical power" and scrupulosity. It respects autonomy by preserving the patient's control of the manner, method, and timing of death.

b. Against: It undermines the value of, and respect for, all human life. A focus on euthanasia will divert attention from other valuable palliative techniques. If legalized, it is predicted patients will feel a subtle pressure to conform in order to relieve the economic and emotional burdens they impose on family and friends.

9. a. No-code: If a physician has written DNR on the chart of a patient, the patient or surrogate has expressed a wish that there be no attempts to resuscitate the patient in the event of a cardiopulmonary emergency. The nurse must clarify the patient's code status.

b. Comfort measures only: Nurses should be familiar with the forms used to indicate patient preferences about end-of-life care. The goal of a comfort measures only order is to indicate that the goal of treatment is a comfortable, dignified death and that further life-sustaining measures are no longer indicated.

c. Do-not-hospitalize orders: These orders are used by patients in nursing homes and other residential settings who have elected not to be hospitalized for further aggressive treatment. The nursing responsibilities would be the same as for comfort measures only.

d. Terminal weaning: The nurse's role is to participate in the decision-making process by offering helpful information about the benefits and burdens of continued ventilation and a description of what to expect if terminal weaning is initiated.

10. a. Durable power of attorney: Nurses must facilitate dialog about this advance directive, which appoints an agent the person trusts to make decisions in the event of the appointing person's subsequent incapacity.

b. Living will: Nurses must also facilitate dialog about this advance directive, which provides specific instructions about the kinds of healthcare that should be provided or avoided in particular situations.

APPLYING YOUR KNOWLEDGE

REFLECTIVE PRACTICE USING CRITICAL THINKING SKILLS

Sample Answers

1. How might the nurse react to Ms. Malic in a manner that respects her right to privacy while at the same time helping her through the grief process?
The nurse should realize that Ms. Malic is experiencing anticipatory loss and use this knowledge to help her cope with the potential loss of her baby. To develop meaningful communication, the nurse must develop a trusting relationship with the patient. The nurse needs to use open-ended questions to elicit information and listen to Ms. Malic, recognizing both her verbal and nonverbal cues. The nurse should also be encouraging without giving false reassurances. If she agrees to participate, Ms. Malic would benefit from grief counseling.

2. What would be a successful outcome for this patient?
By next visit, Ms. Malic vocalizes her fears for her baby and herself and lists the benefits of grief counseling.

3. What intellectual, technical, interpersonal, and/or ethical/legal competencies are most likely to bring about the desired outcome?
Intellectual: ability to identify the impact that loss, grief, and death and dying have on the patient and his or her family members
Interpersonal: ability to establish trusting relationships, even in times of great crisis related to anticipatory loss
Ethical/Legal: commitment to safety and quality, strong sense of responsibility and accountability, and strong advocacy skills

4. What resources might be helpful for Ms. Malic?
Grief counseling, information on premature babies

PATIENT CARE STUDY

1. Objective data are underlined; subjective data are in boldface.

   LeRoy is a 40-year-old architect whose life partner, Michael, is dying of AIDS. Although both LeRoy and Michael "did the bathhouse scene" in the early 1980s and had multiple unprotected sexual encounters, they have been in a monogamous relationship for the past 14 years. Michael has been in and out of the hospital during the past 3 years and is now dying of end-stage AIDS at home. He is enrolled in a hospice program. LeRoy has been very supportive of Michael throughout the different phases of his illness but at present **seems to be "losing it."** Michael noticed that LeRoy is sleeping at odd times and seems to be losing weight. **He suspects that LeRoy may be drinking more than usual and using recreational drugs.** He also says that **he is "acting strangely;" he seems emotionally withdrawn and unusually uncommunicative. "I don't think he's able to deal with the fact that I am dying,"** Michael tells you. **"He won't let me talk about it at all."** The hospice nurse notes that LeRoy is now rarely home when he comes to visit. When the hospice nurse calls to arrange a meeting with LeRoy, LeRoy informs him that he is **"managing quite well, thank you,"** and that **he has no concerns or problems to discuss.**

2. Nursing Process Worksheet

   Health Problem: Anticipatory grieving

   Etiology: Inability to allow himself to think about what his life will be like without his life partner; history of using denial as a coping mechanism

   Signs and Symptoms: Partner reports that LeRoy is sleeping at odd times and seems to be losing weight. He suspects that LeRoy is drinking more than usual and using recreational drugs. He also says that he is "acting strangely" and that he seems emotionally withdrawn and unusually uncommunicative. LeRoy is now rarely home when the hospice nurse visits. When the nurse called to arrange a meeting with him, LeRoy informed him that he was "managing quite well, thank you" and that he had no concerns or problems to discuss.

   Expected Outcome: LeRoy will openly express his grief over Michael's impending death and participate in decision making for the future.

   Nursing Interventions:

   a. Determine what is making this anticipated loss so "unthinkable."

   b. Encourage patient to share concerns. Normalize the experience of grieving by sharing experiences of other gay partners who have successfully grieved over the death of their friends and loved ones. Respect patient's use of denial to make time to work things through. Let him know you are available to help at a later date, if necessary.

   c. Help the patient explore his usual strategies for adjusting to loss (i.e., denial) and determine how they are serving him now. If he feels they are inadequate, help him develop new strategies.

   d. Promote grief work through each phase of the grieving process: denial, isolation, depression, anger, guilt, fear, rejection. Help Michael understand LeRoy's grief and need to move in and out of each stage at his own pace.

   e. Refer patient to community-based support groups.

   Evaluative Statement: 5/1/11: Goal not met. LeRoy is still denying that he is experiencing any difficulty dealing with Michael's impending death; appears fearful of even discussing this subject. Revision: Reiterated stages of grieving and importance of grief work; offered a listening ear should he decide he wishes to talk about this later.—*C. Taylor, RN*

3. Patient strengths: LeRoy's longstanding relationship with Michael and desire to be present and supportive is a powerful motivator for getting him to address his inability to consciously work through his grief. LeRoy is intelligent and trusts healthcare professionals, with whom he has had good experiences in the past.

   Personal strengths: Knowledge about stages of grief and grief work; strong interpersonal skills; teaching and counseling skills

4. 5/13/11: LeRoy, the patient's life partner and significant other, called today to arrange a time to meet. He noted that he finally had a long talk with Michael and can see that he hasn't been able to deal with his dying in a conscious manner at all: "I guess I just kept hoping that if I didn't think about it, it wouldn't happen." He says he realizes that if he continues in this manner, he won't be able to provide Michael the support he needs. He also admits feeling "totally overwhelmed." Brief discussion of stages of grieving and grief work, and appointment made for follow-up.—*C. Taylor, RN*

CHAPTER 44

PRACTICING FOR NCLEX
MULTIPLE CHOICE QUESTIONS

1. c	**2.** d	**3.** b	**4.** a	**5.** b
6. d	**7.** b			

ALTERNATE-FORMAT QUESTIONS
Multiple Response Questions

1. b, c, e, f
2. c, d, e
3. a, c, e
4. d, e, f
5. a, d, f
6. b, d, f
7. c, e, f

DEVELOPING YOUR KNOWLEDGE BASE

FILL-IN-THE-BLANKS

1. Sensory reception
2. Kinesthesia
3. Stereognosis
4. Impaired memory
5. Sensory deficit

MATCHING EXERCISES

1. h	**2.** d	**3.** a	**4.** c	**5.** b
6. f	**7.** e	**8.** a	**9.** c	**10.** d
11. b	**12.** c	**13.** d	**14.** b	**15.** a

SHORT ANSWER

1. a. A stimulus, an agent, act, or other influence capable of initiating a response by the nervous system
  b. A receptor or sense organ must receive the stimulus and convert it into a nerve impulse.
  c. The nerve impulse must be conducted along a nervous pathway from the receptor or sense organ to the brain.
  d. A particular area in the brain must receive and translate the impulse into a sensation.

2. Sample answers:
  a. Environment: A patient with AIDS in isolation is at high risk for sensory deprivation.
  b. Impaired ability to receive environmental stimuli: A patient who is visually impaired is at high risk for sensory deprivation.
  c. Inability to process environmental stimuli: A patient who is confused cannot process environmental stimuli.

3. a. Perceptual responses: Inaccurate perception of sights, sounds, tastes, smells, and body position; poor coordination and equilibrium; mild to gross distortions in perception, ranging from daydreams to hallucinations
  b. Cognitive responses: Inability to control the direction of thought content; decreased attention span and ability to concentrate; difficulty with memory, problem solving, and task performance
  c. Emotional responses: Inappropriate emotional responses: apathy, anxiety, fear, anger, belligerence, panic, depression; rapid mood changes

4. Sample answers:
  a. A patient is disoriented by the strange sights, odors, and sounds in a CCU.
  b. A burn victim is in constant pain and cannot concentrate on his environment.
  c. A confused patient panics at the sight of doctors and nurses probing his body.

5. Cultural care deprivation is a lack of culturally assistive, supportive, or facilitative acts (e.g., touching is viewed as a natural and welcome custom in certain cultures, while in other cultures it is taboo).

6. Sample answers:
  a. Infant: Soothing sounds, rocking, holding and changing position, changing patterns of light and shade, developing appropriate play

  b. Adult: Use of music, poetry, drama to alleviate boredom
  c. Elderly: Use of art classes or organizing a book club in a nursing home

7. Sample answers:
  a. Patient will report feeling safe and in control of his/her environment.
  b. Patient will verbalize acceptance of the sensory deficit.

8. Sample answer:
This patient is suffering from sensory deprivation. Measures should be taken to stimulate as many senses as possible. The curtains could be opened to allow light into the room; soft music could be played to stimulate auditory functioning; flavorful meals could be prepared to stimulate taste; flowers, cards, and pictures could be displayed to stimulate visual functioning.

9. a. Avoid damage from UV rays.
  b. Use caution with aerosol sprays.
  c. Have regular eye examinations and tests for glaucoma.
  d. Know the danger signals that indicate serious eye problems.

10. Sample answers:
  a. Visual: Read different types of books to the child; limit television watching; plan various outings.
  b. Auditory: Teach the child songs; play records; join a storytelling group.
  c. Olfactory: Have child identify different odors; prepare enticing meals and savor the aromas.
  d. Gustatory: Encourage the child to experiment with different foods with varying colors, tastes, shapes, and textures; introduce finger foods into diet.
  e. Tactile: Use games and sports to increase body contact with child; demonstrate affection by hugging, holding child in lap, and so on.

11. Sample answers:
  a. Developmental considerations: The adult may experience the need to compensate for the loss of one type of stimulation by increasing other sources of sensory stimuli.
  b. Culture and lifestyle: An individual's culture may dictate how much sensory stimulation is considered normal.
  c. Personality: Different personality types demand different levels of stimulation.
  d. Stress: Increased sensory stimulation may be sought during periods of high stress.
  e. Illness and medication: Illness can affect the reception of sensory stimuli; medications that alert or depress the central nervous system may interfere with the perception of sensory stimuli.

12. Sample answers:
  a. Stimulation: Assess for recent changes in sensory stimulation if the type of stimulation present is developmentally appropriate.

b. Reception: Assess for anything that may interfere with sensory reception and prescribe any corrective devices the patient uses for sensory impairment.

c. Transmission–perception–reaction: High-risk patients include confused patients and patients with nervous system impairments. Assess the patient's abilities to transmit, perceive, and react to stimuli during everyday interactions.

13. Sample answers:
a. Visually impaired patients: Acknowledge your presence in the patient's room, identify yourself by name, and speak in a normal tone of voice.
b. Hearing-impaired patients: Avoid excessive noise, avoid excessive cleaning of ears, and know the symptoms of hearing loss.
c. Unconscious patients: Be careful of what is said in the patient's presence, assume the person can hear you, and speak to the person before touching him.

APPLYING YOUR KNOWLEDGE

REFLECTIVE PRACTICE USING CRITICAL THINKING SKILLS

Sample Answers

1. What nursing interventions might be appropriate for Mr. Pirolla?
Sensory deprivation can lead to perceptual, cognitive, and emotional disturbances. Therefore, the nursing plan of care should include sensory stimulation for Mr. and Mrs. Pirolla. The nurse should also investigate if hearing aids would help Mr. Pirolla with his hearing loss. The nurse should assess both Mr. Pirolla and his wife to see how they are coping with the changes in their social environment. Safety in the home and community is also an issue that needs to be addressed. The nurse should incorporate knowledge of the guidelines for communicating both with persons with reduced vision and hearing when developing a teaching plan to assist Mrs. Pirolla in dealing with her husband's condition

2. What would be a successful outcome for this patient?
By next visit, Mr. Pirolla states that he is adapting to his condition and receiving new sensory stimulation from his environment.

3. What intellectual, technical, interpersonal, and/or ethical/legal competencies are most likely to bring about the desired outcome?
Intellectual: knowledge of the arousal mechanism and how the body responds, including sensoristasis and adaptation; ability to integrate knowledge of sensory alterations, including factors contributing to disturbed sensory perceptions
Interpersonal: demonstration of the ability to empathize and communicate with patients with sensory deficits and interact effectively with patients and their caregivers.

4. What resources might be helpful for Mr. Pirolla?
Social services, printed materials on sensory deficits, community services

PATIENT CARE STUDY

1. Objective data are underlined; subjective data are in boldface.
George Gibson, an 81-year-old, married, African American man, reluctantly reports, after much prodding from his wife, that he is not hearing as well as he used to be. **"I don't know what the trouble is,"** he tells you. **"I'm in perfect health, always have been. More and more, people just seem to be mumbling instead of talking."** You notice he is seated on the edge of his chair and bends toward you when you speak to him. His wife reports that he has stopped going out and pretty much stays in his room whenever people come to visit because **he is embarrassed** by his inability to hear. "This is really a shame, because George was always the life of the party," she says. You ask Mr. Gibson if he has ever had his hearing evaluated, and he tells you no, until now, he's been trying **to convince himself that nothing's wrong with his hearing.**

2. Nursing Process Worksheet
Health Problem: Sensory/perceptual alteration: auditory
Etiology: Reluctance to accept that he has an auditory problem and to seek help
Signs and Symptoms: Leans forward to hear speaker; attempts to deny hearing loss and attributes problem to others who are "mumbling"; has greatly reduced opportunities for conversation; has not sought help until now
Expected Outcome: After medical evaluation of hearing loss and treatment, patient demonstrates better coping skills by increasing amount of time he spends socializing.
Nursing Interventions:
a. Explain that hearing loss often accompanies aging and that a medical evaluation is important to provide proper treatment.
b. Help patient make an appointment for evaluation.
c. Explore strategies for improving his communication skills and preventing social isolation.
Evaluative Statement: 12/5/11: Goal partially met—hearing aid has enabled patient to comprehend most one-to-one conversations, but ability to hear well in groups is still impaired. Is willing to investigate possibility of learning to lip-read. No longer avoids company, especially if it is only one or two people.—D. Mason, RN

3. Patient strengths: Healthy until now; wife is supportive; previous history of strong interactional skills
Personal strengths: Recognize significance of sensory/perceptual alterations; able to distinguish changes in perceptual abilities normally related to aging from those indicating treatable medical problems; able to establish trusting relationship with older patients

4. 12/5/11: Patient presents after auditory examination revealed a partial sensorineural loss that was distorting his perception of certain frequencies; partially correctable with amplification. Patient still leans close to speaker, but in a one-to-one conversation, his responses demonstrate his ability to correctly interpret most of what the speaker is saying. He reports that he still has great difficulty listening in groups. His wife notes with delight that he seems "more like his old self" when one or two friends come to visit. He expresses an interest in learning to lip-read.—*D. Mason, RN*

CHAPTER 45

PRACTICING FOR NCLEX
MULTIPLE CHOICE QUESTIONS

1. a	**2.** c	**3.** c	**4.** b	**5.** d
6. c	**7.** b	**8.** b	**9.** c	

ALTERNATE-FORMAT QUESTIONS
Multiple Response Questions

1. a, b, e, f
2. b, c, e
3. c, e, f
4. a, b, f
5. b, d, e
6. c, d, e
7. a, b, e
8. d, e, f

Prioritization Questions

1.

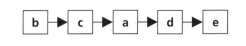

2.

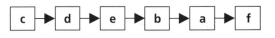

DEVELOPING YOUR KNOWLEDGE BASE

FILL-IN-THE-BLANKS

1. Sexuality
2. Gender identity
3. Sexual orientation
4. Premenstrual syndrome (PMS)
5. Erogenous zones
6. Norplant
7. Transdermal contraceptive

MATCHING EXERCISES

1. d	**2.** a	**3.** h	**4.** b	**5.** g
6. e	**7.** c	**8.** f		

SHORT ANSWER

1. Sample answers:
  a. Chronic pain: Teach altered or modified positions for coitus.

b. Diabetes: Some men may be candidates for a penile prosthesis; pharmacologic management of erectile dysfunction may be indicated.
c. Cardiovascular disease: Teach gradual resumption of sexual activity, comfortable position for affected partner.
d. Loss of body part: Teach acceptance of body image.
e. Spinal cord injury: Promote stimulation of other erogenous zones.
f. Mental illness: Provide counseling for depression
g. Sexually transmitted infections: Educate the public about the prevention and treatment of STIs.

2. a. Follicular phase: Days 4 to 14; a number of follicles mature, but only one produces a mature ovum; at the same time, in the uterus the endometrium is becoming thick and velvety in preparation for the fertilized egg.
  b. Proliferation phase: Ovulation occurs on day 14; the mature ovum ruptures from the follicle and is swept into the fallopian tube. If sperm are present, the ovum is fertilized at this time.
  c. Luteal phase: Days 15 to 28; the empty follicle fills with a yellow pigment and is then called the corpus luteum, which produces hormones that encourage a fertilized egg to grow. If fertilization does not occur, the corpus luteum disintegrates.
  d. Secretory phase: The endometrial lining becomes thick; in the absence of fertilized egg, the corpus luteum dies, and the endometrial lining disintegrates; menses begins on day 28 as a result of the uterus shedding the endometrial lining.

3. a. Excitement phase:
  Female: The breasts of the woman swell and nipples become erect; vaginal lubricant seeps out of body; upper two thirds of vagina expand; clitoris enlarges and emerges slightly from clitoral hood; labia enlarge and turn deep rosy red.
  Male: Erection of the penis caused by increased congestion with blood; scrotum noticeably elevates, thickens, and enlarges. The skin of the penis and scrotum turns deep reddish-purple; male nipples may harden and become erect.
  b. Plateau:
  Female: The clitoris retracts and disappears under clitoral hood; intensity is greater than that of excitement phase but not enough to begin orgasm.
  Male: Secretions from Cowper's glands may appear at the glans of the penis during this phase.
  c. Orgasm:
  Female: The orgasm phase begins with a heightened feeling of physical pleasure followed by overwhelming release and involuntary contractions of the genitals. Loss of muscular control can cause spastic contractions.
  Male: Involuntary spasmodic contractions of the genitals occur in the penis, epididymis, vas deferens, and rectum; most often accompanied by ejaculation.

d. Resolution:

Female: Return to normal body functioning; feelings of relaxation, fatigue, and fulfillment; the woman is physiologically capable of immediate response to sexual stimulation and may achieve multiple orgasms.

Male: Return to normal body functioning accompanied by same feelings as above; men experience a refractory period during which they are incapable of sexual response.

4. a. Any inpatient or outpatient who is receiving care for pregnancy, an STD, infertility, or conception

b. Any patient who is currently experiencing a sexual dysfunction or problem

c. Any patient whose illness will affect sexual functioning and behavior in any way

5. Sample answers:

a. "How would you describe this problem?"

b. "What do you think caused the problem, or what was happening when you first noticed it?"

c. "What have you tried in the past to correct the problem?"

6. a. A change in knowledge

b. A change in patient attitude

c. A change in behavior

7. See table below.

Method	Advantages	Disadvantages
a. Natural family planning	Methods can be effective in avoiding pregnancy if mutual understanding, support, and motivation exist between the woman and her partner. There are no side effects (as in hormonal methods) and no messy devices to insert.	Requires abstinence during ovulation and complete understanding of the signs and symptoms of ovulation.
b. Barrier methods	Condoms help to prevent STDs; appropriate for women with sensitivity to the pill; effective when used correctly; relatively inexpensive methods.	Devices must be applied before intercourse; not all women can wear them; threat of toxic shock syndrome with vaginal sponge.
c. Intrauterine devices	High rate of effectiveness; little care or motivation on part of patient is necessary; excellent method for women who have completed their families but are not ready for sterilization.	Serious side effects and complications.
d. Hormonal methods	Many beneficial noncontraceptive effects, for example, protecting women against development of breast, ovarian, and endometrial cancer; almost 100% effective when taken as directed.	Cost may be prohibitive to some; compliance is necessary; some women should not take the pill due to physiologic disorders or diseases.
e. Sterilization	After initial surgery and recheck, no further compliance is necessary; almost 100% effective.	Should be considered permanent and irreversible.

APPLYING YOUR KNOWLEDGE

REFLECTIVE PRACTICE USING CRITICAL THINKING SKILLS

Sample Answers

1. What issues might the nurse address in the plan of care for Mr. Smith? What patient teaching should be incorporated into the plan of care?

The nurse should review the effects of Mr. Smith's conditions on sexual function and assess his current status, as well as the effect of the medications he is taking to see if they are a contributing factor. The nurse could consult with the primary healthcare provider to see if an adjustment in the medications might alleviate the problem. The nurse should also explore the emotional and psychological effects of the dysfunction on Mr. Smith and his wife and consult with other members of the healthcare team to develop an effective plan of care. Patient teaching could include information about medications to treat impotence and the possibility of having a penile implant.

2. What would be a successful outcome for this patient? Following an adjustment to his medications, Mr. Smith vocalizes an improvement in his sexual functioning.
3. What intellectual, technical, interpersonal, and/or ethical/legal competencies are most likely to bring about the desired outcome?
Intellectual: ability to integrate knowledge about sexual health into nursing care, including the ability to identify areas of sexual dysfunction for the patient with a history of diabetes and hypertension experiencing impotence.
Interpersonal: strong interpersonal skills to establish trusting relationships and build rapport with a patient experiencing impotence.
4. What resources might be helpful for Mr. Smith? Counseling, printed materials on impotence and corrective measures, information on the effect of medications on sexual functioning

PATIENT CARE STUDY

1. Objective data are underlined; subjective data are in boldface.
Anthony Piscatelli, a 6-foot-tall, muscular, healthy 19-year-old college freshman in the School of Nursing, confides to his nursing advisor that **"everything is great"** about college life, with one exception: **"All of a sudden, I find myself questioning the values I learned at home about sex and marriage.** My Mom was really insistent that each of her sons should respect women and that intercourse was something you saved until you were ready to get married. If she told us once, she told us a hundred times, that we'd save ourselves, the girls in our lives, and her and Dad a lot of heartache if we could just learn to control ourselves sexually. Problem is that no one here seems to subscribe to this philosophy. **I feel like I'm abnormal in some way to even think like this.** There's a lot of sexual activity in the dorms, and no one even thinks you're serious if you talk about virginity positively. What do you think? Did my Mom sell me a bill of goods? Is it true that if you take the proper precautions, no one gets hurt and everyone has a good time?" Tony reports that **he is a virgin and that he really misses his close family back home:** **"I do get lonely at times and would love to just cuddle with someone or even give and get a big hug, but no one seems to understand this."**
2. Nursing Process Worksheet
Health Problem: High risk for altered sexuality patterns
Etiology: Discrepancy between his family's values about sex and marriage and those he is discovering in peer group
Signs and Symptoms: "All of a sudden, I find myself questioning the values I learned at home about sex and marriage"; feels like he is "abnormal" in some way to value virginity; lonely—wants intimacy; "Is it true that if you take the proper precautions, no one gets hurt and everyone has a good time?"

Expected Outcome: By next meeting, 11/17/11, patient will report personal satisfaction with the results of his reevaluation of his beliefs/values concerning sex and marriage.
Nursing Interventions:
a. Assess patient's knowledge of sexual development and need for intimacy and belonging, and correct any misinformation.
b. Explore with the patient the source of the beliefs/values he learned at home and assist in determining the role he wants these beliefs/values to play in his life.
c. Compare the options of abstinence and becoming sexually active, and perform related sexual teaching.
d. Refer to appropriate on-campus sexuality classes, counseling center, or seminars, as indicated.
Evaluative Statement: 11/17/11: Goal not met. Patient reports that his confusion has only deepened and he now feels like "my head is warring with my body." Reports sleeping with his girlfriend but feeling very guilty afterward—now ignores this girl. Revision: See if he's willing to talk with a peer or professional counselor regarding sexual concerns.—R. LeBon, RN
3. Patient strengths: Healthy; caring family; ability to voice his concerns; very "likable" person
Personal strengths: Sound knowledge of sexuality; respect for and appreciation of sexuality; understanding of developmental challenges of young adults and self-identity and intimacy needs; ability to create trusting relationships with young adults
4. 11/17/11: Patient states he is "more confused now" than when we last met. He yielded to peer pressure and slept with girlfriend; used condom. While he "enjoyed this experience," he has been "wracked with guilt" ever since. He cannot reconcile this behavior with what he learned at home and continues to feel "unsure" of who he wants to be. He definitely wants some resolution of this conflict and is interested in speaking with a professional sexuality counselor. Referral made.—R. LeBon, RN

CHAPTER 46

PRACTICING FOR NCLEX
MULTIPLE CHOICE QUESTIONS

1. b   **2.** d   **3.** c   **4.** a   **5.** b
6. d   **7.** b   **8.** a

ALTERNATE-FORMAT QUESTIONS
Multiple Response Questions

1. a, b, e
2. a, b, d
3. d, e
4. b, d, e
5. c, d

DEVELOPING YOUR KNOWLEDGE BASE

FILL-IN-THE-BLANKS

1. Alienation
2. Spiritual distress
3. Forgiveness
4. Spiritual guilt
5. Christian Scientist

MATCHING EXERCISES

1. d	**2.** a	**3.** e	**4.** b	**5.** g
6. c	**7.** a	**8.** d	**9.** c	**10.** b
11. a	**12.** d	**13.** c		

SHORT ANSWER

1. **a.** Need for meaning and purpose
   b. Need for love and relatedness
   c. Need for forgiveness
2. Sample answers:
   a. Offering a compassionate presence
   b. Assisting in the struggle to find meaning and purpose in the face of suffering, illness, and death
   c. Fostering relationships with God/humans that nurture the spirit
   d. Facilitating the patient's expression of religious or spiritual beliefs and practices
3. **a.** Life-affirming influences: Enhance life, give meaning and purpose to existence, strengthen feeling of self-worth, encourage self-actualization, and are health giving and life sustaining
   b. Life-denying influences: Restrict or enclose life patterns, limit experiences and associations, place burdens of guilt on individuals, encourage feelings of unworthiness, and are generally health denying and life inhibiting
4. Sample answers:
   a. Many religions prescribe dietary requirements and restrictions.
   b. Some religious faiths restrict birth control practices.
5. Sample answers:
   a. As a guide to daily living: Religions may specify dietary requirements or birth control measures.
   b. As a source of support: It is common for people to seek support from religious faith in times of stress; this support is often vital to the acceptance of an illness. Prayer, devotional reading, and other religious practices often do for the person spiritually what protective exercises do for the body physically.
   c. As a source of strength and healing: People have been known to endure extreme physical distress because of strong faith; patients' families have taken on almost unbelievable rehabilitative tasks because they had faith in the eventual positive results of their effort.
   d. As a source of conflict: There are times when religious beliefs conflict with prevalent health-

care practices; for example, the doctrine of Jehovah's Witnesses prohibits blood transfusions. For some, illness is viewed as punishment for sin and is inevitable.
6. **a.** Developmental considerations: As a child matures, life experiences usually influence and mature his/her spiritual beliefs. With advancing years, the tendency to think about life after death prompts some individuals to reexamine and reaffirm their spiritual beliefs.
   b. Family: A child's parents play a key role in the development of the child's spirituality.
   c. Ethnic background: Religious traditions differ among ethnic groups. There are clear distinctions between Eastern and Western spiritual traditions as well as among those of individual ethnic groups, such as Native Americans.
   d. Formal religion: Each of the major religions has several characteristics in common.
   e. Life events: Both positive and negative life experiences can influence spirituality and in turn are influenced by the meaning a person's spiritual beliefs attribute to them.
7. Answers will vary with student's experiences.
8. **a.** Basis of authority or source of power
   b. Scripture or sacred word
   c. An ethical code that defines right and wrong
   d. A psychology and identity that allows its adherents to fit into a group and the world to be defined by the religion
   e. Aspirations or expectations
   f. Some ideas about what follows death
9. Sample answers:
   a. Spiritual pain: "This seems to be a source of deep pain for you."
   b. Spiritual alienation: "Does it seem like God is far away from your life?"
   c. Spiritual anxiety: "Are you afraid that God might not be there for you when you need Him?"
   d. Spiritual anger: "I sense a great deal of anger in your statements about God taking away your daughter. Can you share more about this?"
   e. Spiritual loss: "Tell me more about how your inability to get to the synagogue is affecting you."
   f. Spiritual despair: "So you are saying that no matter how hard you try, you'll never be able to be close to God?"
10. Diagnosis: Hopelessness related to belief that God doesn't care
    Nursing care plan: The nurse should offer a supportive presence, facilitate the patient's practice of religion, counsel the patient spiritually, or contact a spiritual counselor.
11. Answers will vary with the student's experiences.
12. **a.** The room should be orderly and free of clutter.
    b. There should be a seat for the counselor at the bedside or near the patient.

   c. The top of the bedside table should be free of items and covered with a clean, white cover if a sacrament is to be administered.

   d. The bed curtains should be drawn to provide privacy, or the patient should be moved to a private setting.

13. Sample answers:

   a. Deficit: Meaning and purpose: Explore with the patient what has given his/her life meaning and purpose to the present, sources of meaning for other people, and possible meaning of illness. Refer the patient to a spiritual advisor and appropriate support groups.

   b. Deficit: Love and relatedness: Treat the patient at all times with respect, empathy, and genuine caring.

   c. Deficit: Forgiveness: Offer a supportive presence to the patient that demonstrates your acceptance of him/her. Explore the patient's self-expectations and assist the patient in determining how realistic they are. Explore the importance of learning to accept oneself and others.

APPLYING YOUR KNOWLEDGE

REFLECTIVE PRACTICE USING CRITICAL THINKING SKILLS

Sample Answers

1. How might the nurse use blended nursing skills to provide holistic, competent nursing care for Ms. Zeuner?

Ms. Zeuner is in need of assistance at home to help her care for her husband. The nurse could check with social services or look into community services that would allow her to attend her church services and other community support groups.

2. What would be a successful outcome for this patient?

By next visit, Ms. Zeuner vocalizes a connectedness with her church and community stimulated by receiving help at home with her husband.

3. What intellectual, technical, interpersonal, and/or ethical/legal competencies are most likely to bring about the desired outcome?

Intellectual: Ability to identify spirituality as a source of patient support, strength, or conflict, incorporating this information into the patient's plan of care

Interpersonal: ability to establish trusting relationships, even in times of distress, crisis, and conflict. Ability to demonstrate respect, empathy, and caring for the patient

4. What resources might be helpful to Ms. Zeuner?

Respite care, meals-on-wheels, parish nursing, community support groups

PATIENT CARE STUDY

1. Objective data are underlined; subjective data are in boldface.

Jeffrey Stein, a 31-year-old attorney, is in a step-down unit following his transfer from the cardiac care unit, where he was treated for a massive heart attack. **"Bad hearts run in my family, but I never thought it would happen to me,"** he says. **"I jog several times a week and work out at the gym, eat a low-fat diet, and I don't smoke."** Jeffrey is 5 feet 7 inches tall, weighs about 150 pounds, and is well-built. During his second night in the step-down unit, he is unable to sleep and tells the nurse, **"I've really got a lot on my mind tonight. I can't stop thinking about how close I was to death. If I wasn't with someone who knew how to do CPR when I keeled over, I probably wouldn't be here today."** Gentle questioning reveals that Mr. Stein is worried about what would have happened had he died. **"I don't think I've ever thought seriously about my mortality, and I sure don't think much about God.** My parents were semiobservant Jews, but I don't go to synagogue myself. I celebrate the holidays, **but that's about all. If there is a God, I wonder what he thinks about me."** He asks if there is a rabbi or anyone he can talk with in the morning who could answer some questions for him and perhaps help him get himself back on track. **"For the last couple of years, all I've been concerned about is paying off my school debts and making money. I guess there's a whole lot more to life, and maybe this was my invitation to sort out my priorities."**

2. Nursing Process Worksheet

Health Problem: Spiritual distress: spiritual anxiety

Etiology: Challenged belief and value system

Signs and Symptoms: Recent massive heart attack; unable to sleep; raised in semiobservant Jewish family but, "for the last couple of years all I've been concerned about is paying off my school debts and making money"; questions about afterlife.

Expected Outcome: After meeting with Rabbi White 2/12/11, patient reported feeling "less anxious" about his religious belief system and re-evaluated sense of priorities.

Nursing Interventions:

   a. Encourage patient to continue to share concerns about his religious beliefs and value system.

   b. Arrange for patient to talk with the hospital's Jewish chaplain in the morning.

   c. Normalize this experience by sharing with the patient that serious illness often prompts a life review.

   d. Recommend that the patient begin to list the things in life that are most important to him.

Evaluative Statement: Patient slept last 2 nights after meeting with Rabbi White and reports being "less anxious" about "religion." He says there are some things he wants to change about his life, and that this is a good time to start.—*T. Michael Gray, RN*

3. Patient strengths: Healthy; practices healthy self-care behaviors; strongly motivated to attain life goals. Knows himself well enough to "name his problems" and cares enough about himself to seek the assistance he needs.

Personal strengths: Belief that meeting spiritual needs is an important component of good nursing; excellent rapport with the hospital's pastoral care department; history of establishing therapeutic relationships with patients

4. 2 a.m., 2/14/11: Before patient fell asleep, he thanked me for arranging for him to meet with Rabbi White. "I guess I did what a lot of people do—forget all about God while they try to make a living." He appears less anxious about his religious beliefs and feels that his "recent bout with death" was a timely reminder to evaluate his priorities in life and make some needed changes. Sleeping peacefully at present.—*T. Michael Gray, RN*